Update on X-linked Hypophosphatemia

Update on X-linked Hypophosphatemia

Editors

Yukihiro Hasegawa
Seiji Fukumoto

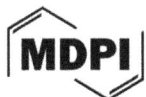

Basel • Beijing • Wuhan • Barcelona • Belgrade • Novi Sad • Cluj • Manchester

Editors
Yukihiro Hasegawa
Tokyo Metropolitan
Children's Medical Center
Tokyo, Japan

Seiji Fukumoto
Tokushima University
Tokushima, Japan

Editorial Office
MDPI
St. Alban-Anlage 66
4052 Basel, Switzerland

This is a reprint of articles from the Special Issue published online in the open access journal *Endocrines* (ISSN 2673-396X) (available at: https://www.mdpi.com/journal/endocrines/special_issues/Hypophosphatemia).

For citation purposes, cite each article independently as indicated on the article page online and as indicated below:

Lastname, A.A.; Lastname, B.B. Article Title. *Journal Name* **Year**, *Volume Number*, Page Range.

ISBN 978-3-0365-9686-0 (Hbk)
ISBN 978-3-0365-9687-7 (PDF)
doi.org/10.3390/books978-3-0365-9687-7

© 2024 by the authors. Articles in this book are Open Access and distributed under the Creative Commons Attribution (CC BY) license. The book as a whole is distributed by MDPI under the terms and conditions of the Creative Commons Attribution-NonCommercial-NoDerivs (CC BY-NC-ND) license.

Contents

Seiji Fukumoto and Yukihiro Hasegawa
Special Issue: "X-Linked Hypophosphatemia"
Reprinted from: *Endocrines* **2023**, *4*, 720–721, doi:10.3390/endocrines4040052 1

Tomoka Hasegawa, Hiromi Hongo, Tomomaya Yamamoto, Takafumi Muneyama, Yukina Miyamoto and Norio Amizuka
Histological Assessment of Endochondral Ossification and Bone Mineralization
Reprinted from: *Endocrines* **2023**, *4*, 66–81, doi:10.3390/endocrines4010006 3

Megumi Koike, Minori Uga, Yuji Shiozaki, Ken-ichi Miyamoto and Hiroko Segawa
Regulation of Phosphate Transporters and Novel Regulator of Phosphate Metabolism
Reprinted from: *Endocrines* **2023**, *4*, 607–615, doi:10.3390/endocrines4030043 19

Tatsuro Nakanishi and Toshimi Michigami
Pathogenesis of FGF23-Related Hypophosphatemic Diseases Including X-linked Hypophosphatemia
Reprinted from: *Endocrines* **2022**, *3*, 303–316, doi:10.3390/endocrines4040052 29

Yasuhisa Ohata and Yasuki Ishihara
Pathogenic Variants of the *PHEX* Gene
Reprinted from: *Endocrines* **2022**, *3*, 498–511, doi:10.3390/endocrines3030040 43

Kento Ikegawa and Yukihiro Hasegawa
Presentation and Diagnosis of Pediatric X-Linked Hypophosphatemia
Reprinted from: *Endocrines* **2023**, *4*, 128–137, doi:10.3390/endocrines4010012 57

Nobuaki Ito
Adult Presentation of X-Linked Hypophosphatemia
Reprinted from: *Endocrines* **2022**, *3*, 375–390, doi:10.3390/endocrines3030030 67

Rena Okawa and Kazuhiko Nakano
Dental Manifestations and Oral Management of X-Linked Hypophosphatemia
Reprinted from: *Endocrines* **2022**, *3*, 654–664, doi:10.3390/endocrines3040056 83

Takuo Kubota
X-Linked Hypophosphatemia Transition and Team Management
Reprinted from: *Endocrines* **2022**, *3*, 411–418, doi:10.3390/endocrines3030032 95

Toshihiro Tajima and Yukihiro Hasegawa
Treatment of X-Linked Hypophosphatemia in Children
Reprinted from: *Endocrines* **2022**, *3*, 522–529, doi:10.3390/endocrines3030042 103

Yasuo Imanishi, Tetsuo Shoji and Masanori Emoto
Complications and Treatments in Adult X-Linked Hypophosphatemia
Reprinted from: *Endocrines* **2022**, *3*, 560–569, doi:10.3390/endocrines3030047 111

Hiroaki Zukeran, Kento Ikegawa, Chikahiko Numakura and Yukihiro Hasegawa
The Possible Outcomes of Poor Adherence to Conventional Treatment in Patients with X-Linked Hypophosphatemic Rickets/Osteomalacia
Reprinted from: *Endocrines* **2023**, *4*, 110–116, doi:10.3390/endocrines4010010 121

Chikahisa Higuchi
Orthopedic Complications and Management in Children with X-Linked Hypophosphatemia
Reprinted from: *Endocrines* **2022**, *3*, 488–497, doi:10.3390/endocrines3030039 129

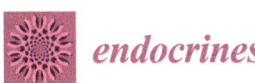

Editorial

Special Issue: "X-Linked Hypophosphatemia"

Seiji Fukumoto [1,*] and Yukihiro Hasegawa [2]

1. Department of Diabetes and Endocrinology, Tamaki-Aozora Hospital, Kitakashiya 56-1, Hayabuchi, Kokufucho, Tokushima 779-3125, Japan
2. Division of Endocrinology and Metabolism, Tokyo Metropolitan Children Medical Center, 2-8-29 Musashidai, Fuchu-shi, Tokyo 183-8561, Japan; yhaset@gmail.com
* Correspondence: fukumoto.tky@gmail.com

Rickets and osteomalacia are associated with impaired mineralization in growth plate cartilage and the bone osteoid. Many cells and factors are involved in this complex process of mineralization (Hasegawa et al. in this Special Issue, Contribution 1). Historically, vitamin D was discovered as an anti-rachitic factor [1], and it cured vitamin-D-deficient rickets/osteomalacia. However, vitamin D deficiency is one of the causes of rickets/osteomalacia, and vitamin-D-resistant rickets was later reported [2]. An investigation of a large family with vitamin-D-resistant rickets indicated the X-linked dominant inheritance of this disease [3].

There were some controversies regarding terminology before the cloning of *X-linked phosphate-regulating endopeptidase homolog* (*PHEX*) [4]; hypophosphatemic rickets and vitamin D-resistant rickets had been used almost synonymously with X-linked hypophosphatemia. Indeed, XLH, which is caused by inactivating mutations of *PHEX*, is the most common type of hypophosphatemic or vitamin D-resistant rickets in which the excessive actions of FGF23 [5] lower serum phosphate by suppressing the expression of sodium–phosphate cotransporters in proximal tubules (Koike et al. in this Special Issue, Contribution 2). In addition, several other diseases have similar clinical and biochemical findings to XLH (Nakanishi et al. in this Special Issue, Contribution 3), indicating the importance of genetic testing in achieving a definite diagnosis of XLH (Ohata et al. in this Special Issue, Contribution 4). However, depending on the methods used, genetic testing cannot detect some mutations.

Since the primary pathophysiology of XLH is due to excessive actions of FGF23 and subsequent chronic hypophosphatemia, patients with XLH present various symptoms and signs involving bone, cartilage, ligament, joint, tooth, and muscle which significantly affect QOL in both child- and adulthood (Ikegawa et al., Contribution 5, Ito, and Okawa et al. in this Special Issue, Contributions 6, 7). Because of this multiorgan involvement and life-long burden, multidisciplinary team management and an appropriate transition are essential issues in managing patients with XLH (Kubota in this Special Issue, Contribution 8).

Patients with XLH have conventionally been treated with phosphate and active vitamin D, which effectively correct some but not all abnormalities (Tajima et al., Imanishi et al. in this Special Issue, Contributions 9,10). This conventional treatment also has some limitations, such as adverse events and poor adherence (Zukeran et al. in this issue, Contribution 11). Recently, burosumab, an anti-FGF23 monoclonal antibody, was approved for XLH in several countries. While burosumab improves some features, it is not known whether burosumab can correct all the abnormalities in XLH (Tajima et al. and Imanishi et al. in this Special Issue, Contributions 9,10). The long-term efficacy and safety of burosumab also require further study, as do the indication of this new therapy. When medical therapy cannot correct bone deformities, various orthopedic approaches remain an option (Higuchi in this Special Issue, Contribution 12).

In this Special Issue concerning X-linked hypophosphatemia, the above-mentioned basic and clinical topics are discussed by several experts in this field. Still, several important

Citation: Fukumoto, S.; Hasegawa, Y. Special Issue: "X-Linked Hypophosphatemia". *Endocrines* 2023, *4*, 720–721. https://doi.org/10.3390/endocrines4040052

Received: 25 September 2023
Accepted: 3 November 2023
Published: 16 November 2023

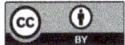

Copyright: © 2023 by the authors. Licensee MDPI, Basel, Switzerland. This article is an open access article distributed under the terms and conditions of the Creative Commons Attribution (CC BY) license (https://creativecommons.org/licenses/by/4.0/).

questions remain, as discussed in the following papers, such as the physiological function of the PHEX protein, the mechanism of FGF23 overexpression via inactivating mutations in *PHEX*, and the pathogenesis of enthesopathy. Furthermore, it is largely unknown whether all the clinical features, including the response to treatment described in patients with XLH, can be similarly observed in other patients with hypophosphatemia caused by FGF23 excess. We hope that this Special Issue, which summarizes up-to-date knowledge concerning XLH, will be helpful not only for clinicians caring for patients with rickets/osteomalacia but also as an inspiration to scientists for future research.

Author Contributions: Writing—original draft preparation, S.F.; writing—review and editing, S.F. and Y.H. All authors have read and agreed to the published version of the manuscript.

Conflicts of Interest: The authors declare no conflict of interest.

List of Contributions

1. Hasegawa, T.; Hongo, H.; Yamamoto, T.; Muneyama, T.; Miyamoto, Y.; Amizuka, N. Histological Assessment of Endochondral Ossification and Bone Mineralization. *Endocrines* **2023**, *4*, 66–81.
2. Koike, M.; Uga, M.; Shiozaki, Y.; Miyamoto, K.I.; Segawa, H. Regulation of Phosphate Transporters and Novel Regulator of Phosphate Metabolism. *Endocrines* **2023**, *4*, 607–615.
3. Nakanishi, T.; Michigami, T. Pathogenesis of FGF23-Related Hypophosphatemic Diseases Including X-linked Hypophosphatemia. *Endocrines* **2022**, *3*, 303–316.
4. Ohata, Y.; Ishihara, Y. Pathogenic Variants of the PHEX Gene. *Endocrines* **2022**, *3*, 498–511.
5. Ikegawa, K.; Hasegawa, Y. Presentation and Diagnosis of Pediatric X-Linked Hypophosphatemia. *Endocrines* **2023**, *4*, 128–137.
6. Ito, N. Adult Presentation of X-Linked Hypophosphatemia. *Endocrines* **2022**, *3*, 375–390.
7. Okawa, R.; Nakano, K. Dental Manifestations and Oral Management of X-Linked Hypophosphatemia. *Endocrines* **2022**, *3*, 654–664.
8. Kubota, T. X-Linked Hypophosphatemia Transition and Team Management. *Endocrines* **2022**, *3*, 411–418.
9. Tajima, T.; Hasegawa, Y. Treatment of X-Linked Hypophosphatemia in Children. *Endocrines* **2022**, *3*, 522–529.
10. Imanishi, Y.; Shoji, T.; Emoto, M. Complications and treatments in adult X-linked hypophosphatemia. *Endocrines* **2022**, *3*, 560–569.
11. Zukeran, H.; Ikegawa, K.; Numakura, C.; Hasegawa, Y. The Possible Outcomes of Poor Adherence to Conventional Treatment in Patients with X-Linked Hypophosphatemic Rickets/Osteomalacia. *Endocrines* **2023**, *4*, 110–116.
12. Higuchi, C. Orthopedic Complications and Management in Children with X-Linked Hypophosphatemia. *Endocrines* **2022**, *3*, 488–497.

References

1. McCollum, E.V.; Simmonds, N.; Becker, J.E.; Shipley, P.G. Studies on experimental rickets. XXI. An experimental demonstration of the existence of a vitamin which promotes calcium deposition. *J. Biol. Chem.* **1922**, *53*, 293–312. [CrossRef]
2. Albright, F.; Butler, A.M.; Bloomberg, E. Rickets resistant to vitamin D therapy. *Am. J. Dis. Child.* **1937**, *54*, 529–547. [CrossRef]
3. Winters, R.W.; Graham, J.B.; Williams, T.F.; McFalls, V.W.; Burnett, C.H. A genetic study of familial hypophosphatemia and vitamin D-resistant rickets with a review of the literature. *Medicine* **1958**, *37*, 97–142. [CrossRef] [PubMed]
4. The HYP Consortium. A gene (PEX) with homologies to endopeptidases is mutated in patients with X-linked hypophosphatemic rickets. *Nat. Genet.* **1995**, *11*, 130–136. [CrossRef] [PubMed]
5. ADHR Consortium. Autosomal dominant hypophosphatemic rickets is associated with mutations in FGF23. *Nat. Genet.* **2000**, *26*, 345–348. [CrossRef] [PubMed]

Disclaimer/Publisher's Note: The statements, opinions and data contained in all publications are solely those of the individual author(s) and contributor(s) and not of MDPI and/or the editor(s). MDPI and/or the editor(s) disclaim responsibility for any injury to people or property resulting from any ideas, methods, instructions or products referred to in the content.

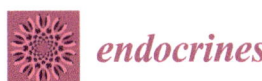

Review

Histological Assessment of Endochondral Ossification and Bone Mineralization

Tomoka Hasegawa [1], Hiromi Hongo [1], Tomomaya Yamamoto [1,2], Takafumi Muneyama [1], Yukina Miyamoto [1] and Norio Amizuka [1,*]

[1] Developmental Biology of Hard Tissue, Faculty of Medicine, Hokkaido University, Sapporo 060-8586, Japan
[2] Northern Army Medical Unit, Camp Makomanai, Japan Ground Self-Defense Forces, Sapporo 005-8543, Japan
* Correspondence: amizuka@den.hokudai.ac.jp; Tel.: +81-11-706-4223

Abstract: Finely tuned cartilage mineralization, endochondral ossification, and normal bone formation are necessary for normal bone growth. Hypertrophic chondrocytes in the epiphyseal cartilage secrete matrix vesicles, which are small extracellular vesicles initiating mineralization, into the intercolumnar septa but not the transverse partitions of the cartilage columns. Bone-specific blood vessels invade the unmineralized transverse septum, exposing the mineralized cartilage cores. Many osteoblast precursors migrate to the cartilage cores, where they synthesize abundant bone matrices, and mineralize them in a process of matrix vesicle-mediated bone mineralization. Matrix vesicle-mediated mineralization concentrates calcium (Ca) and inorganic phosphates (Pi), which are converted into hydroxyapatite crystals. These crystals grow radially and are eventually get out of the vesicles to form spherical mineralized nodules, leading to collagen mineralization. The influx of Ca and Pi into the matrix vesicle is regulated by several enzymes and transporters such as TNAP, ENPP1, PiT1, PHOSPHO1, annexins, and others. Such matrix vesicle-mediated mineralization is regulated by osteoblastic activities, synchronizing the synthesis of organic bone material. However, osteocytes reportedly regulate peripheral mineralization, e.g., osteocytic osteolysis. The interplay between cartilage mineralization and vascular invasion during endochondral ossification, as well as that of osteoblasts and osteocytes for normal mineralization, appears to be crucial for normal bone growth.

Keywords: matrix vesicle; mineralization; bone; endochondral ossification; osteoblast

1. Introduction

The growth of long bone depends on endochondral ossification, which can be sequentially divided into cartilage matrix mineralization, vascular invasion into the epiphyseal cartilage to expose the mineralized cartilage matrix, osteoblastic migration into the mineralized cartilage cores, and bone deposition to form the primary trabeculae. Hypertrophic chondrocytes play a key role in normal cartilage mineralization, and subsequently in endochondral ossification. These hypertrophic chondrocytes secrete matrix vesicles, extracellular small vesicles that initiate mineralization, and also produce vascular endothelial growth factor (VEGF) allowing the vascular endothelial cells to invade the epiphyseal cartilage. Cartilage mineralization is involved in the modeling of long bones and their changes of shape and size, i.e., the development and growth of the metaphyseal trabeculae. Finely tuned interplays among chondrocytes, vascular endothelial cells, osteoclasts (chondroclasts), and osteoblasts is apparently necessary for adequate endochondral ossification [1].

Bone is a mineralized tissue composed of calcium phosphates and organic materials such as collagen and proteoglycans. There are two phases of bone mineralization: primary and secondary. Primary mineralization is achieved by osteoblasts. Osteoblasts also produce a large amount of matrix vesicles, which mineralize in nodules (globular assemblies of hydroxyapatite crystals) and then extend into the collagen fibrils secreted by the osteoblasts. In contrast to primary mineralization, secondary mineralization is the process whereby the mineral density of bone increases after primary mineralization. It is postulated that secondary mineralization is regulated through physical crystal maturation, and by the cellular activities of osteocytes embedded in the bone matrix. However, the exact mechanism of secondary mineralization is not yet fully understood.

Histological processes of primary mineralization in the bones can be divided into two phases: matrix vesicle-mediated mineralization and collagen mineralization. In matrix vesicle-mediated mineralization, osteoblasts appear to regulate the secretion speed and the amount of matrix vesicle according to the synthesis of bone matrix. The discovery of matrix vesicles was a breakthrough in the field of bone mineralization [2–8], and many membrane transporters and enzymes related to matrix vesicle-mediated mineralization have recently been discovered. In addition to matrix vesicle-mediated mineralization, recent reports have suggested that osteocytes putatively regulate the mineralization in the periphery. As osteoblasts and osteocytes are directly connected to each other by means of their cytoplasmic processes, bone mineralization may be regulated by the interplay of osteoblasts and osteocytes. Updated knowledge of the matrix vesicles and osteocytic network in bone mineralization may deepen the understanding of mineral metabolism in bones.

In this review, we present the ultrastructural and histological aspects of endochondral ossification, matrix vesicle-mediated mineralization, and osteocytic regulation of bone mineralization.

2. Histological Aspects on Endochondral Ossification

2.1. Cartilage Mineralization by Hypertrophic Chondrocytes

Epiphyseal cartilage can be divided into three distinctive zones: resting, proliferating, and hypertrophic zones. Chondrocytes form the longitudinal columns in the proliferative and hypertrophic zones, but the proliferative chondrocytes synchronously enlarge in the hypertrophic phenotype [1]. Parathyroid hormone (PTH)-related peptide (PTHrP) has been reported to regulate hypertrophic differentiation of chondrocytes by mediating the Indian hedgehog (IHH)/PTHrP negative feedback [9]. IHH expressed in the prehypertrophic zone (the upper region of the hypertrophic zone) stimulates PTHrP expression in the early differentiation stage of chondrocytes. PTHrP promotes the proliferation activity of chondrocytes by binding to the common receptor of PTH and PTHrP (PTH/PTHrP receptor) in the proliferative zone. PTHrP alternatively inhibits the hypertrophic phenotype of chondrocytes, and IHH expression is then turned off. In addition to IHH/PTHrP negative feedback, another important regulatory factor in chondrocyte proliferation is fibroblast growth factor receptor 3 (FGFR3). Point mutations in FGFR3 cause achondroplasia and thanatophoric dysplasia by continuous activation of the transcription factor Stat1 [10,11]. FGFR3 signaling has also been proposed to increase the pool of proliferating cells by stimulating chondrocytes in the resting zone and promoting their transit to the proliferative zone [12,13]. Thus, the action of IHH/PTHrP and FGFR3 may be essential for chondrocyte proliferation and differentiation [14]. Hypertrophic chondrocytes have large and translucent cell bodies and produce type I and X collagens, tissue nonspecific alkaline phosphatase (TNAP), proteoglycan, and osteopontin [15–19]. Hypertrophic chondrocytes do not proliferate but acquire mineralization ability in the cartilage matrix. Hypertrophic chondrocytes also reportedly secrete VEGF, an angiogenic molecule that has been implicated in matrix metabolism enabling vascular invasion of the epiphyseal cartilage [20]. Hypertrophic chondrocytes of the epiphyseal cartilage secrete matrix vesicles, in which crystalline calcium phosphates appear, forming hydroxyapatite crystals that grow and eventually break through the membrane to form mineralized nodules in the cartilage matrix. Hypertrophic chondrocytes deposit matrix vesicles in the intercolumnar septae but not in the transverse partitions, consequently forming mineralized longitudinal septae and unmineralized transverse partitions. The regular distribution of mineralized cartilage matrix in the longitudinal intercolumnar septum allows the vertical invasion of vascular endothelial cells, which infiltrate into the cartilage by penetrating the unmineralized transverse partitions. After the formation of these calcified cartilage cores exposed to bone tissues, many osteoblast precursors migrate and attach to the mineralized cartilage cores to deposit abundant organic bone matrices including type I collagen, osteocalcin, osteopontin, and so forth, thereby forming the primary trabeculae. Thus, the process of endochondral ossification involves a well-defined series of events which include the invasion of vascular endothelial cells, osteogenic cell migration, new bone deposition onto the cartilage core, and the formation of primary trabeculae.

2.2. Vascular Invasion at the Chondro-Osseous Junction

Vascular endothelial cells can invade the epiphyseal cartilage by piercing the incompletely calcified transverse partition of the columns. We demonstrated endomucin-reactive blood vessels invading the chondrocyte lacunae at the chondro-osseous junction [21]. Transmission electron microscopic (TEM) observation verified that the vascular endothelial cells, present in blood vessels close to the cartilaginous matrix, extend their fine cytoplasmic processes into the matrix. The tips of the extended cytoplasmic processes showed fine finger-like structures facing the cartilaginous matrix, suggesting that the apical region of the invading endothelial cells may be partially open. In some observations, cell debris was present inside the blood vessels facing the cartilaginous columns at the chondro-osseous junction, while erythrocytes were found outside the blood vessels. Since the apical region of invading blood vessels might be open, blood vessels could presumably invade the cartilaginous matrix and exclude unnecessary impeditive materials (mainly cellular debris) to avoid accumulation at the junction (Figure 1).

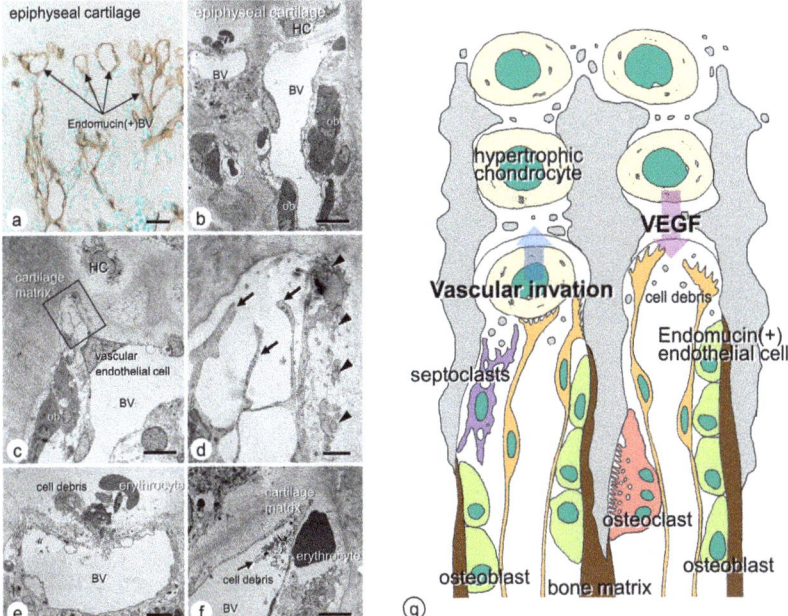

Figure 1. Vascular endothelial cells at the chondro-osseous junction. (**a**) Endomucin-immunoreactive (brown color) blood vessels at the chondro-osseous junction under light microscope. (**b–f**) TEM images of blood vessels at the chondro-osseous junction. Invading blood vessels are seen beneath the chondrocytic lacunae. (**c,d**) When observed under higher magnification as shown in panel c, fine cytoplasmic processes (arrows) are seen extending from the vascular endothelial cell, with invaginations of the cell membranes in the superficial layer of the cartilaginous matrix. (**e,f**) Panel e demonstrates cell debris, including erythrocytes from the blood vessels, and panel f reveals an erythrocyte outside the vessel and cell debris in the vessels. (**g**) Schematic design of vascular invasion at the chondro-osseous junction. HP: hypertrophic chondrocyte; BV: blood vessel, ob: osteoblast. Bar, (**a**) 20 μm, (**b**) 10 μm, (**c,e,f**) 5 μm, (**d**) 1 μm.

2.3. Osteoclasts' Function at the Chondro-Osseous Junction

It is well known that osteoclasts, also referred to as chondroclasts, accumulate in the chondro-osseous junction. Osteoclasts at the chondro-osseous junction show intense matrix metalloproteinase (MMP)-9 immunoreactivity [22]. Additionally, MMP-9 immunoreactivity is exhibited in the tips of the vascular endothelial cells facing the cartilaginous matrix, unlike the other areas distant from the chondro-osseous junction [20]. Therefore, osteoclasts and vascular endothelial cells apparently synthesize MMP-9, which dissolves the cartilaginous matrix [23,24]. Vascular invasion rather than osteoclastic resorption seems essential during endochondral ossification. Studies have found that op/op mice, c-$fos^{-/-}$ mice, and receptor activator of nuclear factor κβ ligand ($Rankl$)$^{-/-}$ mice preserve similar lengths of long bones to those seen in their wild-type counterparts in murine models that lack osteoclasts. However, without osteoclasts, the primary trabeculae form a disorganized but highly connected meshwork in the long bones. As described by Marks and Odgren [25], it seems likely that osteoclastic activity during endochondral ossification resorbs the excess mineralized cartilage matrices and scattered islets of mineralized cartilage in the chondro-osseous junction, enabling the longitudinal arrangement of primary trabeculae. Furthermore, another cell type, septoclasts, also referred to as perivascular cells, may also be involved in vascular invasion during endochondral ossification [26–28]. Septoclasts are positive for Dolichos biflorus agglutinin lectin histochemistry [26] and E-FABP [29,30], featuring well-developed Golgi apparatus and several cytoplasmic lysosomes filled with abundant cathepsin B [27]. We speculate that one major function of septoclasts is to remove excess extracellular organic (non-mineralized) debris that would otherwise interrupt the vascular invasion path into the cartilage, and it is unlikely that osteoclasts are designated to resorb the excess mineralized matrices in the cartilage.

3. Ultrastructural Aspects of Matrix Vesicle-Mediated Mineralization in Bone

3.1. Formation of Crystalline Calcium Phosphates in Matrix Vesicles

The primary trabeculae resulting from endochondral ossification can be mineralized by osteoblasts. Osteoblasts secrete matrix vesicles enveloped by a plasma membrane (ranging 30–1000 nm in diameter) into the osteoid (incompletely mineralized areas beneath the osteoblasts) [3]. Matrix vesicles are equipped with several enzymes and membrane transporters on the plasma membrane and inside the vesicles, enabling calcium phosphate nucleation and subsequent crystal growth. A crystalline calcium phosphate such as hydroxyapatite crystal [$Ca_{10}(PO_4)_6(OH)_2$] appears inside the matrix vesicles and grows radially, eventually breaking out of the vesicle membrane to form mineralized nodules in a globular assembly of radially oriented hydroxyapatite crystals with a small ribbon-like structure approximately 25 nm wide, 10 nm high, and 50 nm long [31,32].

It seems likely that crystal nucleation begins on the inner leaflet of the vesicle membrane, because the deposition of amorphous mineral crystals is initially observed on the inner leaflet. Acidic phospholipids such as phosphatidylserine and phosphatidylinositol, which have a high affinity for Ca^{2+}, are abundantly present in the matrix vesicles and consequently form a stable calcium phosphate–phospholipid complex associated with the inner leaflet of the vesicle membrane [8]. Therefore, it is possible that such complexes may play important roles in crystal nucleation in the matrix vesicles.

3.2. Mineralized Nodules Develop from Matrix Vesicles

After crystal formation, matrix vesicles develop mineralized nodules in a globular assembly of needle-like hydroxyapatite crystals (Figure 2). The growth of mineralized nodules appears to be regulated by a large amount of extracellular Ca/Pi and organic materials in the osteoid. To allow the growth of mineralized nodules, many enzymes and transporters on the vesicle membrane may participate in the accumulation of Ca and Pi on the mineralized nodules. However, osteopontin and osteocalcin are suited to the function of regulating mineralization, because they effectively inhibit calcium phosphate nucleation and crystal growth [33,34]. Osteopontin is localized in the periphery of mineralized nodules, where it might block excessive mineralization [35]. Osteocalcin includes γ-carboxyglutamic acid, which binds to mineral crystals [36–38]. When warfarin, an inhibitor of glutamine residue γ-carboxylation, was administered in our previous study, numerous fragments of needle-shaped mineral crystals were dispersed throughout the osteoid [39] (Figure 3), and γ-carboxylase-deficient mice demonstrated similar abnormality, showing disassembled and scattered crystal minerals in the bones [40]. It seems feasible that γ-carboxylated osteocalcin may bind hydroxyapatite crystals to form and maintain the mineralized nodules.

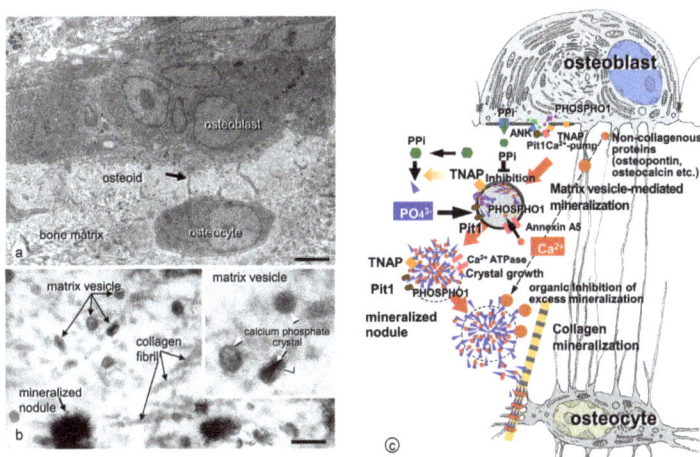

Figure 2. Matrix vesicle-mediated bone mineralization by osteoblasts. (**a**,**b**) TEM observation of osteoblasts, osteocytes, and matrix vesicles. (**a**) Mature osteoblasts located on the bone surface (osteoid) connected to osteocytes with their cytoplasmic processes (black arrow). (**b**) At a higher magnification, many matrix vesicles and mineralized nodules are observed. Note the lipid bilayer of the vesicles (white arrowheads) and calcium phosphate crystals (white arrow) in the inset. (**c**) Schematic design of matrix vesicle-mediated bone mineralization. Bar, (**a**) 3 mm, (**b**) 400 nm. Panel C is modified from ref [41].

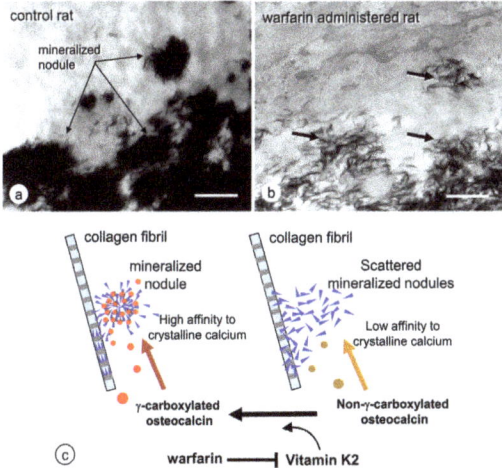

Figure 3. Ultrastructure of dispersed mineral crystals in rats administered with warfarin. (**a**) TEM image of mineralized nodules with globular assembled mineral crystals in the control rats. (**b**) The rats administrated with warfarin demonstrate many dispersed mineral crystals (arrows) in the osteoid under TEM. (**c**) Schematic design of forming mineralized nodules by osteocalcin. Bar, 2 mm. Panel C is modified from ref [42].

3.3. Enzymes and Membrane Transporter Necessary for Matrix Vesicle-Mediated Mineralization in Bone

Matrix vesicles enable the influx of Ca^{2+} and phosphate ions (PO_4^{3-}) by a variety of enzymes and membrane transporters such as tissue nonspecific alkaline phosphatase (TNAP) [6,43–50], ectonucleotide pyrophosphatase/phosphodiesterase 1(ENPP1) [51–53], ankylosis (ANK) [54,55], phosphoethanolamine/phosphocholine phosphatase 1 (PHOSPHO1) [54–61], and annexins [62]. TNAP, a glycosylphosphatidylinositol-anchored enzyme on the cell membrane, is one of the most important enzymes to initiate mineralization. In bones and cartilages, ENPP1 cleaves the extracellular ATPs into AMPs and pyrophosphate (PPi), and then TNAP hydrolyzes PPi, a phosphorus oxyanion with two phosphorus atoms in a P-O-P linkage, consequently producing PO_4^{3-}. The resultant PO_4^{3-} is transported into the matrix vesicles through sodium/phosphate co-transporter type III, also referred to as PiT1. Alternatively, Ca^{2+} can be delivered into the matrix vesicles by passage through annexins. TNAP is expressed not only by mature osteoblasts but also by preosteoblasts (osteoblast precursors), and therefore has been used as an osteoblastic lineage marker.

3.3.1. TNAP

TNAP is localized on the cell membranes of hypertrophic chondrocytes, mature osteoblasts, and preosteoblasts, as well as on the plasma membranes of matrix vesicles [43,44]. However, TNAP is not uniformly localized on the cell membranes of mature bone-synthesizing osteoblasts that possess cell polarity with distinct basolateral and secretory (osteoidal) domains. In one study, although Ca^{2+} transport ATPase was restricted to the osteoidal domain of the osteoblasts, TNAP was predominantly seen on the basolateral domain of the cell membranes [63]. Thus, the membranous domains in bone that feature an abundant TNAP are not matched to the region where TNAP actively serves for matrix vesicle-mediated mineralization. *Tnap*$^{-/-}$ mice have previously been generated [64,65] to mimic severe hypophosphatasia, with the implication that TNAP is involved in mineralization. *Tnap*$^{-/-}$ fetuses and neonatal mice have intact bones, but gradually show growth retardation and skeletal deformities. TNAP deficiency not only gives rise to hypomineralization in the skeleton, but also markedly disrupts the alignment of mineral crystals [66]. Thus, TNAP is necessary for normal mineralization and the ultrastructural arrangement of crystalline calcium phosphates in bone. In 2015, the development of the drug asfotase alfa (Strensiq) based on the long-lasting research on TNAP shed a ray of light on the treatment of hypophosphatasia caused by a hereditary mutation of *Tnap* gene [67,68].

3.3.2. ENPP1

ENPP1 cleaves the phosphodiester and pyrophosphate bonds of nucleotides and nucleotide sugars. Analysis of the crystalline structure of ENPP1 showed that nucleotides were accommodated in a pocket formed in the catalytic domain of this molecule, verifying that extracellular ATPs are a substrate for ENPP1 [69]. In bone and cartilage, the catalytic activity of ENPP1 generates PPi, which strongly inhibits mineralization by binding to hydroxyapatite crystals and disrupting their extension [51–53]. However, TNAP cleaves PPi into PO_4^{3-}, which is a component of crystalline calcium phosphates in bone. Therefore, balanced interplay between ENPP1 and TNAP seems necessary for bone mineralization [70]. Alternatively, the lack of ENPP1 was proven to be related to the spontaneous mineralization of infantile arteries and periarticular regions [71,72]. In a normal state, therefore, PPi produced by ENPP1 may regulate the growth of hydroxyapatite crystals. In our observations, TNAP was mainly seen in mature osteoblasts and overlying preosteoblasts, while ENPP1 was detected in mature osteoblasts and osteocytes [73]. Genetic ENPP1 dysfunction leading to arterial mineralization may suggest that PPi deficiency or insufficiency can induce osteoblastic differentiation in vascular smooth muscle cells. *Enpp1*$^{-/-}$ mice, also known as tiptoe walking (*ttw*) mice, undergo ossification of the posterior longitudinal ligament of the spine (OPLL) including progressive ankylosing intervertebral and peripheral joint hyperostosis, as well as articular cartilage mineralization [74–78]. Despite the ectopic mineralization, $Enpp1^{-/-}$ mice show reduced serum concentrations of Ca^{2+} and PO_4^{3-} as well as significantly elevated serum levels of fibroblast growth factor 23 (FGF23) [78,79]. FGF23 is an osteocyte-derived molecule that inhibits phosphate reabsorption and 1α-hydroxylase synthesis in the kidney [80–82]. Hence, in $Enpp1^{-/-}$ mice, the induction of Fgf23 mRNA expression, which increases the concentration of serum FGF23, may lead to reductions in the concentrations of Ca^{2+} and PO_4^{3-}.

3.3.3. ANK

ENPP1 can be found not only on the cell surface but also in cytoplasmic regions, generating PPi in both locations. ANK reportedly transports intracellular PPi to the extracellular milieu, i.e., serves as a transmembrane PPi-channeling protein [54,55]. Therefore, it is feasible that ANK-mediated extracellular PPi levels may provide an equivalent balance by disallowing excessive or ectopic mineralization or hypomineralization in various tissues. In previous reports, infants with Ank gene mutations exhibited a three to five-fold decrease in extracellular PPi [54], while calcium pyrophosphate (CPP) crystal deposition (CPPD) was elevated in the synovial fluid by gain-of-function mutations in human ANK genes [83]. Thus, local PPi production naturally inhibits hydroxyapatite deposition, blocking undesirable mineralization in articular cartilage and other tissues. However, with the loss of ANK activity, extracellular PPi levels attenuate, intracellular PPi levels rise, and unregulated mineralization occurs.

3.3.4. PHOSPHO1

PHOSPHO1 is an enzyme abundantly present in bone-forming mature osteoblasts and hypertrophic chondrocytes [56]. Roberts et al. documented that PHOSPHO1 is restricted to the mineralizing regions of the bone and growth plate and plays a role in the initiation of matrix vesicle-mediated mineralization [57]. PHOSPHO1 is reportedly present not only in the cytoplasmic regions of bone-forming osteoblasts and hypertrophic chondrocytes but also in the matrix vesicles. PHOSPHO1 inside the matrix vesicles cleaves PO_4^{3-} from phosphatidylcholine and phosphoethanolamine at the inner leaflet of the vesicles' plasma membranes [56–58]. A recent report suggested that phospholipase A2 as well as ENPP6 are also included in matrix vesicles, acting in sequence to produce phosphocholine, which PHOSPHO1 subsequently hydrolyzes into PO_4^{3-} [84]. Thus, PHOSPHO1 plays a pivotal role in the increased concentration of PO_4^{3-} by cooperating with the PO_4^{3-} supply by means of ENPP1/TNAP interplay. Neonatal $Phospho1^{-/-}$ mice demonstrated incomplete mineralization of the bone, often with spontaneous greenstick fractures [59,60]. Millán's team demonstrated that PHOSPHO1 controls TNAP expression in mineralizing cells and is essential for mechanically competent mineralization [59,61]. Taken together, the PO_4^{3-} supplementation necessary for matrix vesicle-mediated mineralization appears to be derived at least in part from TNAP/ENPP1 interaction outside the matrix vesicles as well as PHOSPHO1 activity inside the vesicles.

3.3.5. Annexins

Annexins are a group of proteins that show high affinity for Ca^{2+} and lipids, serving as ion channels for the transport of Ca^{2+} into the matrix vesicles. Three annexins, annexin A2, A5, and A6, that are abundantly present in vascular endothelial cells, heart, and skeletal muscles, have been discovered in matrix vesicles [62,85–87]. In the initial process of matrix vesicle-mediated mineralization, amorphous calcium phosphates are formed associated with the inner leaflet of the plasma membranes of the matrix vesicles. The annexin A5 might serve as a Ca^{2+} ion channel inside the matrix vesicles. Consequently, transported Ca^{2+} showed strong binding to phosphatidylserine in the inner leaflet of the membrane enclosing the matrix vesicle, which is enriched with anionic lipids [88,89]. Thus, it is feasible that annexin A5 might play an important role in Ca^{2+} transport and subsequent Ca^{2+}-dependent phosphatidylserine binding in the matrix vesicles. It is a possibility that the Pi transported through PiT1 present in the membrane could also bind to Ca^{2+} trapped on the inner leaflet, to form amorphous calcium phosphates. Unexpectedly, *Annexin a5*$^{-/-}$ mice did not show skeletal deformity or reduced mineralization, suggesting that other annexins could compensate for the functions of annexin A5. However, further examination is necessary to clarify the precise role of annexins in bone mineralization.

4. Regulation of Bone Mineralization by Osteocyte
4.1. Erosion of Bone Minerals in the Vicinity of Osteocytes

Osteocytes are located in bone cavities known as osteocytic lacunae, and connect to neighboring osteocytes and osteoblasts on the bone surfaces via fine cytoplasmic processes that run through osteocytic canaliculi [90]. Osteocytes interconnect their cytoplasmic processes via gap junctions, thereby building functional syncytia referred to as the osteocytic lacunar canalicular system (OLCS) [41]. Mature well-mineralized bone develops an OLCS with an orderly arrangement, while immature bone has an irregular and disorganized OLCS [41]. The osteocytic network has been speculated to have roles in multiple processes including mechanical sensing, molecular transport, and regulation of peripheral mineralization [41].

Belanger proposed the concept of osteocytic osteolysis in the 1960s [91], suggesting that osteocytes have the potential not only to erode the peripheral bone minerals but also reversibly to remineralize the bone (Figure 4). This notion was not immediately accepted, however, many researchers have since observed that osteocytes and their canaliculi are involved in the mineral maintenance of the bone matrix [92–99]. The occurrence of osteocytic osteolysis has been reported in cases of PTH administration, including hyperparathyroidism [100,101], during lactation [96,102], in vitamin D receptor deficiency [103], and with sclerostin treatment [104]. During lactation, osteocytes reportedly erode the surrounding bone matrix by exhibiting a pattern of gene expression similar to that of osteoclasts during bone resorption, e.g., an elevation in tartrate-resistant acid phosphatase, cathepsin K, carbonic anhydrase, Na^+/H^+ exchanger, ATPase H^+ transporting lysosomal subunits, and matrix metalloproteinase [96]. Using synchrotron X-ray microscopy, Nango et al. analyzed the degree of bone mineralization in mouse cortical bone around the lacunar canalicular network and reported the dissolution of bone mineral along the osteocyte canaliculi [105]. However, one criticism of the osteocytic osteolysis concept might be that the proteolytic enzymes and acids secreted from the bone-resorbing osteoclasts pass through the osteocytic canaliculi to reach distant osteocytes. Recently, using *Rankl*$^{-/-}$ mice, we have obtained microscopic findings that support the idea of osteocytic osteolysis [106]; osteocytic osteolysis is independent of osteoclastic activity and is discernible in mature cortical bone showing a regular distribution of the osteocytic network (Figure 5).

However, several reports have cautioned that (1) large osteocytic lacunae do not always represent the signs of osteocytic osteolysis [107], (2) the vitamin D receptor is not associated with osteocytic osteolysis [108], and (3) despite considerable research, osteocytic osteolysis has continued to be looked upon with skepticism [109]. Nevertheless, many researchers have attempted to elucidate whether osteocytic osteolysis would affect the mechanical properties of bone, and to extend the concept from including merely osteolysis to encompass a remodeling of the osteocytic network's peripheral bone matrix. Recently, Kaya et al. reported that changes in bone mechanical properties induced by lactation and recovery appear to depend predominantly on the volume of osteocytic lacunae and canaliculi, suggesting that tissue-level mechanical properties of cortical bone are rapidly and reversibly modulated by osteocytes in response to physiological challenges [110]. Emami et al. have consistently reported notable canalicular changes following fracture that could affect mechanical properties of bone [111]. Vahidi et al. reported that femoral fracture in mice induced morphological changes of the canalicular network in the contralateral limb, suggesting decreased rates of bone formation and mineralization in the osteocytic lacunar canaliculi. They proposed that changes in canalicular remodeling by osteocytes involve utilization of the mineral from the bones for callus formation and bone repair after a fracture, but this process may also lessen bone quality and systemically elevate the fracture risk [112]. Osteocytes are the most abundant cells in bone, and the total area of osteocytes and their cytoplasmic processes is much larger than the areas of bone-forming osteoblasts or bone-resorbing osteoclasts. Therefore, osteocytes might be involved in the regulation of mineralization.

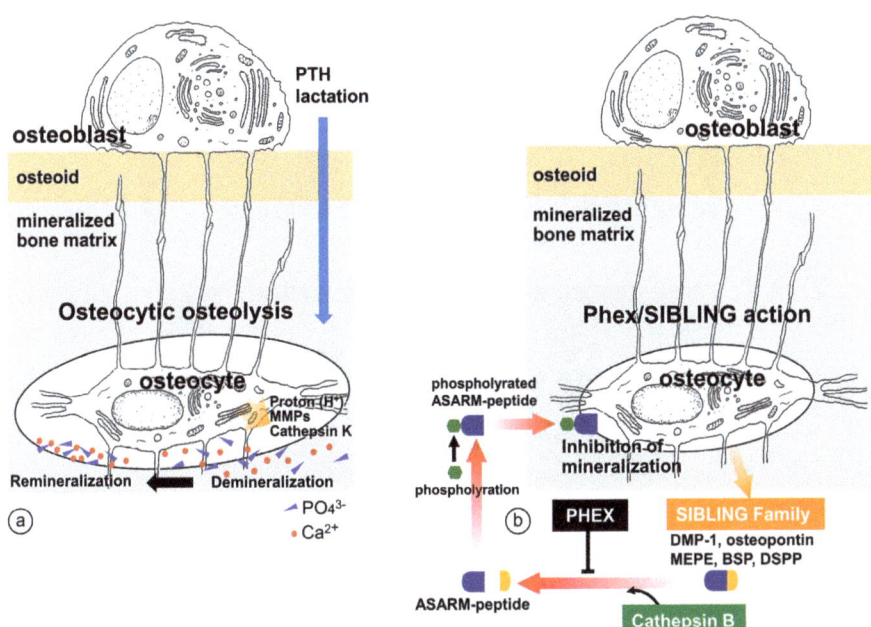

Figure 4. Schematic representations of the two hypotheses: (**a**) osteocytic osteolysis and (**b**) regulation of bone mineralization by PHEX/SIBLINGs. During PTH administration or lactation, osteocytes secrete acids and proteolytic enzymes such as cathepsin K and MMPs to erode the surrounding bone. However, osteocytic osteolysis is reversible, so once-eroded bone can be remineralized. In contrast, SIBLINGs such as MEPE, DMP-1, and osteopontin are cleaved by cathepsin B to generate ASARM, which is then phosphorylated to inhibit mineralization. Alternatively, PHEX blocks the inhibition of mineralization.

4.2. Regulation of Mineralization by Mediating SIBLING Family

Osteocytes are known to produce many important extracellular molecules, including fibroblast growth factor 23 (FGF23), small integrin-binding ligand N-linked glycoprotein (SIBLING) family proteins, and phosphate-regulating gene with homologies to endopeptidases on the X chromosome (PHEX). Through these molecules, osteocytes can regulate bone mineralization in two different manners: (1) systemic regulation of serum Pi by FGF23 in the kidney; and (2) local regulation of mineral crystal growth by PHEX/SIBLING family.

For systemic regulation of serum Pi, FGF23 secreted from osteocytes is circulated to reach the kidneys, where it binds to the receptor complex of fibroblast growth factor receptor Ic (FGFR1c) and αklotho expressed in the proximal renal tubules, to inhibit sodium/phosphate co-transporter type IIa/IIc (NaPi IIa/IIc). Since NaPi IIa/IIc reabsorb phosphate ions in the proximal renal tubules, FGF23 reduces the serum Pi concentration [80–82]. Human X-linked hypophosphatemia (XLH), one of the FGF23-related causes of hypophosphatemic rickets or osteomalacia in children and osteomalacia in adults, is caused by loss-of-function mutations in PHEX resulting in the elevated circulation of FGF23 and markedly decreased bone mineralization. This may indicate that the osteocyte-derived hormone FGF23, along with its function in the kidneys, may play a pivotal role in the systemic regulation of bone mineralization.

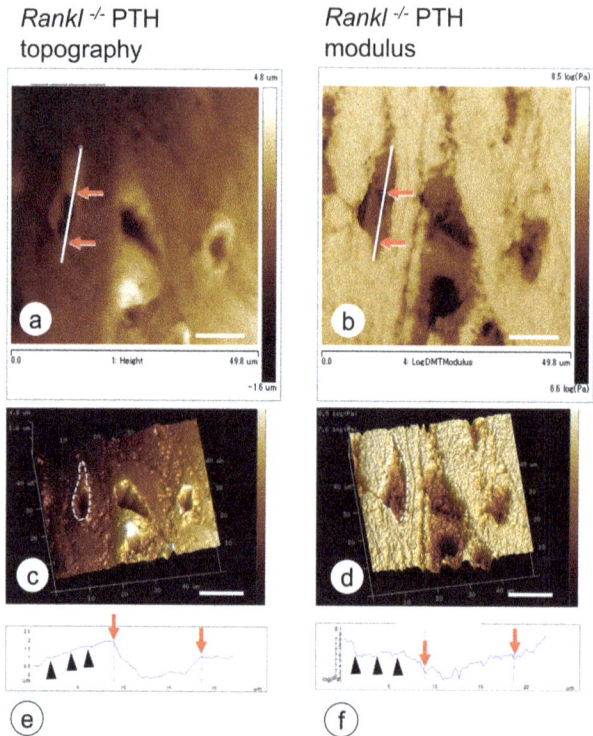

Figure 5. Nano-indentation by atomic force microscopy on bone matrix surrounding osteocytic lacunae. (**a**,**c**) Topography of osteocytic lacunae in the femoral cortical bone of the PTH-administered *Rankl*$^{-/-}$ mice. (**b**,**d**) Elastic modulus of the osteocytic lacunae in the femoral cortical bone of the PTH-administered *Rankl*$^{-/-}$ mice. Red arrows along the white lines in a and b are matched with the red arrows in the graphs (**e**,**f**). Note the slightly expanded diameters in the three-dimensional images of the elastic modulus (compare the dotted circles in (**c**,**d**)), and that the index of the elastic modulus is lower than the topography in the graph (black arrowheads). Bar, 20 mm.

In contrast to systemic regulation of serum Pi and bone mineralization, osteocytes appear to regulate mineralization in the periphery of the osteocytic lacunae. Dentin matrix protein-1 (DMP-1), which is secreted by osteocytes, has high potential to bind Ca^{2+} and is postulated to play a role in the mineralization of the peripheral bone matrix of osteocytes [113]. The SIBLING family includes DMP-1, matrix extracellular phosphoglycoprotein (MEPE), osteopontin, bone sialoprotein (BSP), and dentin sialophosphoprotein (DSPP), which are encoded by a gene located on human chromosome 4q21 and mouse chromosome 5q21 [114,115]. We considered the possibility that the interaction between PHEX and the SIBLING family might regulate mineralization in the periphery of the osteocytic lacunae (Figure 4). For instance, MEPE secreted by osteocytes is cleaved by cathepsin B to release the carboxy terminal region, a novel functional domain referred to as the acidic serine-rich and aspirate-rich motif (ASARM) [116,117]. The resultant ASARM peptides are then phosphorylated to inhibit bone mineralization [117]. However, MEPE also binds to PHEX, forming the MEPE-PHEX complex. In this situation, cathepsin B is unable to cleave the MEPE-PHEX complex, which therefore blocks the synthesis of ASARM, so no phosphorylated ASARM inhibits mineralization, and normal mineralization is thereby attained [118]. It has been reported that the phosphorylated ASARM peptide of osteopontin inhibits mineralization in a phosphorylation-dependent manner, and PHEX disturbs the inhibition of mineralization [119]. These findings implicate the possibility that osteocyte-derived SIBLINGs may regulate peripheral bone mineralization by cooperating with PHEX.

This idea is supported by the observation that the absence of DMP-1 results in rickets or osteomalacia in mice [120] and autosomal recessive hypophosphatemic rickets or osteomalacia (ARHR) in human patients [121]. However, PHEX/SIBLINGs are usually associated with congenital deformities, rickets, and osteomalacia, and therefore it is necessary to elucidate whether PHEX/SIBLINGs play an important role in the physiological regulation of bone mineralization in a healthy state.

5. Conclusions

During endochondral ossification, hypertrophic chondrocytes secrete matrix vesicles into the intercolumnar septa but not the transverse partitions of the cartilage columns; this allows vascular invasion into the epiphyseal cartilage and subsequent osteoblastic bone formation in the mineralized cartilage core. Thus, endochondral ossification is finely tuned by the cellular interplay at the chondro-osseous junction. To achieve matrix vesicle-mediated mineralization, many enzymes and membrane transporters including TNAP, ENPP1, PiT1, PHOSPHO1, annexins, and others are involved in the influx of Ca^{2+}/Pi and the regulation of calcium phosphate crystal growth. In addition to their role in osteoblastic primary mineralization, osteocytes have recently been shown to regulate bone mineralization, presumably by controlling the synthesis of PHEX/SIBLING, as well as osteocytic osteolysis. Thus, normal mineralization is maintained by the orchestrated activities of bone cells.

Author Contributions: Conceptualization, writing—original draft preparation, T.H.; investigation; T.H., H.H., T.H., T.Y., T.M. and Y.M.; writing—review and editing, N.A.; supervision and funding acquisition, T.H. and N.A. All authors have read and agreed to the published version of the manuscript.

Funding: This study was partially supported by grants from the Japanese Society for the Promotion of Science (JSPS, 22K09911 to T.H., 21K16928 to H.H., and 21H03103 to N.A.) and a grant-in-aid for young scientists provided by the Uehara Memorial Foundation (202110102 to T.H.).

Institutional Review Board Statement: Not applicable.

Informed Consent Statement: Not applicable.

Data Availability Statement: Not applicable.

Conflicts of Interest: The authors declare no conflict of interest.

References

1. Amizuka, N.; Hasegawa, T.; Oda, K.; Freitas, P.H.L.; Hoshi, K.; Li, M.; Ozawa, H. Histology of epiphyseal cartilage calcification and endochondral ossification. *Front. Biosci.* **2012**, *4*, 2085–2100. [CrossRef]
2. Ali, S.Y.; Sajdera, S.W.; Anderson, H.C. Isolation and characterization of calcifying matrix vesicles from epiphyseal cartilage. *Proc. Natl. Acad. Sci. USA* **1970**, *67*, 1513–1520. [CrossRef]
3. Anderson, H.C. Vesicles associated with calcification in the matrix of epiphyseal cartilage. *J. Cell Biol.* **1969**, *41*, 59–72. [CrossRef]
4. Bonucci, E. Fine structure of early cartilage calcification. *J. Ultrastruct. Res.* **1967**, *20*, 33–50. [CrossRef] [PubMed]
5. Bonucci, E. Fine structure and histochemistry of "calcifying globules" in epiphyseal cartilage. *Z. Zellforsch. Mikrosk. Anat.* **1970**, *103*, 192–217. [CrossRef]
6. Ozawa, H.; Yamada, M.; Yajima, T. The ultrastructural and cytochemical aspects of matrix vesicles and calcification processes. In *Formation and Calcification of Hard Tissues*; Talmage, R.V., Ozawa, H., Eds.; Shakai Hoken Pub: Tokyo, Japan, 1978; pp. 9–57.
7. Ozawa, H.; Yamada, M.; Yamamoto, T. Ultrastructural observations on the location of lead and calcium in the mineralizing dentine of rat incisor. In *Matrix Vesicles*; Ascenzi, A., Bonucci, E., de Bernard, B., Eds.; Wiching Editore srl: Milano, Italy, 1981; pp. 179–187.
8. Wuthier, R.E. Lipid composition of isolated epiphyseal cartilage cells, membranes and matrix vesicles. *Biochim. Biophys. Acta* **1975**, *409*, 128–143. [CrossRef] [PubMed]
9. Ohba, S. Hedgehog Signaling in Skeletal Development: Roles of Indian Hedgehog and the Mode of Its Action. *Int. J. Mol. Sci.* **2020**, *21*, 6665. [CrossRef] [PubMed]
10. Tavormina, P.L.; Shiang, R.; Thompson, L.M.; Zhu, Y.Z.; Wilkin, D.J.; Lachman, R.S.; Wilcox, W.R.; Rimoin, D.L.; Cohn, D.H.; Wasmuth, J.J. Thanatophoric dysplasia (types I and II) caused by distinct mutations in fibroblast growth factor receptor 3. *Nat. Genet.* **1995**, *9*, 321–328. [CrossRef] [PubMed]
11. Su, W.C.; Kitagawa, M.; Xue, N.; Xie, B.; Garofalo, S.; Cho, J.; Deng, C.; Horton, W.A.; Fu, X.Y. Activation of Stat1 by mutant fibroblast growth-factor receptor in thanatophoric dysplasia type II dwarfism. *Nature* **1997**, *386*, 288–292. [CrossRef]

12. Peters, K.; Ornitz, D.; Werner, S.; Williams, L. Unique expression pattern of the FGF receptor 3 gene during mouse organogenesis. *Dev. Biol.* **1993**, *155*, 423–430. [CrossRef]
13. Deng, C.; Wynshaw-Boris, A.; Zhou, F.; Kuo, A.; Leder, P. Fibroblast growth factor receptor 3 is a negative regulator of bone growth. *Cell* **1996**, *84*, 911–921. [CrossRef] [PubMed]
14. Amizuka, N.; Davidson, D.; Liu, H.; Valverde-Franco, G.; Chai, S.; Maeda, T.; Ozawa, H.; Hammond, V.; Ornitz, D.M.; Goltzman, D.; et al. Signalling by fibroblast growth factor receptor 3 and parathyroid hormone-related peptide coordinate cartilage and bone development. *Bone* **2004**, *34*, 13–25. [CrossRef]
15. Greenspan, J.S.; Blackwood, H.J. Histochemical studies of chondrocyte function in the cartilage of the mandibular codyle of the rat. *J. Anat.* **1966**, *100*, 615–626. [PubMed]
16. Ikeda, T.; Nomura, S.; Yamaguchi, A.; Suda, T.; Yoshiki, S. In situ hybridization of bone matrix proteins in undecalcified adult rat bone sections. *J. Histochem. Cytochem.* **1992**, *40*, 1079–1088. [CrossRef]
17. Oshima, O.; Leboy, P.S.; McDonald, S.A.; Tuan, R.S.; Shapiro, I.M. Developmental expression of genes in chick growth cartilage detected by in situ hybridization. *Calcif. Tissue Int.* **1989**, *45*, 182–192. [CrossRef] [PubMed]
18. Poole, A.R.; Pidoux, I.; Rosenberg, L. Role of proteoglycans in endochondral ossification: Immunofluorescent localization of link protein and proteoglycan monomer in bovine fetal epiphyseal growth plate. *J. Cell Biol.* **1982**, *92*, 249–260. [CrossRef]
19. Schmid, T.M.; Linsenmayer, T.F. Immunohistochemical localization of short chain cartilage collagen (type X) in avian tissues. *J. Cell Biol.* **1985**, *100*, 598–605. [CrossRef]
20. Gerber, H.P.; Vu, T.H.; Ryan, A.M.; Kowalski, J.; Werb, Z.; Ferrara, N. VEGF couples hypertrophic cartilage remodeling, ossification and angiogenesis during endochondral bone formation. *Nat. Med.* **1999**, *5*, 623–628. [CrossRef]
21. Tsuchiya, E.; Hasegawa, T.; Hongo, H.; Yamamoto, T.; Abe, M.; Yoshida, T.; Zhao, S.; Tsuboi, K.; Udagawa, N.; Freitas, P.H.L.; et al. Histochemical assessment on the cellular interplay of vascular endothelial cells and septoclasts during endochondral ossification in mice. *Microscopy* **2021**, *70*, 201–214. [CrossRef]
22. Kojima, T.; Hasegawa, T.; Freitas, P.H.L.; Yamamoto, T.; Sasaki, M.; Horiuchi, K.; Hongo, H.; Yamada, T.; Sakagami, N.; Saito, N.; et al. Histochemical aspects of the vascular invasion at the erosion zone of the epiphyseal cartilage in MMP-9-deficient mice. *Biomed. Res.* **2013**, *34*, 119–128. [CrossRef]
23. Vu, T.H.; Shipley, J.M.; Bergers, G.; Berger, J.E.; Helms, J.A.; Hanahan, D.; Shapiro, S.D.; Senior, R.M.; Werb, Z. MMP-9/gelatinase B is a key regulator of growth plate angiogenesis and apoptosis of hypertrophic chondrocytes. *Cell* **1998**, *93*, 411–422. [CrossRef] [PubMed]
24. Engsig, M.T.; Chen, Q.J.; Vu, T.H.; Pedersen, A.C.; Therkidsen, B.; Lund, L.R.; Henriksen, K.; Lenhard, T.; Foged, N.T.; Werb, Z.; et al. Matrix metalloproteinase 9 and vascular endothelial growth factor are essential for osteoclast recruitment into developing long bones. *J. Cell Biol.* **2000**, *151*, 879–889. [CrossRef]
25. Marks, S.C., Jr.; Odgren, P.R. The structure and development of the skeleton. In *Principles of Bone Biology*; Bilezikian, J.P., Raisz, L.G., Rodan, G.A., Eds.; Academic Press: New York, NY, USA, 2002; pp. 3–15.
26. Nakamura, H.; Ozawa, H. Ultrastructural, enzyme-, lectin, and immunohistochemical studies of the erosion zone in rat tibiae. *J. Bone Miner. Res.* **1996**, *11*, 1158–1164. [CrossRef] [PubMed]
27. Lee, E.R.; Lamplugh, L.; Shepard, N.L.; Mort, J.S. The septoclast, a cathepsin B-rich cell involved in the resorption of growth plate cartilage. *J. Histochem. Cytochem.* **1995**, *43*, 525–536. [CrossRef]
28. Gartland, A.; Mason-Savas, A.; Yang, M.; MacKay, C.A.; Birnbaum, M.J.; Odgren, P.R. Septoclast deficiency accompanies postnatal growth plate chondrodysplasia in the toothless (tl) osteopetrotic, colony-stimulating factor-1 (CSF-1)-deficient rat and is partially responsive to CSF-1 injections. *Am. J. Pathol.* **2009**, *175*, 2668–2675. [CrossRef]
29. Bando, Y.; Yamamoto, M.; Sakiyama, K.; Inoue, K.; Takizawa, S.; Owada, Y.; Iseki, S.; Kondo, H.; Amano, O. Expression of epidermal fatty acid binding protein (E-FABP) in septoclasts in the growth plate cartilage of mice. *J. Mol. Histol.* **2014**, *45*, 507–518. [CrossRef]
30. Bando, Y.; Yamamoto, M.; Sakiyama, K.; Sakashita, H.; Taira, F.; Miyake, G.; Iseki, S.; Owada, Y.; Amano, O. Retinoic acid regulates cell-shape and -death of E-FABP (FABP5)-immunoreactive septoclasts in the growth plate cartilage of mice. *Histochem. Cell Biol.* **2017**, *148*, 229–238. [CrossRef] [PubMed]
31. Weiner, S. Organization of extracellularly mineralized tissues: A comparative study of biological crystal growth. *CRC Crit. Rev. Biochem.* **1986**, *20*, 365–408. [CrossRef] [PubMed]
32. Ozawa, H. Ultrastructural Concepts on Biological Calcification; Focused on Matrix Vesicles. *J. Oral Biosci.* **1985**, *27*, 751–774.
33. Bosky, A.L.; Maresca, M.; Ullrich, W.; Doty, S.B.; Butler, W.T.; Prince, C.W. Osteopontin-hydroxyapatite interactions in vitro: Inhibition of hydroxyapatite formation and growth in a gelatin-gel. *Bone Miner.* **1993**, *22*, 147–159. [CrossRef]
34. Hunter, G.K.; Hauschka, P.V.; Poole, A.R.; Rosenberg, L.C.; Goldberg, H.A. Nucleation and inhibition of hydroxyapatite formation by mineralized tissue proteins. *Biochem. J.* **1996**, *317*, 59–64. [CrossRef]
35. Mark, M.P.; Butler, W.T.; Prince, C.W.; Finkleman, R.D.; Ruch, J.V. Developmental expression of 44-kDa phosphoprotein (osteopontin) and bone-carboxyglutamic acid (Gla)-containing protein (osteocalcin) in calcifying tissues of rat. *Differentiation* **1988**, *37*, 123–136. [CrossRef] [PubMed]
36. Hall, J.G.; Pauli, R.M.; Wilson, K.M. Maternal and fetal sequelae of anti-coagulation during pregnancy. *Am. J. Med.* **1980**, *68*, 122–140. [CrossRef]

37. Hauschka, P.V.; Lian, J.B.; Gallop, P.M. Direct identification of the calcium-binding amino acid, gamma-carboxyglutamate, in mineralized tissue. *Proc. Natl. Acad. Sci. USA* **1975**, *72*, 3925–3929. [CrossRef]
38. Price, P.A.; Otsuka, A.A.; Poser, J.W.; Kristaponis, J.; Raman, N. Characterization of a gamma-carboxyglutamic acid-containing protein from bone. *Proc. Natl. Acad. Sci. USA* **1976**, *73*, 1447–1451. [CrossRef]
39. Amizuka, N.; Li, M.; Hara, K.; Kobayashi, M.; Freitas, P.H.L.; Ubaidus, S.; Oda, K.; Akiyama, Y. Warfarin administration disrupts the assembly of mineralized nodules in the osteoid. *J. Electron. Microsc.* **2009**, *58*, 55–65. [CrossRef]
40. Azuma, K.; Shiba, S.; Hasegawa, T.; Ikeda, K.; Urano, T.; Horie-Inoue, K.; Ouchi, Y.; Amizuka, N.; Inoue, S. Osteoblast-specific γ-glutamyl carboxylase-deficient mice display enhanced bone formation with aberrant mineralization. *J. Bone Miner. Res.* **2015**, *30*, 1245–1254. [CrossRef] [PubMed]
41. Hasegawa, T.; Hongo, H.; Yamamoto, T.; Abe, M.; Yoshino, H.; Haraguchi-Kitakamae, M.; Ishizu, H.; Shimizu, T.; Iwasaki, N.; Amizuka, N. Matrix vesicle-mediated mineralization and osteocytic regulation of bone mineralization. *Int. J. Mol. Sci.* **2022**, *23*, 9941. [CrossRef]
42. Hasegawa, T. Ultrastructure and biological function of matrix vesicles in bone mineralization. *Histochem. Cell Biol.* **2018**, *149*, 289–304. [CrossRef] [PubMed]
43. de Bernard, B.; Bianco, P.; Bonucci, E.; Costantini, M.; Lunazzi, G.C.; Martinuzzi, P.; Modricky, C.; Moro, L.; Panfili, E.; Pollesello, P. Biochemical and immunohistochemical evidence that in cartilage an alkaline phosphatase is a Ca^{2+}-binding glycoprotein. *J. Cell Biol.* **1986**, *103*, 1615–1623. [CrossRef]
44. Matsuzawa, T.; Anderson, H.C. Phosphatases of epiphyseal cartilage studied by electron microscopic cytochemical methods. *J. Histochem. Cytochem.* **1971**, *19*, 801–808. [CrossRef] [PubMed]
45. Yamada, M. Ultrastructural and cytochemical studies on the calcification of the tendon-bone joint. *Arch. Histol. Jap.* **1976**, *39*, 347–378. [CrossRef]
46. Hoshi, K.; Ejiri, S.; Ozawa, H. Localizational alterations of calcium, phosphorus, and calcification-related organics such as proteoglycans and alkaline phosphatase during bone calcification. *J. Bone Miner. Res.* **2001**, *16*, 289–298. [CrossRef]
47. Schmitz, J.P.; Schwartz, Z.; Sylvia, V.L.; Dean, D.D.; Calderon, F.; Boyan, B.D. Vitamin D3 regulation of stromelysin-1 (MMP-3) in chondrocyte cultures is mediated by protein kinase C. *J. Cell Physiol.* **1996**, *168*, 570–579. [CrossRef]
48. Fleish, H.; Neuman, W.F. Mechanisms of calcification: Role of collagen, polyphosphates, and phosphatase. *Am. J. Physiol.* **1961**, *200*, 1296–1300. [CrossRef] [PubMed]
49. Fleish, H.; Neuman, W. The role of phosphatase and polyphosphates in calcification of collagen. *Helv. Physiol. Pharmacol. Acta* **1961**, *19*, C17–C18. [CrossRef] [PubMed]
50. Takano, Y.; Ozawa, H.; Crenshaw, M.A. Ca-ATPase and ALPase activities at the initial calcification sites of dentine and enamel in the rat incisor. *Cell Tissue Res.* **1986**, *243*, 91–99. [CrossRef]
51. Terkeltaub, R.; Rosenbach, M.; Fong, F.; Goding, J. Causal link between nucleotide pyrophosphohydrolase overactivity and increased intracellular inorganic pyrophosphate generation demonstrated by transfection of cultured fibroblasts and osteoblasts with plasma cell membrane glycoprotein-1. *Arthritis Rheum.* **1994**, *37*, 934–941. [CrossRef] [PubMed]
52. Johnson, K.; Vaingankar, S.; Chen, Y.; Moffa, A.; Goldring, M.B.; Sano, K.; Jin-Hua, P.; Sali, A.; Goding, J.; Terkeltaub, R. Differential mechanisms of inorganic pyrophosphate production by plasma cell membrane glycoprotein-1 and B10 in chondrocytes. *Arthritis Rheum.* **1999**, *42*, 1986–1997. [CrossRef]
53. Johnson, K.; Moffa, A.; Chen, Y.; Pritzker, K.; Goding, J.; Terkeltaub, R. Matrix vesicle plasma membrane glycoprotein-1 regulates mineralization by murine osteoblastic MC3T3 cells. *J. Bone Miner. Res.* **1999**, *14*, 883–892. [CrossRef]
54. Ho, A.M.; Johnson, M.D.; Kingsley, D.M. Role of the mouse ank gene in control of tissue calcification and arthritis. *Science* **2000**, *289*, 265–270. [CrossRef]
55. Szeri, F.; Niaziorimi, F.; Donnelly, S.; Fariha, N.; Tertyshnaia, M.; Patel, D.; Lundkvist, S.; van de Wetering, K. The Mineralization Regulator ANKH Mediates Cellular Efflux of ATP, Not Pyrophosphate. *J. Bone Miner. Res.* **2022**, *37*, 1024–1031. [CrossRef]
56. Houston, B.; Stewart, A.J.; Farquharson, C. PHOSPHO1-A novel phosphatase specifically expressed at sites of mineralisation in bone and cartilage. *Bone* **2004**, *34*, 629–637. [CrossRef]
57. Roberts, S.; Narisawa, S.; Harmey, D.; Millán, J.L.; Farquharson, C. Functional involvement of PHOSPHO1 in matrix vesicle–mediated skeletal mineralization. *J. Bone. Miner. Res.* **2007**, *22*, 617–627. [CrossRef]
58. Ciancaglini, P.; Yadav, M.C.; Simão, A.M.; Narisawa, S.; Pizauro, J.M.; Farquharson, C.; Hoylaerts, M.F.; Millán, J.L. Kinetic analysis of substrate utilization by native and TNAP-, NPP1-, or PHOSPHO1-deficient matrix vesicles. *J. Bone. Miner. Res.* **2010**, *25*, 716–723. [CrossRef]
59. Huesa, C.; Yadav, M.C.; Finnilä, M.A.; Goodyear, S.R.; Robins, S.P.; Tanner, K.E.; Aspden, R.M.; Millán, J.L.; Farquharson, C. PHOSPHO1 is essential for mechanically competent mineralization and the avoidance of spontaneous fractures. *Bone* **2011**, *48*, 1066–1074. [CrossRef] [PubMed]
60. Boyde, A.; Staines, K.A.; Javaheri, B.; Millan, J.L.; Pitsillides, A.A.; Farquharson, C. A distinctive patchy osteomalacia characterizes PHOSPHO1-deficient mice. *J. Anat.* **2017**, *231*, 298–308. [CrossRef] [PubMed]
61. Yadav, M.C.; Simão, A.M.S.; Narisawa, S.; Huesa, C.; McKee, M.D.; Farquharson, C.; Millán, J.L. Loss of skeletal mineralization by the simultaneous ablation of PHOSPHO1 and alkaline phosphatase function—A unified model of the mechanisms of initiation of skeletal calcification. *J. Bone Miner. Res.* **2011**, *26*, 286–297. [CrossRef] [PubMed]

62. Kirsch, T.; Nah, H.D.; Shapiro, I.M.; Pacifici, M. Regulated production of mineralization-competent matrix vesicles in hypertrophic chondrocytes. *J. Cell Biol.* **1997**, *137*, 1149–1160. [CrossRef]
63. Nakano, Y.; Beertsen, W.; van den Bos, T.; Kawamoto, T.; Oda, K.; Takano, Y. Site-specific localization of two distinct phosphatases along the osteoblast plasma membrane: Tissue non-specific alkaline phosphatase and plasma membrane calcium ATPase. *Bone* **2004**, *35*, 1077–1085. [CrossRef]
64. Narisawa, S.; Fröhlander, N.; Millian, J.L. Inactivation of two mouse alkaline phosphatase genes and establishment of a model of infantile hypophosphatasia. *Dev. Dyn.* **1997**, *208*, 432–446. [CrossRef]
65. Waymire, K.G.; Mahuren, J.D.; Jaje, J.M.; Guilarte, T.R.; Coburn, S.P.; MacGregor, G.R. Mice lacking tissue non-specific alkaline phosphatase die from seizures due to defective metabolism of vitamin B-6. *Nat. Genet.* **1995**, *11*, 45–51. [CrossRef] [PubMed]
66. Tesch, W.; Vandenbos, T.; Roschgr, P.; Fratzl-Zelman, N.; Klaushofer, K.; Beertsen, W.; Fratzl, P. Orientation of mineral crystallites and mineral density during skeletal development in mice deficient in tissue nonspecific alkaline phosphatase. *J. Bone Miner. Res.* **2003**, *18*, 117–125. [CrossRef] [PubMed]
67. Hofmann, C.; Jakob, F.; Seefried, L.; Mentrup, B.; Graser, S.; Plotkin, H.; Girschick, H.J.; Liese, J. Recombinant enzyme replacement therapy in hypophosphatasia. *Subcell. Biochem.* **2015**, *76*, 323–341. [PubMed]
68. Whyte, M.P.; Rockman-Greenberg, C.; Ozono, K.; Riese, R.; Moseley, S.; Melian, A.; Thompson, D.D.; Bishop, N.; Hofmann, C. Asfotase alfa treatment improves survival for perinatal and infantile hypophosphatasia. *J. Clin. Endocrinol. Metab.* **2016**, *101*, 334–342. [CrossRef] [PubMed]
69. Kato, K.; Nishimasu, H.; Okudaira, S.; Mihara, E.; Ishitani, R.; Takagi, J.; Aoki, J.; Nureki, O. Crystal structure of Enpp1, an extracellular glycoprotein involved in bone mineralization and insulin signaling. *Proc. Natl. Acad. Sci. USA* **2012**, *109*, 16876–16881. [CrossRef]
70. Andrilli, L.H.S.; Sebinelli, H.G.; Favarin, B.Z.; Cruz, M.A.E.; Ramos, A.P.; Bolean, M.; Millán, J.L.; Bottini, M.; Ciancaglini, P. NPP1 and TNAP hydrolyze ATP synergistically during biomineralization. *Purinergic. Signal.* 2022; in press. [CrossRef]
71. Rutsch, F.; Vaingankar, S.; Johnson, K.; Goldfine, I.; Maddux, B.; Schauerte, P.; Kalhoff, H.; Sano, K.; Boisvert, W.A.; Superti-Furga, A.; et al. PC-1 Nucleoside triphosphate pyrophosphohydrolase deficiency in idiopathic infantile arterial calcification. *Am. J. Pathol.* **2001**, *158*, 543–554. [CrossRef]
72. Rutsch, F.; Ruf, N.; Vaingankar, S.; Toliat, M.R.; Suk, A.; Höhne, W.; Schauer, G.; Lehmann, M.; Roscioli, T.; Schnabel, D.; et al. Mutations in ENPP1 are associated with 'idiopathic' infantile arterial calcification. *Nat. Genet.* **2003**, *34*, 379–381. [CrossRef]
73. Yamamoto, T.; Hasegawa, T.; Mae, T.; Hongo, H.; Yamamoto, T.; Abe, M.; Nasoori, A.; Morimoto, Y.; Maruoka, H.; Kubota, K.; et al. Comparative immunolocalization of tissue nonspecific alkaline phosphatase and ectonucleotide pyrophosphatase/phosphodiesterase 1 in murine bone. *J. Oral Biosci.* **2021**, *63*, 259–264. [CrossRef]
74. Okawa, A.; Nakamura, I.; Goto, S.; Moriya, H.; Nakamura, Y.; Ikegawa, S. Mutation in Npps in a mouse model of ossification of the posterior longitudinal ligament of the spine. *Nat. Genet.* **1998**, *19*, 271–273. [CrossRef]
75. Johnson, K.; Pritzker, K.; Goding, J.; Terkeltaub, R. The nucleoside triphosphate pyrophosphohydrolase isozyme PC-1 directly promotes cartilage calcification through chondrocyte apoptosis and increased calcium precipitation by mineralizing vesicles. *J. Rheumatol.* **2001**, *28*, 2681–2691. [PubMed]
76. Johnson, K.; Hashimoto, S.; Lotz, M.; Pritzker, K.; Goding, J.; Terkeltaub, R. Up-regulated expression of the phosphodiesterase nucleotide pyrophosphatase family member PC-1 is a marker and pathogenic factor for knee meniscal cartilage matrix calcification. *Arthritis Rheum.* **2001**, *44*, 1071–1081. [CrossRef]
77. Johnson, K.; Goding, J.; Van Etten, D.; Sali, A.; Hu, S.I.; Farley, D.; Krug, H.; Hessle, L.; Millán, J.L.; Terkeltaub, R. Linked deficiencies in extracellular PP(i) and osteopontin mediate pathologic calcification associated with defective PC-1 and ANK expression. *J. Bone Miner. Res.* **2003**, *18*, 994–1004. [CrossRef] [PubMed]
78. Mackenzie, N.C.; Zhu, D.; Milne, E.M.; van 't Hof, R.; Martin, A.; Darryl Quarles, L.; Millán, J.L.; Farquharson, C.; MacRae, V.E. Altered bone development and an increase in FGF-23 expression in Enpp1(-/-) mice. *PLoS ONE* **2012**, *7*, e32177. [CrossRef]
79. Nam, H.K.; Emmanouil, E.; Hatch, N.E. Deletion of the pyrophosphate generating enzyme ENPP1 rescues craniofacial abnormalities in the TNAP-/- mouse model of Hypophosphatasia and reveals FGF23 as a marker of phenotype severity. *Front. Dent. Med.* **2022**, *3*, 846962. [CrossRef]
80. Bergwitz, C.; Juppner, H. FGF23 and syndromes of abnormal renal phosphate handling. *Adv. Exp. Med. Biol.* **2012**, *728*, 41–64.
81. Ho, B.B.; Bergwitz, C. FGF23 signalling and physiology. *J. Mol. Endocrinol.* **2021**, *66*, R23–R32. [CrossRef]
82. Lederer, E. Regulation of serum phosphate. *J. Physiol.* **2014**, *592*, 3985–3995. [CrossRef]
83. Abhishek, A.; Doherty, M. Pathophysiology of articular chondrocalcinosis–role of ANKH. *Nat. Rev. Rheumatol.* **2011**, *7*, 96–104. [PubMed]
84. Stewart, A.J.; Leong, D.T.K.; Farquharson, C. PLA 2 and ENPP6 may act in concert to generate phosphocholine from the matrix vesicle membrane during skeletal mineralization. *FASEB J.* **2018**, *32*, 20–25. [CrossRef]
85. Cao, X.; Genge, B.R.; Wu, L.N.; Buzzi, W.R.; Showman, R.M.; Wuthier, R.E. Characterization, cloning and expression of the 67-kDA annexin from chicken growth plate cartilage matrix vesicles. *Biochem. Biophys. Res. Commun.* **1993**, *197*, 556–561. [CrossRef]
86. Kirsch, T.; Nah, H.D.; Demuth, D.R.; Harrison, G.; Golub, E.E.; Adams, S.L.; Pacifici, M. Annexin V-mediated calcium flux across membranes is dependent on the lipid composition: Implications for cartilage mineralization. *Biochemistry* **1997**, *36*, 3359–3367. [CrossRef] [PubMed]

87. Kirsch, T.; Claassen, H. Matrix vesicles mediate mineralization of human thyroid cartilage. *Calcif. Tissue Int.* **2000**, *66*, 292–297. [CrossRef] [PubMed]
88. Majeska, R.J.; Holwerda, D.L.; Wuthier, R.E. Localization of phosphatidylserine in isolated chick epiphyseal cartilage matrix vesicles with trinitrobenzenesulfonate. *Calcif. Tissue Int.* **1979**, *27*, 41–46. [CrossRef]
89. Taylor, M.G.; Simkiss, K.; Simmons, J.; Wu, L.N.; Wuthier, R.E. Structural studies of a phosphatidyl serine-amorphous calcium phosphate complex. *Cell. Mol. Life Sci.* **1998**, *54*, 196–202. [CrossRef]
90. Hasegawa, T.; Yamamoto, T.; Hongo, H.; Qiu, Z.; Abe, M.; Kanesaki, T.; Tanaka, K.; Endo, T.; Freitas, P.H.L.; Li, M. Three-dimensional ultrastructure of osteocytes assessed by focused ion beam-scanning electron microscopy (FIB-SEM). *Histochem. Cell Biol.* **2018**, *149*, 423–432. [CrossRef] [PubMed]
91. Bélanger, L.F. Osteocytic osteolysis. *Calcif. Tissue. Res.* **1969**, *4*, 1–12. [CrossRef] [PubMed]
92. Bai, L.; Collins, J.F.; Xu, H.; Xu, L.; Ghishan, F.K. Molecular cloning of a murine type III sodium-dependent phosphate cotransporter (Pit-2) gene promoter. *Biochim. Biophys. Acta* **2001**, *1522*, 42–45. [CrossRef]
93. Qing, H.; Bonewald, L.F. Osteocyte remodeling of perilacunar and pericanalicular matrix. *Int. J. Oral Sci.* **2009**, *1*, 59–65. [CrossRef]
94. Teit, A.; Zallone, A. Do osteocytes contribute to bone mikneral homeostasis? Osteocytic osteolysis revisited. *Bone* **2009**, *44*, 11–16. [CrossRef]
95. Bonewald, L.F. The amazing osteocyte. *J. Bone Miner. Res.* **2011**, *26*, 229–238. [CrossRef]
96. Qing, H.; Ardeshirpour, L.; Pajevic, P.D.; Dusevich, V.; Jähn, K.; Kato, S.; Wysolmerski, J.; Bonewald, L.F. Demonstration of osteocytic perilacunar/canalicular remodeling in mice during lactation. *J. Bone Miner. Res.* **2012**, *27*, 1018–1029. [CrossRef]
97. Whysolmerski, J.J. Osteocytic osteolysis: Time for a second look? *BoneKEy Rep.* **2012**, *1*, 229. [CrossRef]
98. Whysolmerski, J.J. Osteocytes remove and replace perilacunar minewral during reproductive cycles. *Bone* **2013**, *54*, 230–236. [CrossRef]
99. Sano, H.; Kikuta, J.; Furuya, M.; Kondo, N.; Endo, N.; Ishii, M. Intravital bone imaging by two-photon excitation microscopy to identify osteocytic osteolysis in vivo. *Bone* **2015**, *74*, 134–139. [CrossRef] [PubMed]
100. Bonucci, E.; Gherardi, G.; Faraggiana, T. Bone changes in hemodialyzed uremic subjects. Comparative light and electron microscope investigations. *Virchows Arch. A Pathol. Anat. Histol.* **1976**, *371*, 183–198. [CrossRef] [PubMed]
101. Mosekilde, L.; Melsen, F. A tetracycline-based histomorphometric evaluation of bone resorption and bone turnover in hyperthyroidism and hyperparathyroidism. *Acta Med. Scand.* **1978**, *204*, 97–102. [CrossRef] [PubMed]
102. Jähn, K.; Kelkar, S.; Zhao, H.; Xie, Y.; Tiede-Lewis, L.M.; Dusevich, V.; Dallas, S.L.; Bonewald, L.F. Osteocytes acidify their microenvironment in response to PTHrP in vitro and in lactating mice in vivo. *J. Bone Miner. Res.* **2017**, *32*, 1761–1772. [CrossRef] [PubMed]
103. Rolvien, T.; Krause, M.; Jeschke, A.; Yorgan, T.; Püschel, K.; Schinke, T.; Busse, B.; Demay, M.B.; Amling, M. Vitamin D regulates osteocyte survival and perilacunar remodeling in human and murine bone. *Bone* **2017**, *103*, 78–87. [CrossRef]
104. Kogawa, M.; Wijenayaka, A.R.; Ormsby, R.T.; Thomas, G.P.; Anderson, P.H.; Bonewald, L.F.; Findlay, D.M.; Atkins, G.J. Sclerostin regulates release of bone mineral by osteocytes by induction of carbonic anhydrase 2. *J. Bone Miner. Res.* **2013**, *28*, 2436–2448. [CrossRef]
105. Nango, N.; Kubota, S.; Hasegawa, T.; Yashiro, W.; Momose, A.; Matsuo, K. Osteocyte-directed bone demineralization along canaliculi. *Bone* **2016**, *84*, 279–288. [CrossRef]
106. Hongo, H.; Hasegawa, T.; Saito, M.; Tsuboi, K.; Yamamoto, T.; Sasaki, M.; Abe, M.; de Freitas, P.H.L.; Yurimoto, H.; Udagawa, N.; et al. Osteocytic osteolysis in PTH-treated wild-type and *Rankl*-/- mice examined by transmission electron microscopy, atomic force microscopy, and isotope microscopy. *J. Histochem. Cytochem.* **2020**, *68*, 651–668. [CrossRef] [PubMed]
107. Jandl, N.M.; von Kroge, S.; Stürznickel, J.; Baranowsky, A.; Stockhausen, K.E.; Mushumba, H.; Beil, F.T.; Püschel, K.; Amling, M.; Rolvien, T. Large osteocyte lacunae in iliac crest infantile bone are not associated with impaired mineral distribution or signs of osteocytic osteolysis. *Bone* **2020**, *135*, 115324. [CrossRef] [PubMed]
108. Misof, B.M.; Blouin, S.; Hofstaetter, J.G.; Roschger, P.; Zwerina, J.; Erben, R.G. No role of osteocytic osteolysis in the development and recovery of the bone phenotype induced by severe secondary hyperparathyroidism in vitamin D receptor deficient mice. *Int. J. Mol. Sci.* **2020**, *21*, 7989. [CrossRef] [PubMed]
109. Ryan, B.A.; Kovacs, C.S. The puzzle of lactational bone physiology: Osteocytes masquerade as osteoclasts and osteoblasts. *J. Clin. Investig.* **2019**, *129*, 3041–3044. [CrossRef] [PubMed]
110. Kaya, S.; Basta-Pljakic, J.; Seref-Ferlengez, Z.; Majeska, R.J.; Cardoso, L.; Bromage, T.G.; Zhang, Q.; Flach, C.R.; Mendelsohn, R.; Yakar, S.; et al. Lactation-induced changes in the volume of osteocyte lacunar-canalicular space alter mechanical properties in cortical bone tissue. *J. Bone Miner. Res.* **2017**, *32*, 688–697. [CrossRef]
111. Emami, A.J.; Sebastian, A.; Lin, Y.Y.; Yee, C.S.; Osipov, B.; Loots, G.G.; Alliston, T.; Christiansen, B.A. Altered canalicular remodeling associated with femur fracture in mice. *J. Orthop. Res.* **2022**, *40*, 891–900. [CrossRef]
112. Vahidi, G.; Rux, C.; Sherk, V.D.; Heveran, C.M. Lacunar-canalicular bone remodeling: Impacts on bone quality and tools for assessment. *Bone* **2021**, *143*, 115663. [CrossRef]
113. Sasaki, M.; Hasegawa, T.; Yamada, T.; Hongo, H.; de Freitas, P.H.; Suzuki, R.; Yamamoto, T.; Tabata, C.; Toyosawa, S.; Yamamoto, T.; et al. Altered distribution of bone matrix proteins and defective bone mineralization in klotho-deficient mice. *Bone* **2013**, *57*, 206–219. [CrossRef]

114. Liu, S.; Rowe, P.S.; Vierthaler, L.; Zhou, J.; Quarles, L.D. Phosphorylated acidic serine-aspartate-rich MEPE-associated motif peptide from matrix extracellular phosphoglycoprotein inhibits phosphate regulating gene with homologies to endopeptidases on the X-chromosome enzyme activity. *J. Endocrinol.* **2007**, *192*, 261–267. [CrossRef]
115. Staines, K.A.; MacRae, V.E.; Farquharson, C. The importance of the SIBLING family of proteins. *J. Endocrinol.* **2012**, *214*, 241–255. [CrossRef]
116. Rowe, P.S.; de Zoysa, P.A.; Dong, R.; Wang, H.R.; White, K.E.; Econs, M.J.; Oudet, C.L. MEPE, a new gene expressed in bone marrow and tumors causing osteomalacia. *Genomics* **2000**, *67*, 54–68. [CrossRef]
117. Rowe, P.S.; Kumagai, Y.; Gutierrez, G.; Garrett, I.R.; Blacher, R.; Rosen, D.; Cundy, J.; Navvab, S.; Chen, D.; Drezner, M.K.; et al. MEPE has the properties of an osteoblastic phosphatonin and minhibin. *Bone* **2004**, *34*, 303–319. [CrossRef] [PubMed]
118. Rowe, P.S.; Garrett, I.R.; Schwarz, P.M.; Carnes, D.L.; Lafer, E.M.; Mundy, G.R.; Gutierrez, G.E. Surface plasmon resonance (SPR) confirms that MEPE binds to PHEX via the MEPE-ASARM motif: A model for impaired mineralization in X-linked rickets (HYP). *Bone* **2005**, *36*, 33–46. [CrossRef] [PubMed]
119. Addison, W.N.; Masica, D.L.; Gray, J.J.; McKee, M.D. Phosphorylation-dependent inhibition of mineralization by osteopontin ASARM peptides is regulated by PHEX cleavage. *J. Bone Miner. Res.* **2010**, *25*, 695–705. [CrossRef] [PubMed]
120. Feng, J.Q.; Ward, L.M.; Liu, S.; Lu, Y.; Xie, Y.; Yuan, B.; Yu, X.; Rauch, F.; Davis, S.I.; Zhang, S.; et al. Loss of DMP1 causes rickets and osteomalacia and identifies a role for osteocytes in mineral metabolism. *Nat. Genet.* **2006**, *38*, 1310–1315. [CrossRef]
121. Mäkitie, O.; Pereira, R.C.; Kaitila, I.; Turan, S.; Bastepe, M.; Laine, T.; Kröger, H.; Cole, W.G.; Jüppner, H. Long-term clinical outcome and carrier phenotype in autosomal recessive hypophosphatemia caused by a novel DMP1 mutation. *J. Bone Miner. Res.* **2010**, *25*, 2165–2174. [CrossRef] [PubMed]

Disclaimer/Publisher's Note: The statements, opinions and data contained in all publications are solely those of the individual author(s) and contributor(s) and not of MDPI and/or the editor(s). MDPI and/or the editor(s) disclaim responsibility for any injury to people or property resulting from any ideas, methods, instructions or products referred to in the content.

Communication

Regulation of Phosphate Transporters and Novel Regulator of Phosphate Metabolism

Megumi Koike [1], Minori Uga [1], Yuji Shiozaki [1], Ken-ichi Miyamoto [1,2] and Hiroko Segawa [1,*]

[1] Department of Applied Nutrition, Institute of Biomedical Sciences, Tokushima University Graduate School, 3-18-15 Kuramoto-cho, Tokushima 770-8503, Japan; megmilk.yt@gmail.com (M.K.); ugaminori@gmail.com (M.U.); shiozaki.yuji@tokushima-u.ac.jp (Y.S.); kmiyamoto@agr.ryukoku.ac.jp (K.-i.M.)
[2] Graduate School of Agriculture, Ryukoku University, 1-5 Yokotani, Seta Oe-cho, Otsu 520-2194, Shiga, Japan
* Correspondence: segawa@tokushima-u.ac.jp; Tel./Fax: +81-88-633-7082

Abstract: Phosphorus is essential for all living organisms. It plays an important role in maintaining biological functions, such as energy metabolism, cell membrane formation, and bone mineralization. Various factors in the intestine, kidneys, and bones regulate the homeostasis of the inorganic phosphate (Pi) concentration in the body. X-linked hypophosphatemia (XLH), the most common form of hereditary hypophosphatemic rickets, is characterized by an impaired mineralization of the bone matrix, hypertrophic chondrocytes with hypophosphatemia, and active vitamin D resistance in childhood. Phosphate-regulating gene with homologies to endopeptidases on the X chromosome was recognized as the responsible gene for XLH. XLH is classified as fibroblast growth factor 23 (FGF23)-related hypophosphatemic rickets. The enhanced FGF23 stimulates renal phosphate wasting by downregulating sodium-dependent Pi cotransporters, NaPi2a and NaPi2c proteins, in the proximal tubules. Recently, transmembrane protein (Tmem) 174 has been identified as a novel regulator of phosphate transporters. This review introduces the role of Tmem174 in the Pi homeostasis in the body.

Keywords: phosphate transporter; *SLC34*; Tmem174; kidney; bone; FGF23

1. Introduction

Phosphorus is available in many foods in both organic and inorganic forms [1–4]. Organic phosphate is naturally present in foods, whereas inorganic phosphate (Pi) is added to processed foods. The absorption rate is approximately 60% for organic phosphate and approximately 90% for inorganic phosphate [2,3].

In adults, approximately 85% of the body's phosphorus is stored in the bones and teeth, with an additional 10% found in skeletal muscle. Phosphorus accounts for about 1% of body weight. Pi is an essential nutrient for several biological functions, including intracellular signal transduction, cell membrane formation, function, and energy exchange in the body [5]. The regulation of blood Pi levels depends on the coordinated activity of three major organs: intestines, kidneys, and bones. Furthermore, a transport system is necessary to transfer Pi across hydrophobic cell membranes to achieve these functions [5].

Intestinal Pi absorption, bone formation, and renal Pi reabsorption maintain phosphorus balance. Factors such as dietary phosphorus amount, active vitamin D (1,25(OH)$_2$D), parathyroid hormone (PTH), and fibroblast growth factor 23 (FGF23) regulate Pi absorption/reabsorption [5]. Low Pi diets increase intestinal and renal Pi reabsorption. Active vitamin D stimulates intestinal Pi absorption. In contrast, a high Pi diet promotes the secretion of PTH from the parathyroid gland and FGF23 from the bone. In the kidney, PTH binds to PTH receptors, and FGF23 binds to alfa-Klotho and FGF receptor 1 to inhibit Pi resorption and stimulate urinary Pi excretion. In addition, FGF23 inhibits 1-α-hydroxylase (*cyp27b1*) expression and decreases active vitamin D synthesis by increasing 24-hydroxylase (*cyp24a1*) expression, thereby inhibiting intestinal Pi absorption.

As mentioned above, bone acts as a reservoir of Pi. Pi can be resorbed from bone into the extracellular space to maintain blood Pi level [6,7]. The release of phosphate into the blood from bone resorption is thought to play a role in supporting the amount of substrate needed to sustain ATP turnover in skeletal muscle and help maintain the high rate of muscle protein synthesis and turnover [6]. This intestinal–kidney–bone–parathyroid pathway contributes to regulating blood Pi levels [5].

The blood Pi concentration regulates the intracellular Pi in various tissues. Energy metabolism factors, such as adenosine triphosphate/nicotinamide adenine dinucleotide, are thought to contribute to Pi regulation. In this regard, hormones such as insulin and glucagon regulate the tissue transfer of Pi, thereby affecting the blood Pi concentration. Furthermore, the circadian rhythm of the blood Pi concentration has been reported to be regulated by renal nicotinamide adenine dinucleotide metabolism, which is dependent on food intake [8–10]. Pi absorption/reabsorption and movement of Pi into and out of the cells are promoted by increasing or decreasing the expression levels of Pi transporters localized at cell membranes.

2. Phosphate Transporter Classification in the Body

To date, 65 solute carrier (SLC) families are identified as being highly expressed in critical metabolic organs contributing to homeostasis by regulating the transmembrane transportation of nutrients and metabolites (http://slc.bioparadigms.org/ accessed on 19/08/2023) [11]. The *SLC20, 34, 37,* and *53* families are involved in the inorganic monophosphate transport (Table 1).

Table 1. Phosphate transporters in SLC family.

Name	Function	Substrates
SLC20	Na+-phosphate cotransporter	Phosphate
SLC34	Na+-phosphate cotransporter	Phosphate
SLC37	Sugar-phosphate/phosphate exchanger	Glucose-6-phosphate/phosphate
SLC53	Phosphate carriers	Phosphate
SLC62	Pyrophosphate transporter	Pyrophosphate
SLC63	Sphingosine-phosphate transporter	Sphingosine-phosphate

SLC; solute carrier.

The *SLC20* family of transporters includes PiT1 (*SLC20A1*) and PiT2 (*SLC20A2*). These proteins were initially described as a family of cell surface receptors for the gibbon ape leukemia virus and murine amphotropic retrovirus and are distributed throughout the body [5].

The *SLC20* family of transporters includes PiT1 (*SLC20A1*) and PiT2 (*SLC20A2*). These proteins were initially described as a family of cell surface receptors for the gibbon ape leukemia virus and murine amphotropic retrovirus and are distributed throughout the body [5].

The *SLC34* family of transporters includes NaPi2a (*SLC34A1*), NaPi2b (*SLC34A2*), and NaPi2c (*SLC34A3*). NaPi2a and NaPi2c mainly play a role in renal Pi reabsorption, whereas NaPi2b plays a role in intestinal Pi absorption and in several organs, including the lung and placenta [5,10].

The *SLC37* family includes four proteins, *SLC37A1–4*. In the *SLC37* family, *SLC37A4* is known as glucose-6-phosphate transporter 1 (G6PT1) that is strongly expressed in the liver, kidney, and hematopoietic progenitor cells [12–15]. *SLC37A4* is a glucose-6-phosphate (Glc-6P)/Pi exchanger that is required to transport Glc-6P into the endoplasmic reticulum. Gene mutations of *SLC37A4* cause the glycogen storage disease non-1A type. However, whether *SLC37* is involved in Pi homeostasis in the cells and body remains unclear.

SLC53A1 (xenotropic and polytropic retrovirus receptor 1, XPR1) is thought to be a Pi exporter and is ubiquitously expressed. Several studies have reported a correlation between altered XPR1 expression/function and placental calcification, familial brain calcification, and Fanconi syndrome [16–21]. However, how XPR1 is also involved in regulating Pi metabolism in cells and the body is unclear. Furthermore, XPR1 localization in the small intestine and kidney is still unknown.

Previous studies have demonstrated that the *SLC34* family regulates blood Pi levels, whereas the *SLC20* family is involved in bone and tissue calcification [5,10,18]. Further studies are needed to investigate the role of other molecules.

3. Pi Transporters and Disease

Defects in *SLC34A1* cause Fanconi syndrome and infantile hypercalcemia [22], and defects in *SLC34A2* cause alveolar microlithiasis, an autosomal recessive genetic disease resulting in calcium phosphate stones in the alveoli [23–27]. NaPi2b is expressed in a broader range of organs and cells than NaPi2a and NaPi2c [5]. However, no abnormal blood Pi and calcium levels have been reported in patients with this gene mutation. Defects in *SLC34A3* cause hypophosphatemic rickets with hereditary hypercalciuria [28–31]. Defects in *SLC20A2* are involved in idiopathic basal ganglia calcification [32,33], and XPR1 is associated with primary familial brain calcification [34].

The average Pi concentration in the blood is 2.5–4.5 mg/dL in adults, and proper bone calcification occurs when maintained at this level [4,35–37]. Infants have a 50% higher blood phosphate concentration than adults, and children have a 30% higher concentration [4,38]. This is likely because phosphate-dependent processes play a crucial role in growth. Blood Pi levels below 2.5 mg/dL (hypophosphatemia) are associated with rickets and renal stone disease, whereas Pi levels above 4.5 mg/dL (hyperphosphatemia) increase the risk of vascular calcification [4,35,36]. Various factors contribute to abnormal Pi metabolism [35,36]. FGF23 overactivity causes hypophosphatemia, and conversely, a decreased FGF23 activity causes hyperphosphatemia [18,35,36]. The primary target of the phosphaturic factor FGF23 is NaPi2a and NaPi2c in the kidney [18,35,36,39,40].

The main relationship between phosphate metabolism and α-Klotho is that membrane-bound α-Klotho acts as a co-receptor for FGFR. In the absence of Klotho, the FGF23 signaling pathway becomes disrupted, leading to hyperphosphatemia. In α-Klotho mutant mice, the expression of NaPi2a and NaPi2c is upregulated at both the transcriptional and protein levels [41]. On the other hand, in the small intestine of α-Klotho mutant mice, NaPi2b is transcriptionally suppressed but its protein expression is increased [41]. In α-Klotho knockout (KO) mice, an increase in the expression of NaPi2a and NaPi2c, or specifically an upregulation of NaPi2c expression, has been reported [42–44]. In the small intestine of α-Klotho KO mice, there is an observed increase in the expression of Pi transporters, not only NaPi2b, but also PiT1, PiT2, and NaPi2c mRNA levels [42]. The exact mechanism underlying these differences in Pi transporter expression between α-Klotho mutant mice and α-Klotho knockout mice remains unclear.

The direct relationship between Pi transporters NaPi2a, NaPi2b, and membrane-bound α-Klotho has also been reported in electrophysiological studies using *Xenopus* oocytes [45]. When NaPi2a or NaPi2b and full-length α-Klotho (membrane form) were expressed in oocytes, the electrophysiological phosphate transport activity was significantly inhibited. Furthermore, α-Klotho has been detected not only as a membrane-bound form, but also as a soluble protein secreted into blood, urine, and cerebrospinal fluid. The secreted soluble form of α-Klotho has been reported to function as a hormone with various roles, including antioxidant stress, anti-inflammatory, and anti-aging effects, in different tissues [46]. The relationship between the secreted form of α-Klotho and NaPi2a has been investigated through studies using opossum kidney (OK) cells and brush border membrane vesicles (BBMVs) [47]. In these studies, recombinant α-Klotho was added to either OK cells or BBMV to examine the expression and Pi transport activity of NaPi2a. The results indicated that the secreted form of α-Klotho directly induced the endocytosis of NaPi2a, leading to a decrease in phosphate transport activity. These reports suggest that α-Klotho may regulate NaPi2a or NaPi2b directly, independent of FGF23 or active vitamin D signaling. However, the direct relationship between the expression and functional activity of NaPi transporters and α-Klotho has not been fully elucidated yet.

Chronic kidney disease (CKD) leads to hyperphosphatemia due to inadequate Pi excretion by the kidneys. In addition, the mineral dysregulation associated with CKD induces a pathological accumulation of Pi, leading to vascular calcification (VC) [48]. PiT-1 and PiT-2 Pi transporters are involved in developing vascular calcification caused by hyperphosphatemia during CKD [46,49]. VC is a severe complication of hyperphosphatemia, causing cardiovascular morbidity and mortality. In previous studies, PiT-1 and PiT-2 have been reported to regulate vascular smooth muscle cell (VSMCs) depolarization, Ca^{2+} influx, oxidative stress, and calcium changes. Recently, the uptake of Pi into mitochondria via the mitochondrial phosphate carrier protein (PiC), which SLC25A3 encodes in humans, has been revealed as a critical molecular mechanism mediating pathological calcification changes and superoxide generation in mitochondria [50].

Therefore, treating hyperphosphatemia in patients with CKD and dialysis is essential because hyperphosphatemia affects patient outcomes. The target of hyperphosphatemia treatment is intestinal Pi absorption. Intestinal NaPi2b, PiT1, and PiT2 inhibitors have been developed [51–53]. EOS789, a pan-Pi transporter inhibitor, inhibits Pi absorption in the intestine through a distinct mechanism compared to Pi binders, with low absorption, minimal body accumulation, and potential for inhibiting Pi transport inhibition at low doses [38–41]. Additionally, drugs that inhibit NaPi2a are specifically developed to treat hereditary and acquired hyperphosphatemia [54,55].

4. A Novel Regulator of Phosphate Metabolism

Previous studies on patients with X-linked hypophosphatemia (XLH) and a murine model of XLH (Hyp mice) classified XLH as FGF23-related hypophosphatemic rickets [35,36]. Enhanced FGF23 stimulates renal Pi wasting by downregulating the Na^+-dependent Pi cotransporters, NaPi2a and NaPi2c, in the proximal tubules [56–58]. Downstream signaling from FGF23 disrupts the binding of NaPi2a by phosphorylating NHERF1 or Ezrin, allowing it to enter the clathrin-coated vesicle system and induce endocytosis and reducing NaPi2a protein expression [5,59]. This NaPi2a regulatory mechanism is rapid and may be responsible for the rapid response that is essential for the regulation of blood Pi levels [5]. This regulation of NaPi2a degradation has not been observed for NaPi2c. Not all of this mechanism has been clarified.

Recently, transmembrane protein (Tmem) 174 has been reported as a novel regulator of NaPi2a degradation [60]. Tmem174 was identified as a molecule associated with slc34a1 and slc34a3 gene expression through in silico analysis. Tmem174 had already been identified, but its function details were unclear [49–51]. The mRNA sequences of human (NM_153217), rat (NM_00102429), and mouse (NM_026685.2) were reported in the NCBI database. The Tmem174 protein consists of 243 amino acids and has two transmembrane domains (Figure 1A). Mouse Tmem174 mRNA was significantly higher in the kidney than in other tissues (Figure 1B), and the protein is localized to the apical membrane of the renal proximal tubules (Figure 1C) [60]. However, the Tmem174 function and role have not been clarified. Tmem174 knockout mice fed with standard mouse chow showed an oversecretion of PTH and FGF23 despite normal Pi levels in the blood and urinary Pi excretion (Figure 2A–D) [60]. Renal NaPi2a expression was not suppressed, although NaPi2c expression was markedly reduced in Tmem174 knockout mice compared with wild-type (WT) mice (Figure 2E). Tmem174 binds to NaPi2a, but not to NHERF1 without NaPi2a, and Tmem174 deficiency is limited to the control function of NaPi2a [60]. Tmem174 KO mice were shown to lead to PTH/FGF23 resistance in renal NaPi2a. For example, vitamin D administration for Hyp mice restores serum Pi levels by causing FGF23 resistance to NaPi2a/NHERF1 [45,46]. In Tmem174 KO mice, dietary Pi loading caused marked hyperphosphatemia and high levels of FGF23 compared to WT mice [48]. These abnormal blood Pi and FGF23 levels in Tmem174 KO mice might be due to disrupted NaPi2a internalization.

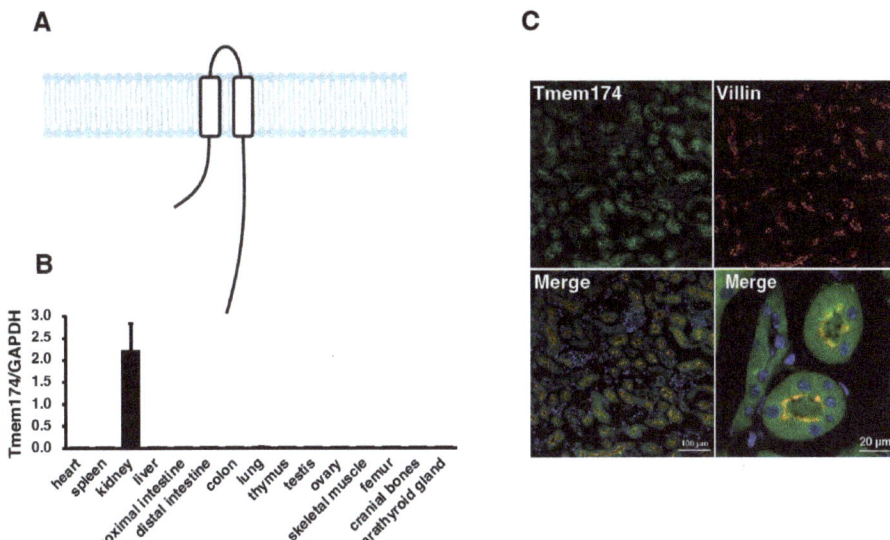

Figure 1. Tissue expression and renal localization of mouse transmembrane protein 174 (Tmem174). (**A**) The Tmem174 protein has 243 amino acids and is putatively 2 transmembrane domains. (**B**) Real-time PCR of Tmem174 mRNA levels in several wild-type (WT) mice tissues. Internal control was glyceraldehyde-3-phosphate dehydrogenase (GAPDH). Values are indicated as mean ± standard error (SE). (**C**) Tmem174 (green), DAPI (blue), and Villin (red) immunofluorescence staining in kidney sections of WT mice. Sections were prepared from mouse kidneys embedded in an optimal cutting temperature compound and frozen. 1B and 1C are modified by Sasaki et al. [60], and there are no issues with copyright.

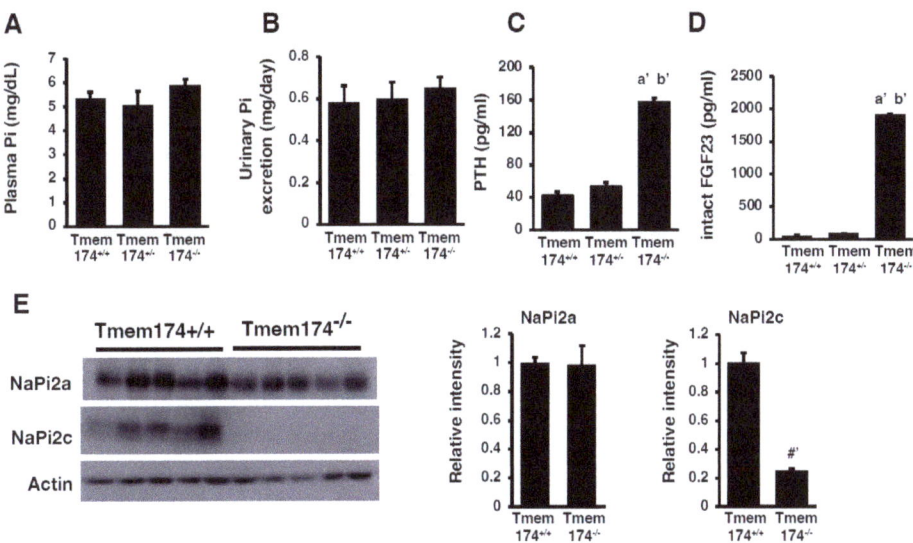

Figure 2. Characterization of Tmem174 knockout mice fed standard mouse chow. (**A**) Plasma Pi, (**B**) urinary Pi excretion, (**C**) plasma intact PTH, and (**D**) serum intact FGF23 levels of male Tmem174 knockout mice fed standard mouse chow. Values are presented as mean ± SE. a' $p < 0.01$ vs. Tmem174$^{+/+}$ mice. b' $p < 0.01$ vs. Tmem174$^{+/-}$ mice. (**E**) Immunoblotting analysis of NaPi2 transporters

protein expression in Tmem174$^{+/+}$ and Tmem174$^{-/-}$ mice (8-week-old mice, n = 5 each). A 20 µg brush border membrane vesicle was loaded in each lane. Actin was used as an internal control. Values are presented as mean ± SE. #' $p < 0.01$. All figures are modified from Sasaki et al. [60], and there are no issues with copyright.

Tmem174 KO mice had an enhanced FGF23 induction from bone [48]. High serum FGF23 levels cause the abnormal bone morphology observed in the Hyp mice, but Tmem174 KO mice did not show them. The reason may be that Tmem174 KO mice do not develop hypophosphatemia. Further detailed studies are needed to elucidate the function of Tmem174 in bone physiology. Tmem174 in the kidney is a novel regulator of Pi metabolism that plays a demanding role in regulating NaPi2a protein expression and PTH and FGF23 secretion, which are important for regulating blood Pi levels. However, how Tmem174 is involved in NaPi2a degradation and how it is involved in PTH and FGF23 secretion are still unclear. A detailed analysis of this new network linking the kidneys (Tmem174), bones (FGF23), and parathyroid glands (PTH) is still being conducted. Around the same time, Tmem174 was discovered by Miyazaki-Anzai et al. using RNA-seq and RT-qPCR analysis as a new Pi homeostasis regulator interacting with NPT2A [61]. Their analysis of knockout mice yielded results similar to our report but showed vascular calcification in Tmem174 knockout mice. However, in our analysis, no vascular calcification was observed in the knockout mice. The predicted role of Tmem174 in regulating plasma Pi concentrations is summarized in Figure 3.

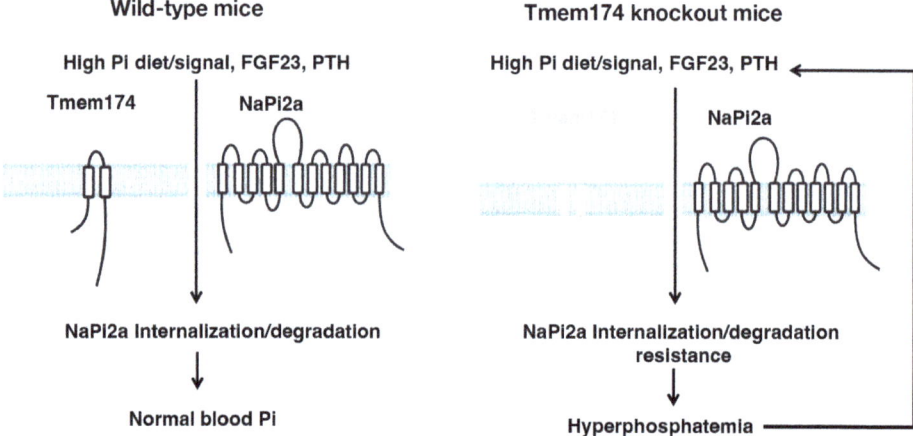

Figure 3. Summary: The putative role of Tmem174 in the regulation of plasma Pi concentrations. Phosphaturic hormones, PTH, and FGF23 are secreted in response to Pi load and act on the kidney to promote Pi excretion. The NaPi2a/NHERF1 complex is predicted to play an important role in regulating PTH and FGF23 responsiveness by modulating NaPi2a localization levels at the apical membrane of the proximal tubule in response to Pi deficiency or excess by Tmem174. The figure is modified from Sasaki et al. [60], and there are no issues with copyright.

5. Conclusions

Since identifying Pi transporters in the late 1990s, extensive research has focused on clarifying the underlying mechanisms regulating blood Pi levels and NaPi transporters. Pi plays a variety of important functions in the body. Thus, the regulating mechanisms of Pi transporters in energy production, signal transduction, and cell differentiation and proliferation are important areas of focus for future research. Understanding the role of Tmem174 may help treat hypophosphatemia, including XLH, and other diseases associated with abnormal Pi metabolism.

Author Contributions: Writing, M.K., M.U., Y.S. and H.S.; review and editing, K.-i.M. and H.S. All authors have read and agreed to the published version of the manuscript.

Funding: This work was supported by JSPS KAKENHI Grants (JP17H04190 and JP20K08637 to K.M. and JP21H03375 to H.S.).

Institutional Review Board Statement: All procedures involving the use of animals were subjected to approval from Tokushima University School of Medicine (T2019-126) ethics committee.

Data Availability Statement: No new data were generated in this manuscript. All data presented in the figures were previously published, and there were no issues with copyright.

Conflicts of Interest: The authors declare no conflict of interest.

References

1. Erem, S.; Razzaque, M.S. Dietary Phosphate Toxicity: An Emerging Global Health Concern. *Histochem. Cell Biol.* **2018**, *150*, 711–719. [CrossRef] [PubMed]
2. Kalantar-Zadeh, K.; Gutekunst, L.; Mehrotra, R.; Kovesdy, C.P.; Bross, R.; Shinaberger, C.S.; Noori, N.; Hirschberg, R.; Benner, D.; Nissenson, A.R.; et al. Understanding Sources of Dietary Phosphorus in the Treatment of Patients with Chronic Kidney Disease. *Clin. J. Am. Soc. Nephrol.* **2010**, *5*, 519–530. [CrossRef] [PubMed]
3. Uribarri, J. Phosphorus Homeostasis in Normal Health and in Chronic Kidney Disease Patients with Special Emphasis on Dietary Phosphorus Intake. *Semin. Dial.* **2007**, *20*, 295–301. [CrossRef] [PubMed]
4. Qadeer, H.A.; Bashir, K. Physiology, Phosphate. In *StatPearls*; StatPearls Publishing LLC.: Treasure Island, FL, USA, 2023.
5. Hernando, N.; Gagnon, K.; Lederer, E. Phosphate Transport in Epithelial and Nonepithelial Tissue. *Physiol. Rev.* **2021**, *101*, 1–35. [CrossRef]
6. Klein, G.L. The Role of the Musculoskeletal System in Post-Burn Hypermetabolism. *Metabolism* **2019**, *97*, 81–86. [CrossRef]
7. Goretti Penido, M.; Alon, U.S. Phosphate Homeostasis and its Role in Bone Health. *Pediatr. Nephrol.* **2012**, *27*, 2039–2048. [CrossRef]
8. Miyagawa, A.; Tatsumi, S.; Takahama, W.; Fujii, O.; Nagamoto, K.; Kinoshita, E.; Nomura, K.; Ikuta, K.; Fujii, T.; Hanazaki, A.; et al. The Sodium Phosphate Cotransporter Family and Nicotinamide Phosphoribosyltransferase Contribute to the Daily Oscillation of Plasma Inorganic Phosphate Concentration. *Kidney Int.* **2018**, *93*, 1073–1085. [CrossRef]
9. Nomura, K.; Tatsumi, S.; Miyagawa, A.; Shiozaki, Y.; Sasaki, S.; Kaneko, I.; Ito, M.; Kido, S.; Segawa, H.; Sano, M.; et al. Hepatectomy-Related Hypophosphatemia: A Novel Phosphaturic Factor in the Liver-Kidney Axis. *J. Am. Soc. Nephrol.* **2014**, *25*, 761–772. [CrossRef]
10. Tatsumi, S.; Katai, K.; Kaneko, I.; Segawa, H.; Miyamoto, K.I. Nad Metabolism and the Slc34 Family: Evidence for a Liver-Kidney Axis Regulating Inorganic Phosphate. *Pflug. Arch.* **2019**, *471*, 109–122. [CrossRef]
11. Pizzagalli, M.D.; Bensimon, A.; Superti-Furga, G. A Guide to Plasma Membrane Solute Carrier Proteins. *FEBS J.* **2021**, *288*, 2784–2835. [CrossRef]
12. Bartoloni, L.; Antonarakis, S.E. The Human Sugar-Phosphate/Phosphate Exchanger Family Slc37. *Pflug. Arch.* **2004**, *447*, 780–783. [CrossRef]
13. Cappello, A.R.; Curcio, R.; Lappano, R.; Maggiolini, M.; Dolce, V. The Physiopathological Role of the Exchangers Belonging to the Slc37 Family. *Front. Chem.* **2018**, *6*, 122. [CrossRef] [PubMed]
14. Chou, J.Y.; Mansfield, B.C. The Slc37 Family of Sugar-Phosphate/Phosphate Exchangers. *Curr. Top. Membr.* **2014**, *73*, 357–382. [CrossRef]
15. Chou, J.Y.; Sik Jun, H.; Mansfield, B.C. The Slc37 Family of Phosphate-Linked Sugar Phosphate Antiporters. *Mol. Aspects Med.* **2013**, *34*, 601–611. [CrossRef] [PubMed]
16. Xu, X.; Sun, H.; Luo, J.; Cheng, X.; Lv, W.; Luo, W.; Chen, W.J.; Xiong, Z.Q.; Liu, J.Y. The Pathology of Primary Familial Brain Calcification: Implications for Treatment. *Neurosci. Bull.* **2023**, *39*, 659–674. [CrossRef] [PubMed]
17. Balck, A.; Schaake, S.; Kuhnke, N.S.; Domingo, A.; Madoev, H.; Margolesky, J.; Dobricic, V.; Alvarez-Fischer, D.; Laabs, B.H.; Kasten, M.; et al. Genotype-Phenotype Relations in Primary Familial Brain Calcification: Systematic Mdsgene Review. *Mov. Disord.* **2021**, *36*, 2468–2480. [CrossRef]
18. Chande, S.; Bergwitz, C. Role of Phosphate Sensing in Bone and Mineral Metabolism. *Nat. Rev. Endocrinol.* **2018**, *14*, 637–655. [CrossRef]
19. Jiang, Y.; Li, X.; Feng, J.; Li, M.; Wang, O.; Xing, X.P.; Xia, W.B. The Genetic Polymorphisms of Xpr1 and Scl34a3 Are Associated with Fanconi Syndrome in Chinese Patients of Tumor-Induced Osteomalacia. *J. Endocrinol. Investig.* **2021**, *44*, 773–780. [CrossRef]
20. Xu, X.; Li, X.; Sun, H.; Cao, Z.; Gao, R.; Niu, T.; Wang, Y.; Ma, T.; Chen, R.; Wang, C.; et al. Murine Placental-Fetal Phosphate Dyshomeostasis Caused by an Xpr1 Deficiency Accelerates Placental Calcification and Restricts Fetal Growth in Late Gestation. *J. Bone Miner. Res.* **2020**, *35*, 116–129. [CrossRef]
21. Ansermet, C.; Moor, M.B.; Centeno, G.; Auberson, M.; Hu, D.Z.; Baron, R.; Nikolaeva, S.; Haenzi, B.; Katanaeva, N.; Gautschi, I.; et al. Renal Fanconi Syndrome and Hypophosphatemic Rickets in the Absence of Xenotropic and Polytropic Retroviral Receptor in the Nephron. *J. Am. Soc. Nephrol.* **2017**, *28*, 1073–1078. [CrossRef]

22. Magen, D.; Berger, L.; Coady, M.J.; Ilivitzki, A.; Militianu, D.; Tieder, M.; Selig, S.; Lapointe, J.Y.; Zelikovic, I.; Skorecki, K. A Loss-of-Function Mutation in Napi-IIa and Renal Fanconi's Syndrome. *N. Engl. J. Med.* **2010**, *362*, 1102–1109. [CrossRef] [PubMed]
23. Al-Sardar, H.; Al-Habbo, D.J.; Al-Hayali, R.M. Pulmonary Alveolar Microlithiasis: Report of Two Brothers with the Same Illness and Review of Literature. *BMJ Case Rep.* **2014**, *2014*. [CrossRef]
24. Dandan, S.; Yuqin, C.; Wei, L.; Ziheng, P.; Dapeng, Z.; Jianzhu, Y.; Xin, X.; Yonghong, L.; Fengjun, T. Novel Deletion of Slc34a2 in Chinese Patients of Pam Shares Mutation Hot Spot with Fusion Gene Slc34a2-Ros1 in Lung Cancer. *J. Genet.* **2018**, *97*, 939–944. [CrossRef] [PubMed]
25. Erel, F.; Güngör, C.; Sarıoğlu, N.; Aksu, G.D.; Turan, G.; Demirpolat, G. Spontaneous Pneumomediastinum and Subcutaneous Emphysema Secondary to Pulmonary Alveolar Microlithiasis. *Tuberk. Toraks* **2021**, *69*, 416–420. [CrossRef]
26. Ma, T.; Ren, J.; Yin, J.; Ma, Z. A Pedigree with Pulmonary Alveolar Microlithiasis: A Clinical Case Report and Literature Review. *Cell Biochem. Biophys.* **2014**, *70*, 565–572. [CrossRef] [PubMed]
27. Saito, A.; Nikolaidis, N.M.; Amlal, H.; Uehara, Y.; Gardner, J.C.; LaSance, K.; Pitstick, L.B.; Bridges, J.P.; Wikenheiser-Brokamp, K.A.; McGraw, D.W.; et al. Modeling Pulmonary Alveolar Microlithiasis by Epithelial Deletion of the Npt2b Sodium Phosphate Cotransporter Reveals Putative Biomarkers and Strategies for Treatment. *Sci. Transl. Med.* **2015**, *7*, 313ra181. [CrossRef]
28. Bergwitz, C.; Miyamoto, K.I. Hereditary Hypophosphatemic Rickets with Hypercalciuria: Pathophysiology, Clinical Presentation, Diagnosis and Therapy. *Pflug. Arch.* **2019**, *471*, 149–163. [CrossRef] [PubMed]
29. Bergwitz, C.; Roslin, N.M.; Tieder, M.; Loredo-Osti, J.C.; Bastepe, M.; Abu-Zahra, H.; Frappier, D.; Burkett, K.; Carpenter, T.O.; Anderson, D.; et al. Slc34a3 Mutations in Patients with Hereditary Hypophosphatemic Rickets with Hypercalciuria Predict a Key Role for the Sodium-Phosphate Cotransporter Napi-Iic in Maintaining Phosphate Homeostasis. *Am. J. Hum. Genet.* **2006**, *78*, 179–192. [CrossRef]
30. Ichikawa, S.; Sorenson, A.H.; Imel, E.A.; Friedman, N.E.; Gertner, J.M.; Econs, M.J. Intronic deletions in the Slc34a3 Gene Cause Hereditary Hypophosphatemic Rickets with Hypercalciuria. *J. Clin. Endocrinol. Metab.* **2006**, *91*, 4022–4027. [CrossRef]
31. Lorenz-Depiereux, B.; Benet-Pages, A.; Eckstein, G.; Tenenbaum-Rakover, Y.; Wagenstaller, J.; Tiosano, D.; Gershoni-Baruch, R.; Albers, N.; Lichtner, P.; Schnabel, D.; et al. Hereditary Hypophosphatemic Rickets with Hypercalciuria is Caused by Mutations in the Sodium-Phosphate Cotransporter Gene Slc34a3. *Am. J. Hum. Genet.* **2006**, *78*, 193–201. [CrossRef]
32. Inden, M.; Iriyama, M.; Zennami, M.; Sekine, S.I.; Hara, A.; Yamada, M.; Hozumi, I. The Type Iii Transporters (Pit-1 and Pit-2) Are the Major Sodium-Dependent Phosphate Transporters in the Mice and Human Brains. *Brain Res.* **2016**, *1637*, 128–136. [CrossRef] [PubMed]
33. Wagner, C.A. Pharmacology of Mammalian Na(+)-Dependent Transporters of Inorganic Phosphate. In *Handbook of Experimental Pharmacology*; Springer: Berlin/Heidelberg, Germany, 2023.
34. Carecchio, M.; Mainardi, M.; Bonato, G. The Clinical and Genetic Spectrum of Primary Familial Brain Calcification. *J. Neurol.* **2023**, *270*, 3270–3277. [CrossRef] [PubMed]
35. Bergwitz, C.; Jüppner, H. Fgf23 and Syndromes of Abnormal Renal Phosphate Handling. *Adv. Exp. Med. Biol.* **2012**, *728*, 41–64. [CrossRef] [PubMed]
36. Christov, M.; Jüppner, H. Phosphate Homeostasis Disorders. *Best. Pract. Res. Clin. Endocrinol. Metab.* **2018**, *32*, 685–706. [CrossRef] [PubMed]
37. Vanessa, H. Calcium, Phosphate and Magnesium Disorders. In *Fluid and Electrolyte Disorders*; Usman, M., Ed.; IntechOpen: Rijeka, Croatia, 2018.
38. Peacock, M. Phosphate Metabolism in Health and Disease. *Calcif. Tissue Int.* **2021**, *108*, 3–15. [CrossRef]
39. Tomoe, Y.; Segawa, H.; Shiozawa, K.; Kaneko, I.; Tominaga, R.; Hanabusa, E.; Aranami, F.; Furutani, J.; Kuwahara, S.; Tatsumi, S.; et al. Phosphaturic Action of Fibroblast Growth Factor 23 in Npt2 Null Mice. *Am. J. Physiol. Renal Physiol.* **2010**, *298*, F1341–F1350. [CrossRef] [PubMed]
40. Segawa, H.; Kawakami, E.; Kaneko, I.; Kuwahata, M.; Ito, M.; Kusano, K.; Saito, H.; Fukushima, N.; Miyamoto, K. Effect of Hydrolysis-Resistant Fgf23-R179q on Dietary Phosphate Regulation of the Renal Type-Ii Na/Pi Transporter. *Pflug. Arch.* **2003**, *446*, 585–592. [CrossRef]
41. Segawa, H.; Yamanaka, S.; Ohno, Y.; Onitsuka, A.; Shiozawa, K.; Aranami, F.; Furutani, J.; Tomoe, Y.; Ito, M.; Kuwahata, M.; et al. Correlation between Hyperphosphatemia and Type Ii Na-Pi Cotransporter Activity in Klotho Mice. *Am. J. Physiol. Renal Physiol.* **2007**, *292*, F769–F779. [CrossRef]
42. Hanazaki, A.; Ikuta, K.; Sasaki, S.; Sasaki, S.; Koike, M.; Tanifuji, K.; Arima, Y.; Kaneko, I.; Shiozaki, Y.; Tatsumi, S.; et al. Role of Sodium-Dependent Pi Transporter/Npt2c on Pi Homeostasis in Klotho Knockout Mice Different Properties between Juvenile and Adult Stages. *Physiol. Rep.* **2020**, *8*, e14324. [CrossRef]
43. Nakatani, T.; Sarraj, B.; Ohnishi, M.; Densmore, M.J.; Taguchi, T.; Goetz, R.; Mohammadi, M.; Lanske, B.; Razzaque, M.S. In Vivo Genetic Evidence for Klotho-Dependent, Fibroblast Growth Factor 23 (Fgf23)-Mediated Regulation of Systemic Phosphate Homeostasis. *FASEB J.* **2009**, *23*, 433–441. [CrossRef]
44. Nakatani, T.; Ohnishi, M.; Razzaque, M.S. Inactivation of Klotho Function Induces Hyperphosphatemia Even in Presence of High Serum Fibroblast Growth Factor 23 Levels in a Genetically Engineered Hypophosphatemic (Hyp) Mouse Model. *FASEB J.* **2009**, *23*, 3702–3711. [CrossRef]

45. Dërmaku-Sopjani, M.; Sopjani, M.; Saxena, A.; Shojaiefard, M.; Bogatikov, E.; Alesutan, I.; Eichenmüller, M.; Lang, F. Downregulation of Napi-IIa and Napi-IIb Na-Coupled Phosphate Transporters by Coexpression of Klotho. *Cell Physiol. Biochem.* **2011**, *28*, 251–258. [CrossRef] [PubMed]
46. Prud'homme, G.J.; Kurt, M.; Wang, Q. Pathobiology of the Klotho Antiaging Protein and Therapeutic Considerations. *Front. Aging* **2022**, *3*, 931331. [CrossRef] [PubMed]
47. Hu, M.C.; Shi, M.; Zhang, J.; Pastor, J.; Nakatani, T.; Lanske, B.; Razzaque, M.S.; Rosenblatt, K.P.; Baum, M.G.; Kuro-o, M.; et al. Klotho: A Novel Phosphaturic Substance Acting as an Autocrine Enzyme in the Renal Proximal Tubule. *FASEB J.* **2010**, *24*, 3438–3450. [CrossRef] [PubMed]
48. Turner, M.E.; Rowsell, T.S.; Lansing, A.P.; Jeronimo, P.S.; Lee, L.H.; Svajger, B.A.; Zelt, J.G.; Forster, C.M.; Petkovich, M.P.; Holden, R.M. Vascular Calcification Maladaptively Participates in Acute Phosphate Homeostasis. *Cardiovasc. Res.* **2023**, *119*, 1077–1091. [CrossRef]
49. Nguyen, N.T.; Nguyen, T.T.; Ly, D.D.; Xia, J.-B.; Qi, X.-F.; Lee, I.-K.; Cha, S.-K.; Park, K.-S. Oxidative Stress by Ca^{2+} Overload Is Critical for Phosphate-Induced Vascular Calcification. *Am. J. Physiol. Heart Circ. Physiol.* **2020**, *319*, H1302–H1312. [CrossRef]
50. Seifert, E.L.; Ligeti, E.; Mayr, J.A.; Sondheimer, N.; Hajnóczky, G. The Mitochondrial Phosphate Carrier: Role in Oxidative Metabolism, Calcium Handling and Mitochondrial Disease. *Biochem. Biophys. Res. Commun.* **2015**, *464*, 369–375. [CrossRef]
51. Hill Gallant, K.M.; Stremke, E.R.; Trevino, L.L.; Moorthi, R.N.; Doshi, S.; Wastney, M.E.; Hisada, N.; Sato, J.; Ogita, Y.; Fujii, N.; et al. EOS789, a Broad-Spectrum Inhibitor of Phosphate Transport, is Safe with an Indication of Efficacy in a Phase 1b Randomized Crossover Trial in Hemodialysis Patients. *Kidney Int.* **2021**, *99*, 1225–1233. [CrossRef]
52. Tsuboi, Y.; Ichida, Y.; Murai, A.; Maeda, A.; Iida, M.; Kato, A.; Ohtomo, S.; Horiba, N. Eos789, Pan-Phosphate Transporter Inhibitor, Ameliorates the Progression of Kidney Injury in anti-GBM-Induced Glomerulonephritis Rats. *Pharmacol. Res. Perspect.* **2022**, *10*, e00973. [CrossRef]
53. Tsuboi, Y.; Ohtomo, S.; Ichida, Y.; Hagita, H.; Ozawa, K.; Iida, M.; Nagao, S.; Ikegami, H.; Takahashi, T.; Horiba, N. Eos789, a Novel Pan-Phosphate Transporter Inhibitor, is Effective for the Treatment of Chronic Kidney Disease-Mineral Bone Disorder. *Kidney Int.* **2020**, *98*, 343–354. [CrossRef]
54. Filipski, K.J.; Sammons, M.F.; Bhattacharya, S.K.; Panteleev, J.; Brown, J.A.; Loria, P.M.; Boehm, M.; Smith, A.C.; Shavnya, A.; Conn, E.L.; et al. Discovery of Orally Bioavailable Selective Inhibitors of the Sodium-Phosphate Cotransporter Napi2a (Slc34a1). *ACS Med. Chem. Lett.* **2018**, *9*, 440–445. [CrossRef]
55. Clerin, V.; Saito, H.; Filipski, K.J.; Nguyen, A.H.; Garren, J.; Kisucka, J.; Reyes, M.; Jüppner, H. Selective Pharmacological Inhibition of the Sodium-Dependent Phosphate Cotransporter NPT2a Promotes Phosphate Excretion. *J. Clin. Investig.* **2020**, *130*, 6510–6522. [CrossRef]
56. Tenenhouse, H.S.; Martel, J.; Gauthier, C.; Segawa, H.; Miyamoto, K. Differential Effects of Npt2a Gene Ablation and X-Linked Hyp Mutation on Renal Expression of Npt2c. *Am. J. Physiol. Renal Physiol.* **2003**, *285*, F1271–F1278. [CrossRef] [PubMed]
57. Kaneko, I.; Segawa, H.; Ikuta, K.; Hanazaki, A.; Fujii, T.; Tatsumi, S.; Kido, S.; Hasegawa, T.; Amizuka, N.; Saito, H.; et al. Eldecalcitol Causes Fgf23 Resistance for Pi Reabsorption and Improves Rachitic Bone Phenotypes in the Male Hyp Mouse. *Endocrinology* **2018**, *159*, 2741–2758. [CrossRef] [PubMed]
58. Martins, J.S.; Liu, E.S.; Sneddon, W.B.; Friedman, P.A.; Demay, M.B. 1,25-Dihydroxyvitamin D Maintains Brush Border Membrane Napi2a and Attenuates Phosphaturia in Hyp Mice. *Endocrinology* **2019**, *160*, 2204–2214. [CrossRef]
59. Friedman, P.A.; Sneddon, W.B.; Mamonova, T.; Montanez-Miranda, C.; Ramineni, S.; Harbin, N.H.; Squires, K.E.; Gefter, J.V.; Magyar, C.E.; Emlet, D.R.; et al. Rgs14 Regulates Pth-and Fgf23-Sensitive Npt2a-Mediated Renal Phosphate Uptake Via Binding to the Nherf1 Scaffolding Protein. *J. Biol. Chem.* **2022**, *298*, 101836. [CrossRef] [PubMed]
60. Sasaki, S.; Shiozaki, Y.; Hanazaki, A.; Koike, M.; Tanifuji, K.; Uga, M.; Kawahara, K.; Kaneko, I.; Kawamoto, Y.; Wiriyasermkul, P.; et al. Tmem174, a Regulator of Phosphate Transporter Prevents Hyperphosphatemia. *Sci. Rep.* **2022**, *12*, 6353. [CrossRef]
61. Miyazaki-Anzai, S.; Keenan, A.L.; Blaine, J.; Miyazaki, M. Targeted Disruption of a Proximal Tubule-Specific Tmem174 Gene in Mice Causes Hyperphosphatemia and Vascular Calcification. *J. Am. Soc. Nephrol.* **2022**, *33*, 1477–1486. [CrossRef]

Disclaimer/Publisher's Note: The statements, opinions and data contained in all publications are solely those of the individual author(s) and contributor(s) and not of MDPI and/or the editor(s). MDPI and/or the editor(s) disclaim responsibility for any injury to people or property resulting from any ideas, methods, instructions or products referred to in the content.

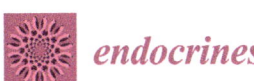

Review

Pathogenesis of FGF23-Related Hypophosphatemic Diseases Including X-linked Hypophosphatemia

Tatsuro Nakanishi [1,2] and Toshimi Michigami [1,*]

1. Department of Bone and Mineral Research, Research Institute, Osaka Women's and Children's Hospital, Izumi 594-1101, Japan; tnrebo@wch.opho.jp
2. Department of Pediatrics, Osaka University Graduate School of Medicine, Suita 565-0871, Japan
* Correspondence: michigami@wch.opho.jp; Tel.: +81-725-56-1220

Abstract: Since phosphate is indispensable for skeletal mineralization, chronic hypophosphatemia causes rickets and osteomalacia. Fibroblast growth factor 23 (FGF23), which is mainly produced by osteocytes in bone, functions as the central regulator of phosphate metabolism by increasing the renal excretion of phosphate and suppressing the production of 1,25-dihydroxyvitamin D. The excessive action of FGF23 results in hypophosphatemic diseases, which include a number of genetic disorders such as X-linked hypophosphatemic rickets (XLH) and tumor-induced osteomalacia (TIO). Phosphate-regulating gene homologous to endopeptidase on the X chromosome (PHEX), dentin matrix protein 1 (DMP1), ectonucleotide pyrophosphatase phosphodiesterase-1, and family with sequence similarity 20c, the inactivating variants of which are responsible for FGF23-related hereditary rickets/osteomalacia, are highly expressed in osteocytes, similar to FGF23, suggesting that they are local negative regulators of FGF23. Autosomal dominant hypophosphatemic rickets (ADHR) is caused by cleavage-resistant variants of FGF23, and iron deficiency increases serum levels of FGF23 and the manifestation of symptoms in ADHR. Enhanced FGF receptor (FGFR) signaling in osteocytes is suggested to be involved in the overproduction of FGF23 in XLH and autosomal recessive hypophosphatemic rickets type 1, which are caused by the inactivation of PHEX and DMP1, respectively. TIO is caused by the overproduction of FGF23 by phosphaturic tumors, which are often positive for FGFR. FGF23-related hypophosphatemia may also be associated with McCune-Albright syndrome, linear sebaceous nevus syndrome, and the intravenous administration of iron. This review summarizes current knowledge on the pathogenesis of FGF23-related hypophosphatemic diseases.

Keywords: phosphate; fibroblast growth factor 23; osteocytes; rickets; osteomalacia

---

1. Introduction

Phosphorus is an essential nutrient that mediates the majority of biological processes, including the integrity of cell membranes, the maintenance and inheritance of genetic information, energy metabolism, and the regulation of protein function by phosphorylation [1]. In vertebrates, phosphorus also contributes to skeletal mineralization as a constituent of hydroxyapatite (calcium-phosphate crystals). In the human adult body, approximately 90% of total phosphorus is stored in bone, while the remainder is present in the soft tissues and less than 1% in extracellular fluid [2]. In serum, the majority of phosphorus exists as free ions of inorganic phosphate (Pi), such as HPO_4^{2-} and $H_2PO_4^{-}$, at a ratio of 4:1 at physiological pH [3]. Serum levels of Pi are influenced by age, dietary intake, serum pH, and so on.

Since phosphate is indispensable for the formation of hydroxyapatite, its chronic deficiency or wasting leads to impaired skeletal mineralization, namely, rickets in children and osteomalacia in adults [4]. At the beginning of this century, fibroblast growth factor 23 (FGF23) was identified as the molecule responsible for autosomal dominant hypophosphatemic rickets (ADHR) and tumor-induced hypophosphatemic osteomalacia (TIO) [5,6].

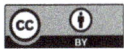

Since then, our understanding of the mechanisms underlying phosphate metabolism and the pathogenesis of various related diseases has increased. This review discusses current concepts on the role of FGF23 in phosphate homeostasis and the pathogenesis of FGF23-related hypophosphatemic diseases.

2. Phosphorus Homeostasis

In mammals, the phosphate balance in postnatal life is maintained by its intestinal absorption, renal excretion, and accumulation in and release from bone and soft tissue [1]. The insufficient absorption, excess renal excretion, or excessive shift of Pi to bone or soft tissue may cause hypophosphatemia [7]. Since phosphate is indispensable for skeletal mineralization, chronic hypophosphatemia leads to rickets and osteomalacia.

Pi absorption in the intestines is mediated by two processes: a passive, paracellular diffusion process and an active, transcellular transport process. The latter is mediated by the type IIb Na^+/Pi co-transporter (NaPi-IIb), which is encoded by the *SLC34A2* gene in humans [8]. The expression of NaPi-IIb in the intestines is up-regulated by the low dietary intake of Pi and 1,25-dihydroxyvitamin D (1,25$(OH)_2$D), an active metabolite of vitamin D [9,10]. A dietary deficiency of phosphate is rare because the majority of foods contain large amounts of phosphate. However, the insufficient action of vitamin D decreases the absorption of Pi in the intestines.

In the kidneys, the majority of Pi filtered in the glomeruli is mainly reabsorbed by type IIa and IIc Na^+/Pi co-transporters (NaPi-IIa and NaPi-IIc) localized at the brush border membrane (BBM) of the proximal tubules [11–13]. NaPi-IIa and NaPi-IIc are encoded by the *SLC34A1* and *SLC34A3* genes, respectively, in humans. Inactivating variants in the *SLC34A3* gene cause hereditary hypophosphatemic rickets with hypercalciuria (HHRH) [14]. HHRH is characterized by renal Pi wasting, hypophosphatemia, increased levels of serum 1,25$(OH)_2$D, and secondary hypocalciuria. On the other hand, inactivating variants in the *SLC34A1* gene have been shown to cause Fanconi renotubular syndrome 2, infantile hypercalciuria 2, and nephrolithiasis/osteoporosis associated with hypophosphatemia [1].

Endocrine factors including 1,25$(OH)_2$D, parathyroid hormone (PTH), and FGF23 play critical roles in phosphate homeostasis. As described above, 1,25$(OH)_2$D increases the intestinal absorption of Pi by up-regulating NaPi-IIb [10]. PTH increases the renal excretion of Pi by decreasing the amounts of NaPi-IIa and NaPi-IIc that localize in the BBM [15–17]. FGF23 functions as the central regulator of phosphate metabolism, as described in the following section.

3. Roles of FGF23 in Mineral Metabolism

FGF23 is a 32-kDa protein that consists of 251 amino acids including a 24-amino acid signal peptide at its N terminus [6]. It is mainly produced by osteoblast lineage cells, particularly osteocytes, which terminally differentiate from osteoblasts and are embedded within the bone matrix [18]. In adult bone, osteocytes make up more than 90% to 95% of all bone cells. Although the location and inaccessibility of osteocytes in the mineralized bone matrix delayed our understanding of their cellular functions, studies conducted in the last few decades have revealed their roles in bone homeostasis. Osteocytes are essential for controlling the bone mass in postnatal life by sensing mechanical strain and regulating the formation and resorption of bone [19]. They also produce sclerostin, an inhibitor of Wnt/β-catenin signaling. Mechanical strain reduces the production of sclerostin by osteocytes, which in turn enhances Wnt/β-catenin signaling and increases bone formation [20]. In addition, mouse studies suggested that the receptor activator of nuclear factor kappa B ligand produced by osteocytes controls the postnatal bone mass [21]. The expression of FGF23 by osteocytes indicates that they also play critical roles in phosphate homeostasis.

FGF23 belongs to the FGF19 subfamily together with FGF19 and FGF21, based on their unique features among FGFs [22]. Members of the FGF19 family exert their effects on distant target organs and tissues in an endocrine manner, and their low binding affinity to heparin/heparan sulfate has been suggested to confer endocrine functions due to less binding to heparan sulfate surrounding their producing cells and their entry into the circulation [22]. Members of the FGF19 subfamily require the single-pass transmembrane protein Klotho, αKlotho for FGF23, and βKlotho for FGF19 and FGF21, for their signal transduction through an FGF receptor (FGFR) [22–24]. A previous study demonstrated that the N-terminal domain of FGF23 bound to FGFR while its C-terminal domain bound to αKlotho [22].

Since FGF23 requires αKlotho together with FGFR to exert its effects, organs and tissues expressing both αKlotho and FGFR, such as the kidneys, parathyroid glands, placenta, and choroid plexus, may be the physiological targets of FGF23 [25,26]. In the kidneys, which are the main target, FGF23 increases urinary Pi excretion by suppressing the expression of NaPi-IIa and NaPi-IIc. In addition, FGF23 decreases the production of $1,25(OH)_2D$ by suppressing the renal expression of *Cyp27b1* encoding 25-hydroxyvitamin D 1α-hydroxylase and increasing that of *Cyp24a1* encoding 25-hydroxyvitamin D-24-hydroxylase, which leads to a reduction in the absorption of Pi in the intestines [6] (Figure 1).

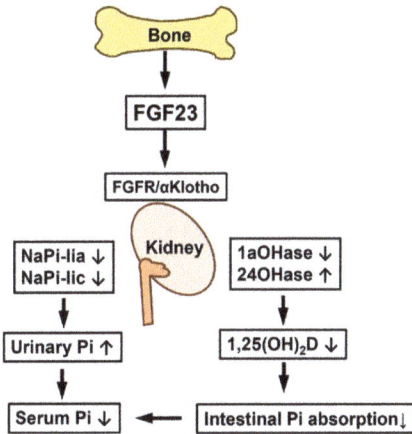

Figure 1. Effects of FGF23 on kidneys. FGF23 produced in bone binds to FGFR and αKlotho in the kidneys and suppresses the renal expression of NaPi-IIa and NaPi-IIc Na^+/Pi co-transporters, which increases urinary Pi excretion and reduces serum Pi levels. In addition, FGF23 decreases the production of $1,25(OH)_2D$ by the down-regulation of 25-hydroxyvitamin D-1α-hydroxylase (1αOHase) and up-regulation of 25-hydroxyvitamin D-24-hydroxylase (24OHase), which reduces the intestinal absorption of Pi and further lowers serum Pi levels.

The findings of animal studies have suggested that FGF23 suppresses the production and secretion of PTH in both αKlotho-dependent and -independent manners [27,28]. Since $1,25(OH)_2D$ and PTH have been shown to increase the expression of FGF23 [29–32], these factors counter-regulate with FGF23 to maintain phosphate homeostasis. The findings of mouse studies have indicated that maternal FGF23 exerts its effects on the placenta to increase the expression of *Cyp24a1*; however, it does not alter placental Pi transport [33].

FGF23 is inactivated by cleavage between Arg^{179} and Ser^{180} via a subtilisin-like proprotein convertase, which recognizes the motif $R^{176}XXR^{179}/S^{180}$ [34]. FGF23 is O-glycosylated at Thr^{178} by the enzyme UDP-N-acetyl-α-D-galactosamine:polypeptide N-acetylgalactosaminyltransferase 3 (GalNAc-T3), which is suggested to prevent cleavage by the subtilisin-like proprotein convertase [35]. Inactivating mutations in the *GALNT3* gene encoding GalNAc-T3 result in the cleavage of intact FGF23 before secretion, and the resultant deficiency of intact FGF23 causes hyperphosphatemic familial tumoral calcinosis (HFTC), a rare autosomal recessive disease characterized by hyperphosphatemia, normal or elevated levels of serum $1,25(OH)_2D$, and ectopic calcification [36,37]. Inactivating mutations in the *FGF23* gene itself and the *KLOTHO* gene encoding αKlotho were also found to be responsible for HFTC [38–40].

Both *Fgf23*-knockout mice and *Klotho*-deficient mice exhibit hyperphosphatemia with increased renal Pi reabsorption and elevated serum 1,25(OH)$_2$D levels, which resemble the features in patients with HFTC [25,41]. These mutant mice also show severe growth retardation with abnormal skeletal phenotype and short lifespan. Interestingly, *Fgf23*-knockout mice display a marked accumulation of osteoid despite hyperphosphatemia [41]. Although mechanisms for this counterintuitive observation remain unclear, it may suggest the effects of FGF23 to be independent of phosphate metabolism.

4. Pathogenesis of FGF23-Related Hypophosphatemic Diseases

4.1. FGF23-Related Hypophosphatemic Diseases

Since the FGF23-αKlotho axis plays a central role in phosphate homeostasis, its disruption causes hyperphosphatemic conditions, as described in the previous section. On the other hand, the excessive action of FGF23 underlies various hypophosphatemic diseases, which are characterized by urinary phosphate wasting, hypophosphatemia, and inappropriately low levels of serum 1,25(OH)$_2$D [42,43]. Phosphate is indispensable for skeletal mineralization; therefore, chronic hypophosphatemia due to excessive FGF23 leads to rickets in children and osteomalacia in adults. The impaired production of 1,25(OH)$_2$D contributes to the resistance of FGF23-related hypophosphatemic rickets/osteomalacia to native vitamin D. FGF23-related hypophosphatemic rickets/osteomalacia include various conditions such as genetic diseases (Tables 1 and 2). The following sections will describe the pathogenesis of each condition.

Table 1. FGF23-related hypophosphatemic diseases and their causes.

Disorder	Causes	Incidences
ADHR	Activating variants of *FGF23*	Very rare
XLH	Inactivating variants of *PHEX*	1:20,000 live birth
ARHR1	Inactivating variants of *DMP1*	Very rare
ARHR2	Inactivating variants of *ENPP1*	Very rare
Raine syndrome	Inactivating variants of *FAM20C*	Very rare
Osteoglophonic dysplasia	Activating variants of *FGFR1*	Very rare
Jansen's metaphyseal chondrodysplasia	Activating variants of *PTH1R*	Very rare
TIO	Phosphaturic mesenchymal tumor, *FN1-FGFR1*, *FN1-FGF1* fusion genes	Most frequent among the acquired disorders
McCune-Albright Syndrome	*GNAS* somatic activating variants in bone lesions	Very rare
Linear sebaceous nevus syndrome	*KRAS/HRAS/NRAS* somatic activating variants in skin/bone lesions	Very rare
I.V. administration of iron preparations	Saccharated ferric oxide, iron polymaltose	Very rare

4.2. Autosomal Dominant Hypophosphatemic Rickets (ADHR)

ADHR (OMIM #193100) is caused by missense variants in the FGF23 gene. Since the responsible variants occur at Arg^{176} or Arg^{179} within the RXXR/S motif recognized by subtilisin-like proprotein convertase, the resultant mutant FGF23 protein is resistant to cleavage-mediated inactivation [5]. However, this disease shows incomplete penetrance. Patients with ADHR variants do not always have high serum levels of intact FGF23, and the disease may occur with an early or delayed onset and variable expressivity [44]. Late-onset ADHR primarily manifests in post-pubertal women who are prone to iron deficiency [45]. Serum iron levels were previously shown to negatively correlate with serum levels of both the C-terminal fragment of FGF23 and intact FGF23 in ADHR patients; however, serum iron levels also negatively correlated with C-terminal FGF23 levels in healthy control subjects, whereas no relationship was observed with intact FGF23 levels [45]. Farrow et al. generated FGF23-knock-in mice carrying the R176Q ADHR point mutation (ADHR mice) and found that a low-iron diet increased bone FGF23 mRNA levels and the serum levels of both intact and C-terminal FGF23 with hypophosphatemia in ADHR mice. On the other hand, wild-type mice fed the low-iron diet showed normal serum levels of intact FGF23 and phosphate, but an elevated level of the C-terminal fragment of FGF23 [46]. Furthermore, the chelation of iron up-regulated the expression of *Fgf23* in a cultured osteoblastic cell line, which involved hypoxia-inducible factor 1α. Collectively, these findings suggest that iron deficiency increases the expression of *Fgf23* in bone and also that the FGF23 protein is cleaved in iron deficiency to maintain normal serum levels of FGF23 and normophosphatemia in control subjects, whereas the cleavage resistance of mutant FGF23 leads to the accumulation of intact FGF23 and hypophosphatemia in ADHR subjects [46].

Table 2. Clinical features of FGF23-related hypophosphatemic diseases.

Disorder	Clinical Features
ADHR	Renal Pi wasting, hypophosphatemia, low or normal serum 1,25(OH)$_2$D levels, rickets/osteomalacia, incomplete penetrance, often delayed onset
XLH	Renal Pi wasting, hypophosphatemia, low or normal serum 1,25(OH)$_2$D levels, rickets/osteomalacia, short stature, bone deformity, dental problems, enthesopathy
ARHR1	Renal Pi wasting, hypophosphatemia, low or normal serum 1,25(OH)$_2$D levels, rickets/osteomalacia, short stature, bone deformity, dental problems, enthesopathy
ARHR2	Renal Pi wasting, hypophosphatemia, low or normal serum 1,25(OH)$_2$D levels, rickets/osteomalacia, short stature, bone deformity, dental problems, enthesopathy
Raine syndrome	Osteosclerosis of early onset, poor life prognosis in most cases, characteristic face, renal Pi wasting, hypophosphatemia, low or normal serum 1,25(OH)$_2$D levels, rickets/osteomalacia, short stature, bone deformity, dental problems, enthesopathy
Osteoglophonic dysplasia	Multiple radiolucent areas in metaphysis, rhizomelic short stature, characteristic face, renal Pi wasting, hypophosphatemia, low or normal serum 1,25(OH)$_2$D levels
Jansen's metaphyseal chondrodysplasia	Short-limbed short stature, usually hypercalcemia, skull sclerosis, renal Pi wasting, hypophosphatemia, low or normal serum 1,25(OH)$_2$D levels
TIO	Renal Pi wasting, hypophosphatemia, low or normal serum 1,25(OH)$_2$D levels, rickets/osteomalacia, improved by tumor resection
McCune-Albright Syndrome	Fibrous dysplasia, café-au-lait skin pigmentation, endocrinologic abnormalities, renal Pi wasting, hypophosphatemia, low or normal serum 1,25(OH)$_2$D levels
Linear sebaceous nevus syndrome	Linear sebaceous nevus, abnormalities in central nervous system, ocular anomalies, bone defects, renal Pi wasting, hypophosphatemia, low or normal serum 1,25(OH)$_2$D levels
I.V. administration of iron preparations	Renal Pi wasting, hypophosphatemia, low or normal serum 1,25(OH)$_2$D levels, rickets/osteomalacia, improved by discontinuation of the responsible drugs

4.3. X-Linked Hypophosphatemic Rickets (XLH)

XLH (OMIM #307800) is the most common form of hereditary hypophosphatemic rickets. Patients with XLH have elevated serum levels of FGF23, which result in urinary Pi wasting, hypophosphatemia, and inappropriately low levels of 1,25(OH)$_2$D [47]. XLH was initially called vitamin D-resistant rickets because of a poor response to treatment with native vitamin D at dosages that cure vitamin D-deficient rickets. XLH is caused by inactivating variants in the *phosphate-regulating gene homologous to endopeptidase on the X chromosome* (*PHEX*) located at Xp22.1, showing X-linked dominant inheritance [48]. Similar to FGF23, PHEX is expressed in osteoblast lineage cells and is more highly expressed in osteocytes [18,49]. Although its structure suggests that the product of *PHEX* functions as a cell surface-bound, zinc-dependent protease, its physiological substrates remain elusive. In hypophosphatemic *Hyp* mice, which harbor a large deletion in the *Phex* gene and are widely used as a model for XLH, the expression of *Fgf23* in osteocytes was found to be increased [18,50]; however, FGF23 did not serve as a substrate for PHEX [51]. Therefore, the regulation of FGF23 by PHEX may be indirect and involve other molecule(s).

Since PHEX is highly expressed in osteocytes, in an attempt to clarify abnormalities in *Phex*-deficient osteocytes, we previously compared the gene expression profiles of osteoblasts and osteocytes in *Hyp* mice and wild-type littermates [18]. As osteoblasts mature into osteocytes, the expression of *dentin matrix protein 1* (*Dmp1*) and *family with sequence similarity 20c* (*Fam20c*), which are responsible for autosomal recessive hypophosphatemic type 1 (ARHR1) and Raine syndrome (RNS), respectively, increased in both *Hyp* and wild-type cells, and these genes were up-regulated in *Hyp* cells, similar to *Fgf23* [18]. These findings indicated the critical roles of osteocytes in phosphate homeostasis and also suggested complex abnormalities in *Phex*-deficient osteocytes. We found that the expression of the genes encoding canonical FGF ligands (*Fgf1* and *Fgf2*), their receptors (*Fgfr1-3*), and *early growth response 1*, which is a target for FGFR activation, was also up-regulated in *Hyp* osteocytes, indicating enhanced FGFR signaling [18]. Furthermore, Martin et al. suggested enhanced FGFR signaling in *Hyp* bone [52], and Xiao et al. demonstrated that the conditional deletion of *Fgfr1* in osteocytes and mature osteoblasts partially restored the overproduction of FGF23 and ameliorated hypophosphatemia and rickets [53]. The regulation of FGF23 production by FGFR signaling is also supported by osteoglophonic dysplasia, which is a rare skeletal dysplasia caused by activating mutations in *FGFR1* that is frequently associated with elevated serum FGF23 levels and hypophosphatemia [54].

Enhanced FGFR signaling in *Phex*-deficient osteocytes is of interest based on previous findings suggesting that FGFR plays a critical role in the transduction of signaling evoked by increased extracellular Pi [55–57]. In various cell types, treatment with high extracellular Pi activated FGFR for the regulation of gene expression. In an osteoblastic cell line, treatment with an FGFR inhibitor abolished the up-regulation of Dmp1 by increased extracellular Pi [56]. In HEK293 cells, the knockdown of FGFR1 diminished the Pi-induced phosphorylation of ERK1/2 [55]. More recently, the activation of FGFR1 by extracellular Pi was shown to increase the expression of *Galnt3* in bone, leading to an elevated serum level of FGF23 in mice [57]. Collectively, these findings suggest that FGFR1 is involved in the sensing of Pi availability. In consideration of this role of FGFR and enhanced FGFR signaling in the osteocytes of *Hyp* mice, abnormal Pi sensing may be involved in the pathogenesis of XLH.

Matrix extracellular phosphoglycoprotein (MEPE) is a member of the SIBLING (small integrin-binding ligand, N-linked glycoproteins) family, and was initially cloned from the tumor of a patient with TIO [58]. A genome-wide association study proposed MEPE as a factor influencing bone mineral density in humans [59]. MEPE contains an acidic serine-aspartate rich MEPE-associated motif (ASARM) consisting of 23 residues at the C terminus. ASARM peptides released from MEPE by cathepsin-mediated cleavage have been shown to inhibit mineralization. Rowe et al. demonstrated that PHEX bound to the ASARM motif in MEPE and the released ASARM peptide and its serum levels were elevated in *Hyp* mice [60,61]. The ASARM motif is also present in other SIBLING proteins, such as DMP1 and osteopontin, and PHEX may bind to these proteins at these motifs [58]. A previous study implicated ASARM peptides released from these SIBLING proteins in defective mineralization in XLH [62].

Growth retardation is often observed in patients with XLH: however, the underlying mechanisms have not yet been elucidated in detail. A study published by Fuente et al. demonstrated marked alterations in the structure, dynamics, and maturation of growth plate cartilage in growth-retarded young *Hyp* mice [63]. In the growth plates of *Hyp* mice, both proliferation and apoptosis rates of chondrocytes were reduced, and the hypertrophy and maturation of chondrocytes were severely disturbed. The spatial organization of the chondro-osseous junction and the primary spongiosa trabeculae were markedly deformed. These alterations in the growth plates might be the mechanisms for the growth retardation in *Hyp* mice. The authors also found an enhanced activation of the extracellular signal-regulated kinase (ERK)1/2 signaling pathway in the *Hyp* growth plates, implying an involvement of FGF23 in these abnormalities [63]. Reduction in caspase-mediated apoptosis of hypertrophic chondrocytes was also reported in rachitic mice with low-phosphate diet-induced hypophosphatemia as well as in *Hyp* mice, which suggests that hypophosphatemia impairs apoptosis of hypertrophic chondrocytes, leading to rickets [64].

Although chondrocytes do not express αKlotho, which is required for FGF23 to activate its downstream signaling pathways at physiological concentrations, soluble forms of αKlotho are present in serum and cerebrospinal fluid [65] and have been implicated in the regulation of FGF23 signaling in cells without the transmembrane form of αKlotho [66]. We previously demonstrated that FGF23 suppressed the linear growth of mouse metatarsal cartilage in cultures in the presence of soluble αKlotho by decreasing the proliferation of chondrocytes, which suggests that suppressed chondrocyte proliferation by FGF23 plays a causative role in the growth retardation associated with XLH [67].

Since the placenta expresses FGFR1 and αKlotho, high levels of FGF23 in pregnant women with XLH may affect their fetuses. We previously investigated this issue using pregnant *Hyp* female mice [33]. *Hyp* and wild-type female mice were mated with wild-type male mice, and the pregnant mothers and their male fetuses were subjected to analyses. FGF23 levels were higher in *Hyp* mothers than in wild-type mothers. *Hyp* fetuses and wild-type fetuses were obtained from mating between *Hyp* females and wild-type males. FGF23 levels in *Hyp* fetuses were approximately 20-fold higher than in their mothers, while wild-type fetuses from *Hyp* mothers had low levels of FGF23, as did fetuses from wild-type mothers, suggesting that FGF23 does not cross the placenta [33]. The expression of *Cyp24a1* was higher in the placentas of fetuses from *Hyp* mothers than in those of fetuses from wild-type mothers, which resulted in decreased levels of plasma 25-hydroxyvitamin D in fetuses from *Hyp* mothers. Therefore, increased levels of circulating FGF23 in *Hyp* mothers may exert direct effects on the placenta during pregnancy and alter fetal vitamin D metabolism via the regulation of *Cyp24a1* expression [33]. Further studies are needed to clarify whether similar phenomena occur with pregnancy in human patients with XLH.

The enthesis is a tissue that forms at the site of insertion of a tendon to bone and consists of a bony eminence, mineralized fibrocartilage, unmineralized fibrocartilage, and a tendon. It optimizes the transfer of mechanical force from muscle to bone, which is required for efficient movements [68]. Enthesopathy is a pathological change at the insertion of tendons and ligaments. Mineralizing enthesopathy is one of the complications of XLH and other types of FGF23-related hypophosphatemia and accounts for a high morbidity rate in adult patients [69]. Karaplis et al. previously reported that a transgenic mouse model overexpressing a secreted form of the human FGF23[p.R176Q] variant, which is resistant to cleavage, displayed mineralizing enthesopathy of the Achilles and planar facial insertions, suggesting the involvement of FGF23 in the development of mineralizing enthesopathy [70]. More recently, Liu et al. investigated the cellular and molecular mechanisms involved in the development of mineralizing enthesopathy in *Hyp* mice and reported that Achilles tendon entheses of *Hyp* mice showed the expansion of hypertrophic-appearing chondrogenic cells. In comparison with the entheses of wild-type mice, *Hyp* entheses exhibited the expansion of cells expressing the chondrogenic marker gene *Sox9* and enhanced bone morphogenetic protein and Indian hedgehog signaling pathways, both of which play critical roles in chondrocyte differentiation [71]. Although oral phosphate salts and active vitamin D metabolites are administered as conventional medical treatments for XLH to correct their deficiencies, it does not prevent or ameliorate enthesopathies [70]. Burosumab, a humanized monoclonal neutralizing antibody to FGF23, has recently become available as a new treatment for XLH [47]. In Japan, burosumab has been approved for the treatment of all types of FGF23-related hypophosphatemic rickets/osteomalacia. In pediatric patients with XLH, improvements in the severity of rickets and biochemical parameters were greater in patients treated with burosumab than in those who continued conventional therapy [72]. Further studies are needed to clarify the effects of burosumab on the prevention and treatment of enthesopathies.

4.4. Autosomal Recessive Hypophosphatemic Rickets Type 1 (ARHR1)

ARHR1 (OMIM #241520) is caused by inactivating variants of the *DMP1* gene [73,74]. DMP1 is an extracellular matrix protein belonging to the SIBLING family and is highly expressed in osteocytes as well as in dentin. Patients with ARHR1 manifest elevated FGF23 levels, hypophosphatemia, inappropriately low $1,25(OH)_2D$ levels, and skeletal hypomineralization, similar to patients with XLH. *Dmp1*-null mice reproduced the phenotype of ARHR1 and exhibited defective osteocyte maturation and the up-regulated expression of *Fgf23* in osteocytes [73,74]. Although the pathogenesis of ARHR1 remains largely unknown, the findings of studies using *Phex*-deficient *Hyp* mice and *Dmp1*-null mice suggest that the overproduction of FGF23 is attributable to enhanced FGFR signaling in bone in both mouse models [52].

4.5. Autosomal Recessive Hypophosphatemic Rickets Type 2 (ARHR2)

ARHR2 (OMIM #613312) also belongs to FGF23-related hypophosphatemic rickets and is caused by inactivating variants in the *ectonucleotide pyrophosphatase phosphodiesterase-1* (*ENPP1*) gene [75,76]. ENPP1 encodes an enzyme that produces pyrophosphate (PPi), a potent inhibitor of mineralization, and inactivating variants in *ENPP1* are also responsible for hypermineralization disorders, such as generalized arterial calcification in infancy [77]. The ectoenzyme tissue non-specific alkaline phosphatase (TNSALP) facilitates skeletal mineralization by degrading PPi to produce Pi. Although PPi may regulate the production of FGF23, patients with hypophosphatasia, which is caused by inactivating variants in TNSALP, had normal levels of FGF23 despite elevated extracellular levels of PPi [78]. Therefore, the mechanisms by which ENPP1 deficiency results in the overproduction of FGF23 remain unclear. Since inactivating variants in ENPP1 cause conditions characterized by ectopic calcification and FGF23-related hypophosphatemia, a close relationship may exist between ectopic calcification and the overproduction of FGF23.

4.6. Raine Syndrome (RNS)

FAM20C, also known as *DMP4*, encodes a kinase that phosphorylates various secreted proteins. The proteins phosphorylated by FAM20C include FGF23 and members of the SIBLING family, such as DMP1, osteopontin, and MEPE [34,79]. Inactivating variants in the *FAM20C* gene are responsible for RNS (OMIM #259775). RNS is an autosomal recessive disease that is characterized by craniofacial malformation, osteosclerotic bone dysplasia, and a poor prognosis [80]. Surviving patients with mild RNS manifest hypophosphatemia due to elevated levels of FGF23 and dental anomalies [81,82]. *Fam20c*-null mice exhibited elevated levels of serum FGF23, hypophosphatemia, and dental anomalies [83]. These mice also showed low expression levels of *Dmp1* in osteocytes, which suggested that the down-regulated expression of DMP1 plays a causal role in the overproduction of FGF23 in RNS [83]. However, the overexpression of *Dmp1* failed to rescue the defects in *Fam20c*-null mice [84]. A previous study reported that FAM20C phosphorylated FGF23 on Ser^{180}, which inhibited the O-glycosylation of FGF23 on Thr^{178} by GalNAc-T3 and accelerated cleavage [34]. Therefore, inactivating variants in FAM20C may increase FGF23 levels by inhibiting its cleavage.

4.7. Tumor-Induced Osteomalacia (TIO)

TIO is a rare paraneoplastic syndrome characterized by urinary phosphate wasting, hypophosphatemia, and osteomalacia. Responsible tumors are generally benign, slow-growing phosphaturic mesenchymal tumors (PMT) [85]. The overproduction of FGF23 by tumors was previously shown to enhance the renal excretion of Pi and induce hypophosphatemia, low $1,25(OH)_2D$ levels, and osteomalacia, which were cured by the surgical removal of the responsible tumor [6,86]. Lee et al. identified the fusion genes *Fibronectin 1* (*FN1*)-*FGFR1* and *FN1*-*FGF1* in subgroups of PMT and showed that immunoreactivity for FGFR1 was positive in 82% of PMT [87,88]. These findings suggest the involvement of the FGF/FGFR signaling pathway in the development of PMT.

4.8. Other Causes of FGF23-Related Hypophosphatemia

McCune-Albright syndrome (MAS, OMIM #174800) is characterized by polyostotic fibrous dysplasia, café-au-lait skin pigmentation, and precocious puberty, and is caused by a somatic activating variant in *GNAS1* encoding the subunit of the stimulatory G protein. MAS is clinically heterogeneous and may manifest various endocrinological abnormalities. Some patients with MAS exhibit hypophosphatemia, which results from the overproduction of FGF23 by abnormal skeletal progenitor cells in the bone lesions of fibrous dysplasia [89]. Serum levels of FGF23 in MAS patients correlate with disease activity [89], and significant hypophosphatemia only occurs in patients with a severe disease burden. A previous study suggested that the ratio of the C-terminal fragment of FGF23 to intact FGF23 was elevated by accelerated cleavage in the bone lesions of fibrous dysplasia [90].

Linear sebaceous nevus syndrome, also called Schimmelpenning-Feuerstein-Mims (SFM) syndrome (OMIM #163200), is characterized by congenital linear nevus sebaceous and abnormalities in neuroectodermal organs and is caused by somatic variants in *RAS* genes, including *KRAS*, *HRAS*, and *NRAS*, which are detectable in skin lesions [91,92]. Hypophosphatemia due to elevated levels of FGF23 is rarely associated with SFM syndrome. Lim et al. suggested that the source of FGF23 in SFM syndrome was bone lesions carrying *RAS* variants rather than skin lesions [93].

Osteoglophonic dysplasia (OMIM #166250) is a rare autosomal dominant disease characterized by rhizomelic dwarfism, non-ossifying bone lesions, craniosynostosis, and face abnormalities, and is caused by activating variants in the *FGFR1* gene. As discussed earlier, this disease may be associated with FGF23-related hypophosphatemia, indicating the involvement of FGFR1 in the regulation of FGF23 production [54].

Jansen's metaphyseal chondrodysplasia (OMIM #156400) is an autosomal dominant disease caused by an activating variant in the *PTH type 1 receptor* (*PTH1R*) gene [94]. Previous studies reported that FGF23-related hypophosphatemia may be associated with Jansen's metaphyseal chondrodysplasia [95]. This finding suggests that PTH signaling stimulates FGF23 production, which is also supported by the findings of several in vivo and in vitro studies [31,32,96].

FGF23-related hypophosphatemic rickets/osteomalacia may also be associated with the intravenous administration of saccharated ferric oxide or iron polymaltose [97,98]. The mechanisms by which these drugs cause the overproduction of FGF23 remain unclear; however, their discontinuance rapidly restores elevated FGF23 levels and hypophosphatemia.

5. Conclusions

FGF23-related hypophosphatemia is characterized by urinary Pi wasting, hypophosphatemia, and inappropriately low levels of $1,25(OH)_2D$, and includes various types of hereditary rickets/osteomalacia, such as XLH, and acquired diseases, including TIO. The molecules responsible for hereditary rickets/osteomalacia are highly expressed by osteocytes, indicating that these cells play a central role in phosphate homeostasis. Since inactivating variants of PHEX, DMP1, ENPP1, and FAM20C lead to the overproduction of FGF23, these molecules appear to function as negative regulators of FGF23. Although the mechanisms underlying the overproduction of FGF23 remain unclear in most FGF23-related hypophosphatemic diseases, enhanced FGFR signaling may be involved in the overproduction of FGF23 in XLH and ARHR1 as well as in TIO. Since FGFR1 is suggested to be involved in Pi sensing, abnormalities in Pi sensing may play a role in the pathogenesis of these diseases.

Author Contributions: Conceptualization, T.M.; writing—original draft preparation, T.N. and T.M.; writing—review and editing, T.N. and T.M.; supervision, T.M.; funding acquisition, T.M. All authors have read and agreed to the published version of the manuscript.

Funding: The preparation of this review was partly supported by a grant from the Japan Society for the Promotion of Science (JSPS KAKENHI Grant Number 21K07835) to T.M.

Conflicts of Interest: The authors declare no conflict of interest.

References

1. Michigami, T.; Kawai, M.; Yamazaki, M.; Ozono, K. Phosphate as a Signaling Molecule and Its Sensing Mechanism. *Physiol. Rev.* **2018**, *98*, 2317–2348. [CrossRef]
2. Mitchell, H.; Hamilton, T.; Steggerda, F.; Bean, H. The chemical composition of the adult human body and its bearing on the biochemistry of growth. *J. Biol. Chem.* **1945**, *158*, 625–637. [CrossRef]
3. Peters, J.P.; Wakeman, A.M.; Lee, C. Total Acid-Base Eqiilibrium of plasma in health and disease: XI. Hypochloremia and Total Salt Deficiency in Nephritis. *J. Clin. Investig.* **1929**, *6*, 551–575. [CrossRef] [PubMed]
4. Michigami, T.; Ozono, K. Roles of Phosphate in Skeleton. *Front. Endocrinol.* **2019**, *10*, 180. [CrossRef] [PubMed]
5. ADHR-CONSORTIUM. Autosomal dominant hypophosphataemic rickets is associated with mutations in FGF23. *Nat. Genet.* **2000**, *26*, 345–348. [CrossRef] [PubMed]
6. Shimada, T.; Mizutani, S.; Muto, T.; Yoneya, T.; Hino, R.; Takeda, S.; Takeuchi, Y.; Fujita, T.; Fukumoto, S.; Yamashita, T. Cloning and characterization of FGF23 as a causative factor of tumor-induced osteomalacia. *Proc. Natl. Acad. Sci. USA* **2001**, *98*, 6500–6505. [CrossRef] [PubMed]
7. Gaasbeek, A.; Meinders, A.E. Hypophosphatemia: An update on its etiology and treatment. *Am. J. Med.* **2005**, *118*, 1094–1101. [CrossRef] [PubMed]
8. Sabbagh, Y.; O'Brien, S.P.; Song, W.; Boulanger, J.H.; Stockmann, A.; Arbeeny, C.; Schiavi, S.C. Intestinal npt2b plays a major role in phosphate absorption and homeostasis. *J. Am. Soc. Nephrol.* **2009**, *20*, 2348–2358. [CrossRef]
9. Hattenhauer, O.; Traebert, M.; Murer, H.; Biber, J. Regulation of small intestinal Na-P(i) type IIb cotransporter by dietary phosphate intake. *Am. J. Physiol.* **1999**, *277*, G756–G762. [CrossRef]
10. Capuano, P.; Radanovic, T.; Wagner, C.A.; Bacic, D.; Kato, S.; Uchiyama, Y.; St-Arnoud, R.; Murer, H.; Biber, J. Intestinal and renal adaptation to a low-Pi diet of type II NaPi cotransporters in vitamin D receptor- and 1alphaOHase-deficient mice. *Am. J. Physiol. Cell Physiol.* **2005**, *288*, C429–C434. [CrossRef]
11. Hernando, N.; Gagnon, K.; Lederer, E. Phosphate Transport in Epithelial and Nonepithelial Tissue. *Physiol. Rev.* **2021**, *101*, 1–35. [CrossRef]
12. Beck, L.; Karaplis, A.C.; Amizuka, N.; Hewson, A.S.; Ozawa, H.; Tenenhouse, H.S. Targeted inactivation of Npt2 in mice leads to severe renal phosphate wasting, hypercalciuria, and skeletal abnormalities. *Proc. Natl. Acad. Sci. USA* **1998**, *95*, 5372–5377. [CrossRef]
13. Segawa, H.; Kaneko, I.; Takahashi, A.; Kuwahata, M.; Ito, M.; Ohkido, I.; Tatsumi, S.; Miyamoto, K. Growth-related renal type II Na/Pi cotransporter. *J. Biol. Chem.* **2002**, *277*, 19665–19672. [CrossRef]
14. Bergwitz, C.; Roslin, N.M.; Tieder, M.; Loredo-Osti, J.C.; Bastepe, M.; Abu-Zahra, H.; Frappier, D.; Burkett, K.; Carpenter, T.O.; Anderson, D.; et al. SLC34A3 mutations in patients with hereditary hypophosphatemic rickets with hypercalciuria predict a key role for the sodium-phosphate cotransporter NaPi-IIc in maintaining phosphate homeostasis. *Am. J. Hum. Genet.* **2006**, *78*, 179–192. [CrossRef]
15. Bacic, D.; Lehir, M.; Biber, J.; Kaissling, B.; Murer, H.; Wagner, C.A. The renal Na^+/phosphate cotransporter NaPi-IIa is internalized via the receptor-mediated endocytic route in response to parathyroid hormone. *Kidney Int.* **2006**, *69*, 495–503. [CrossRef]
16. Picard, N.; Capuano, P.; Stange, G.; Mihailova, M.; Kaissling, B.; Murer, H.; Biber, J.; Wagner, C.A. Acute parathyroid hormone differentially regulates renal brush border membrane phosphate cotransporters. *Pflugers. Arch.* **2010**, *460*, 677–687. [CrossRef]
17. Segawa, H.; Yamanaka, S.; Onitsuka, A.; Tomoe, Y.; Kuwahata, M.; Ito, M.; Taketani, Y.; Miyamoto, K. Parathyroid hormone-dependent endocytosis of renal type IIc Na-Pi cotransporter. *Am. J. Physiol. Renal Physiol.* **2007**, *292*, F395–F403. [CrossRef]
18. Miyagawa, K.; Yamazaki, M.; Kawai, M.; Nishino, J.; Koshimizu, T.; Ohata, Y.; Tachikawa, K.; Mikuni-Takagaki, Y.; Kogo, M.; Ozono, K.; et al. Dysregulated gene expression in the primary osteoblasts and osteocytes isolated from hypophosphatemic Hyp mice. *PLoS ONE* **2014**, *9*, e93840.
19. Bonewald, L.F. The amazing osteocyte. *J. Bone Miner. Res.* **2011**, *26*, 229–238. [CrossRef]
20. Robling, A.G.; Niziolek, P.J.; Baldridge, L.A.; Condon, K.W.; Allen, M.R.; Alam, I.; Mantila, S.M.; Gluhak-Heinrich, J.; Bellido, T.M.; Harris, S.E.; et al. Mechanical stimulation of bone in vivo reduces osteocyte expression of Sost/sclerostin. *J. Biol. Chem.* **2008**, *283*, 5866–5875. [CrossRef]
21. Nakashima, T.; Hayashi, M.; Fukunaga, T.; Kurata, K.; Oh-Hora, M.; Feng, J.Q.; Bonewald, L.F.; Kodama, T.; Wutz, A.; Wagner, E.F.; et al. Evidence for osteocyte regulation of bone homeostasis through RANKL expression. *Nat. Med.* **2011**, *17*, 1231–1234. [CrossRef] [PubMed]
22. Goetz, R.; Beenken, A.; Ibrahimi, O.A.; Kalinina, J.; Olsen, S.K.; Eliseenkova, A.V.; Xu, C.; Neubert, T.A.; Zhang, F.; Linhardt, R.J.; et al. Molecular insights into the klotho-dependent, endocrine mode of action of fibroblast growth factor 19 subfamily members. *Mol. Cell. Biol.* **2007**, *27*, 3417–3428. [CrossRef] [PubMed]
23. Kurosu, H.; Ogawa, Y.; Miyoshi, M.; Yamamoto, M.; Nandi, A.; Rosenblatt, K.P.; Baum, M.G.; Schiavi, S.; Hu, M.C.; Moe, O.W.; et al. Regulation of fibroblast growth factor-23 signaling by klotho. *J. Biol. Chem.* **2006**, *281*, 6120–6123. [CrossRef] [PubMed]
24. Urakawa, I.; Yamazaki, Y.; Shimada, T.; Iijima, K.; Hasegawa, H.; Okawa, K.; Fujita, T.; Fukumoto, S.; Yamashita, T. Klotho converts canonical FGF receptor into a specific receptor for FGF23. *Nature* **2006**, *444*, 770–774. [CrossRef]
25. Kuro-o, M.; Matsumura, Y.; Aizawa, H.; Kawaguchi, H.; Suga, T.; Utsugi, T.; Ohyama, Y.; Kurabayashi, M.; Kaname, T.; Kume, E.; et al. Mutation of the mouse klotho gene leads to a syndrome resembling ageing. *Nature* **1997**, *390*, 45–51. [CrossRef]

26. Stubbs, J.R.; Liu, S.; Tang, W.; Zhou, J.; Wang, Y.; Yao, X.; Quarles, L.D. Role of hyperphosphatemia and 1,25-dihydroxyvitamin D in vascular calcification and mortality in fibroblastic growth factor 23 null mice. *J. Am. Soc. Nephrol.* **2007**, *18*, 2116–2124. [CrossRef]
27. Ben-Dov, I.Z.; Galitzer, H.; Lavi-Moshayoff, V.; Goetz, R.; Kuro-o, M.; Mohammadi, M.; Sirkis, R.; Naveh-Many, T.; Silver, J. The parathyroid is a target organ for FGF23 in rats. *J. Clin. Investig.* **2007**, *117*, 4003–4008. [CrossRef]
28. Olauson, H.; Lindberg, K.; Amin, R.; Jia, T.; Wernerson, A.; Andersson, G.; Larsson, T.E. Targeted deletion of Klotho in kidney distal tubule disrupts mineral metabolism. *J. Am. Soc. Nephrol.* **2012**, *23*, 1641–1651. [CrossRef]
29. Liu, S.; Tang, W.; Zhou, J.; Stubbs, J.R.; Luo, Q.; Pi, M.; Quarles, L.D. Fibroblast growth factor 23 is a counter-regulatory phosphaturic hormone for vitamin D. *J. Am. Soc. Nephrol.* **2006**, *17*, 1305–1315. [CrossRef]
30. Haussler, M.R.; Livingston, S.; Sabir, Z.L.; Haussler, C.A.; Jurutka, P.W. Vitamin D Receptor Mediates a Myriad of Biological Actions Dependent on Its 1,25-Dihydroxyvitamin D Ligand: Distinct Regulatory Themes Revealed by Induction of Klotho and Fibroblast Growth Factor-23. *JBMR Plus* **2021**, *5*, e10432. [CrossRef]
31. Kawata, T.; Imanishi, Y.; Kobayashi, K.; Miki, T.; Arnold, A.; Inaba, M.; Nishizawa, Y. Parathyroid hormone regulates fibroblast growth factor-23 in a mouse model of primary hyperparathyroidism. *J. Am. Soc. Nephrol.* **2007**, *18*, 2683–2688. [CrossRef]
32. Rhee, Y.; Bivi, N.; Farrow, E.; Lezcano, V.; Plotkin, L.I.; White, K.E.; Bellido, T. Parathyroid hormone receptor signaling in osteocytes increases the expression of fibroblast growth factor-23 in vitro and in vivo. *Bone* **2011**, *49*, 636–643. [CrossRef]
33. Ohata, Y.; Yamazaki, M.; Kawai, M.; Tsugawa, N.; Tachikawa, K.; Koinuma, T.; Miyagawa, K.; Kimoto, A.; Nakayama, M.; Namba, N.; et al. Elevated fibroblast growth factor 23 exerts its effects on placenta and regulates vitamin D metabolism in pregnancy of Hyp mice. *J. Bone Miner. Res.* **2014**, *29*, 1627–1638. [CrossRef]
34. Tagliabracci, V.S.; Engel, J.L.; Wiley, S.E.; Xiao, J.; Gonzalez, D.J.; Nidumanda Appaiah, H.; Koller, A.; Nizet, V.; White, K.E.; Dixon, J.E. Dynamic regulation of FGF23 by Fam20C phosphorylation, GalNAc-T3 glycosylation, and furin proteolysis. *Proc. Natl. Acad. Sci. USA* **2014**, *111*, 5520–5525. [CrossRef]
35. Kato, K.; Jeanneau, C.; Tarp, M.A.; Benet-Pages, A.; Lorenz-Depiereux, B.; Bennett, E.P.; Mandel, U.; Strom, T.M.; Clausen, H. Polypeptide GalNAc-transferase T3 and familial tumoral calcinosis. Secretion of fibroblast growth factor 23 requires O-glycosylation. *J. Biol. Chem.* **2006**, *281*, 18370–18377. [CrossRef]
36. Topaz, O.; Shurman, D.L.; Bergman, R.; Indelman, M.; Ratajczak, P.; Mizrachi, M.; Khamaysi, Z.; Behar, D.; Petronius, D.; Friedman, V.; et al. Mutations in GALNT3, encoding a protein involved in O-linked glycosylation, cause familial tumoral calcinosis. *Nat. Genet.* **2004**, *36*, 579–581. [CrossRef]
37. Ichikawa, S.; Baujat, G.; Seyahi, A.; Garoufali, A.G.; Imel, E.A.; Padgett, L.R.; Austin, A.M.; Sorenson, A.H.; Pejin, Z.; Topouchian, V.; et al. Clinical variability of familial tumoral calcinosis caused by novel GALNT3 mutations. *Am. J. Med. Genet. A* **2010**, *152A*, 896–903. [CrossRef]
38. Benet-Pages, A.; Orlik, P.; Strom, T.M.; Lorenz-Depiereux, B. An FGF23 missense mutation causes familial tumoral calcinosis with hyperphosphatemia. *Hum. Mol. Genet.* **2005**, *14*, 385–390. [CrossRef]
39. Araya, K.; Fukumoto, S.; Backenroth, R.; Takeuchi, Y.; Nakayama, K.; Ito, N.; Yoshii, N.; Yamazaki, Y.; Yamashita, T.; Silver, J.; et al. A novel mutation in fibroblast growth factor 23 gene as a cause of tumoral calcinosis. *J. Clin. Endocrinol. Metab.* **2005**, *90*, 5523–5527. [CrossRef]
40. Ichikawa, S.; Imel, E.A.; Kreiter, M.L.; Yu, X.; Mackenzie, D.S.; Sorenson, A.H.; Goetz, R.; Mohammadi, M.; White, K.E.; Econs, M.J. A homozygous missense mutation in human KLOTHO causes severe tumoral calcinosis. *J. Clin. Investig.* **2007**, *117*, 2684–2691. [CrossRef]
41. Shimada, T.; Kakitani, M.; Yamazaki, Y.; Hasegawa, H.; Takeuchi, Y.; Fujita, T.; Fukumoto, S.; Tomizuka, K.; Yamashita, T. Targeted ablation of Fgf23 demonstrates an essential physiological role of FGF23 in phosphate and vitamin D metabolism. *J. Clin. Investig.* **2004**, *113*, 561–568. [CrossRef] [PubMed]
42. Fukumoto, S.; Ozono, K.; Michigami, T.; Minagawa, M.; Okazaki, R.; Sugimoto, T.; Takeuchi, Y.; Matsumoto, T. Pathogenesis and diagnostic criteria for rickets and osteomalacia-proposal by an expert panel supported by the Ministry of Health, Labour and Welfare, Japan, the Japanese Society for Bone and Mineral Research, and the Japan Endocrine Society. *J. Bone Miner. Metab.* **2015**, *33*, 467–473. [CrossRef] [PubMed]
43. Fukumoto, S. FGF23-related hypophosphatemic rickets/osteomalacia: Diagnosis and new treatment. *J. Mol. Endocrinol.* **2021**, *66*, R57–R65. [CrossRef] [PubMed]
44. Imel, E.A.; Hui, S.L.; Econs, M.J. FGF23 concentrations vary with disease status in autosomal dominant hypophosphatemic rickets. *J. Bone Miner. Res.* **2007**, *22*, 520–526. [CrossRef]
45. Imel, E.A.; Peacock, M.; Gray, A.K.; Padgett, L.R.; Hui, S.L.; Econs, M.J. Iron modifies plasma FGF23 differently in autosomal dominant hypophosphatemic rickets and healthy humans. *J. Clin. Endocrinol. Metab.* **2011**, *96*, 3541–3549. [CrossRef]
46. Farrow, E.G.; Yu, X.; Summers, L.J.; Davis, S.I.; Fleet, J.C.; Allen, M.R.; Robling, A.G.; Stayrook, K.R.; Jideonwo, V.; Magers, M.J.; et al. Iron deficiency drives an autosomal dominant hypophosphatemic rickets (ADHR) phenotype in fibroblast growth factor-23 (Fgf23) knock-in mice. *Proc. Natl. Acad. Sci. USA* **2011**, *108*, E1146–E1155. [CrossRef]
47. Haffner, D.; Emma, F.; Eastwood, D.M.; Duplan, M.B.; Bacchetta, J.; Schnabel, D.; Wicart, P.; Bockenhauer, D.; Santos, F.; Levtchenko, E.; et al. Clinical practice recommendations for the diagnosis and management of X-linked hypophosphataemia. *Nat. Rev. Nephrol.* **2019**, *15*, 435–455. [CrossRef]

48. HYP-CONSORTIUM. A gene (PEX) with homologies to endopeptidases is mutated in patients with X-linked hypophosphatemic rickets. The HYP Consortium. *Nat. Genet.* **1995**, *11*, 130–136. [CrossRef]
49. Beck, L.; Soumounou, Y.; Martel, J.; Krishnamurthy, G.; Gauthier, C.; Goodyer, C.G.; Tenenhouse, H.S. Pex/PEX tissue distribution and evidence for a deletion in the 3′ region of the Pex gene in X-linked hypophosphatemic mice. *J. Clin. Investig.* **1997**, *99*, 1200–1209. [CrossRef]
50. Liu, S.; Zhou, J.; Tang, W.; Jiang, X.; Rowe, D.W.; Quarles, L.D. Pathogenic role of Fgf23 in Hyp mice. *Am. J. Physiol. Endocrinol. Metab.* **2006**, *291*, E38–E49. [CrossRef]
51. Benet-Pages, A.; Lorenz-Depiereux, B.; Zischka, H.; White, K.E.; Econs, M.J.; Strom, T.M. FGF23 is processed by proprotein convertases but not by PHEX. *Bone* **2004**, *35*, 455–462. [CrossRef]
52. Martin, A.; Liu, S.; David, V.; Li, H.; Karydis, A.; Feng, J.Q.; Quarles, L.D. Bone proteins PHEX and DMP1 regulate fibroblastic growth factor Fgf23 expression in osteocytes through a common pathway involving FGF receptor (FGFR) signaling. *FASEB J.* **2011**, *25*, 2551–2562. [CrossRef]
53. Xiao, Z.; Huang, J.; Cao, L.; Liang, Y.; Han, X.; Quarles, L.D. Osteocyte-specific deletion of Fgfr1 suppresses FGF23. *PLoS ONE* **2014**, *9*, e104154. [CrossRef]
54. White, K.E.; Cabral, J.M.; Davis, S.I.; Fishburn, T.; Evans, W.E.; Ichikawa, S.; Fields, J.; Yu, X.; Shaw, N.J.; McLellan, N.J.; et al. Mutations that cause osteoglophonic dysplasia define novel roles for FGFR1 in bone elongation. *Am. J. Hum. Genet.* **2005**, *76*, 361–367. [CrossRef]
55. Yamazaki, M.; Ozono, K.; Okada, T.; Tachikawa, K.; Kondou, H.; Ohata, Y.; Michigami, T. Both FGF23 and extracellular phosphate activate Raf/MEK/ERK pathway via FGF receptors in HEK293 cells. *J. Cell. Biochem.* **2010**, *111*, 1210–1221. [CrossRef]
56. Nishino, J.; Yamazaki, M.; Kawai, M.; Tachikawa, K.; Yamamoto, K.; Miyagawa, K.; Kogo, M.; Ozono, K.; Michigami, T. Extracellular Phosphate Induces the Expression of Dentin Matrix Protein 1 Through the FGF Receptor in Osteoblasts. *J. Cell. Biochem.* **2017**, *118*, 1151–1163. [CrossRef]
57. Takashi, Y.; Kosako, H.; Sawatsubashi, S.; Kinoshita, Y.; Ito, N.; Tsoumpra, M.K.; Nangaku, M.; Abe, M.; Matsuhisa, M.; Kato, S.; et al. Activation of unliganded FGF receptor by extracellular phosphate potentiates proteolytic protection of FGF23 by its O-glycosylation. *Proc. Natl. Acad. Sci. USA* **2019**, *116*, 11418–11427. [CrossRef]
58. Rowe, P.S. The chicken or the egg: PHEX, FGF23 and SIBLINGs unscrambled. *Cell Biochem. Funct.* **2012**, *30*, 355–375. [CrossRef]
59. Hsu, Y.H.; Kiel, D.P. Clinical review: Genome-wide association studies of skeletal phenotypes: What we have learned and where we are headed. *J. Clin. Endocrinol. Metab.* **2012**, *97*, E1958–E1977. [CrossRef]
60. Bresler, D.; Bruder, J.; Mohnike, K.; Fraser, W.D.; Rowe, P.S. Serum MEPE-ASARM-peptides are elevated in X-linked rickets (HYP): Implications for phosphaturia and rickets. *J. Endocrinol.* **2004**, *183*, R1–R9. [CrossRef]
61. Rowe, P.S.; Garrett, I.R.; Schwarz, P.M.; Carnes, D.L.; Lafer, E.M.; Mundy, G.R.; Gutierrez, G.E. Surface plasmon resonance (SPR) confirms that MEPE binds to PHEX via the MEPE-ASARM motif: A model for impaired mineralization in X-linked rickets (HYP). *Bone* **2005**, *36*, 33–46. [CrossRef] [PubMed]
62. Martin, A.; David, V.; Laurence, J.S.; Schwarz, P.M.; Lafer, E.M.; Hedge, A.M.; Rowe, P.S. Degradation of MEPE, DMP1, and release of SIBLING ASARM-peptides (minhibins): ASARM-peptide(s) are directly responsible for defective mineralization in HYP. *Endocrinology* **2008**, *149*, 1757–1772. [CrossRef] [PubMed]
63. Fuente, R.; Gil-Pena, H.; Claramunt-Taberner, D.; Hernandez-Frias, O.; Fernandez-Iglesias, A.; Hermida-Prado, F.; Anes-Gonzalez, G.; Rubio-Aliaga, I.; Lopez, J.M.; Santos, F. Marked alterations in the structure, dynamics and maturation of growth plate likely explain growth retardation and bone deformities of young Hyp mice. *Bone* **2018**, *116*, 187–195. [CrossRef] [PubMed]
64. Sabbagh, Y.; Carpenter, T.O.; Demay, M.B. Hypophosphatemia leads to rickets by impairing caspase-mediated apoptosis of hypertrophic chondrocytes. *Proc. Natl. Acad. Sci. USA* **2005**, *102*, 9637–9642. [CrossRef]
65. Imura, A.; Iwano, A.; Tohyama, O.; Tsuji, Y.; Nozaki, K.; Hashimoto, N.; Fujimori, T.; Nabeshima, Y. Secreted Klotho protein in sera and CSF: Implication for post-translational cleavage in release of Klotho protein from cell membrane. *FEBS Lett.* **2004**, *565*, 143–147. [CrossRef]
66. Shalhoub, V.; Ward, S.C.; Sun, B.; Stevens, J.; Renshaw, L.; Hawkins, N.; Richards, W.G. Fibroblast growth factor 23 (FGF23) and alpha-klotho stimulate osteoblastic MC3T3.E1 cell proliferation and inhibit mineralization. *Calcif. Tissue Int.* **2011**, *89*, 140–150. [CrossRef]
67. Kawai, M.; Kinoshita, S.; Kimoto, A.; Hasegawa, Y.; Miyagawa, K.; Yamazaki, M.; Ohata, Y.; Ozono, K.; Michigami, T. FGF23 suppresses chondrocyte proliferation in the presence of soluble alpha-Klotho both in vitro and in vivo. *J. Biol. Chem.* **2013**, *288*, 2414–2427. [CrossRef]
68. Zelzer, E.; Blitz, E.; Killian, M.L.; Thomopoulos, S. Tendon-to-bone attachment: From development to maturity. *Birth Defects Res. Part C Embryo Today* **2014**, *102*, 101–112. [CrossRef]
69. Carpenter, T.O.; Imel, E.A.; Holm, I.A.; Jan de Beur, S.M.; Insogna, K.L. A clinician's guide to X-linked hypophosphatemia. *J. Bone Miner. Res.* **2011**, *26*, 1381–1388. [CrossRef]
70. Karaplis, A.C.; Bai, X.; Falet, J.P.; Macica, C.M. Mineralizing enthesopathy is a common feature of renal phosphate-wasting disorders attributed to FGF23 and is exacerbated by standard therapy in *hyp* mice. *Endocrinology* **2012**, *153*, 5906–5917. [CrossRef]
71. Liu, E.S.; Martins, J.S.; Zhang, W.; Demay, M.B. Molecular analysis of enthesopathy in a mouse model of hypophosphatemic rickets. *Development* **2018**, *145*, dev163519. [CrossRef]

72. Imel, E.A.; Glorieux, F.H.; Whyte, M.P.; Munns, C.F.; Ward, L.M.; Nilsson, O.; Simmons, J.H.; Padidela, R.; Namba, N.; Cheong, H.I.; et al. Burosumab versus conventional therapy in children with X-linked hypophosphataemia: A randomised, active-controlled, open-label, phase 3 trial. *Lancet* **2019**, *393*, 2416–2427. [CrossRef]
73. Feng, J.Q.; Ward, L.M.; Liu, S.; Lu, Y.; Xie, Y.; Yuan, B.; Yu, X.; Rauch, F.; Davis, S.I.; Zhang, S.; et al. Loss of DMP1 causes rickets and osteomalacia and identifies a role for osteocytes in mineral metabolism. *Nat. Genet.* **2006**, *38*, 1310–1315. [CrossRef]
74. Lorenz-Depiereux, B.; Bastepe, M.; Benet-Pages, A.; Amyere, M.; Wagenstaller, J.; Muller-Barth, U.; Badenhoop, K.; Kaiser, S.M.; Rittmaster, R.S.; Shlossberg, A.H.; et al. DMP1 mutations in autosomal recessive hypophosphatemia implicate a bone matrix protein in the regulation of phosphate homeostasis. *Nat. Genet.* **2006**, *38*, 1248–1250. [CrossRef]
75. Lorenz-Depiereux, B.; Schnabel, D.; Tiosano, D.; Hausler, G.; Strom, T.M. Loss-of-function ENPP1 mutations cause both generalized arterial calcification of infancy and autosomal-recessive hypophosphatemic rickets. *Am. J. Hum. Genet.* **2010**, *86*, 267–272. [CrossRef]
76. Levy-Litan, V.; Hershkovitz, E.; Avizov, L.; Leventhal, N.; Bercovich, D.; Chalifa-Caspi, V.; Manor, E.; Buriakovsky, S.; Hadad, Y.; Goding, J.; et al. Autosomal-recessive hypophosphatemic rickets is associated with an inactivation mutation in the ENPP1 gene. *Am. J. Hum. Genet.* **2010**, *86*, 273–278. [CrossRef]
77. Rutsch, F.; Ruf, N.; Vaingankar, S.; Toliat, M.R.; Suk, A.; Hohne, W.; Schauer, G.; Lehmann, M.; Roscioli, T.; Schnabel, D.; et al. Mutations in ENPP1 are associated with 'idiopathic' infantile arterial calcification. *Nat. Genet.* **2003**, *34*, 379–381. [CrossRef]
78. Linglart, A.; Biosse-Duplan, M. Hypophosphatasia. *Curr. Osteoporos. Rep.* **2016**, *14*, 95–105. [CrossRef]
79. Tagliabracci, V.S.; Engel, J.L.; Wen, J.; Wiley, S.E.; Worby, C.A.; Kinch, L.N.; Xiao, J.; Grishin, N.V.; Dixon, J.E. Secreted kinase phosphorylates extracellular proteins that regulate biomineralization. *Science* **2012**, *336*, 1150–1153. [CrossRef]
80. Simpson, M.A.; Hsu, R.; Keir, L.S.; Hao, J.; Sivapalan, G.; Ernst, L.M.; Zackai, E.H.; Al-Gazali, L.I.; Hulskamp, G.; Kingston, H.M.; et al. Mutations in FAM20C are associated with lethal osteosclerotic bone dysplasia (Raine syndrome), highlighting a crucial molecule in bone development. *Am. J. Hum. Genet.* **2007**, *81*, 906–912. [CrossRef]
81. Rafaelsen, S.H.; Raeder, H.; Fagerheim, A.K.; Knappskog, P.; Carpenter, T.O.; Johansson, S.; Bjerknes, R. Exome sequencing reveals FAM20c mutations associated with fibroblast growth factor 23-related hypophosphatemia, dental anomalies, and ectopic calcification. *J. Bone Miner. Res.* **2013**, *28*, 1378–1385. [CrossRef]
82. Takeyari, S.; Yamamoto, T.; Kinoshita, Y.; Fukumoto, S.; Glorieux, F.H.; Michigami, T.; Hasegawa, K.; Kitaoka, T.; Kubota, T.; Imanishi, Y.; et al. Hypophosphatemic osteomalacia and bone sclerosis caused by a novel homozygous mutation of the FAM20C gene in an elderly man with a mild variant of Raine syndrome. *Bone* **2014**, *67*, 56–62. [CrossRef]
83. Wang, X.; Wang, S.; Li, C.; Gao, T.; Liu, Y.; Rangiani, A.; Sun, Y.; Hao, J.; George, A.; Lu, Y.; et al. Inactivation of a novel FGF23 regulator, FAM20C, leads to hypophosphatemic rickets in mice. *PLoS Genet.* **2012**, *8*, e1002708. [CrossRef]
84. Wang, X.; Wang, J.; Yuan, B.; Lu, Y.; Feng, J.Q.; Qin, C. Overexpression of Dmp1 fails to rescue the bone and dentin defects in Fam20C knockout mice. *Connect. Tissue Res.* **2014**, *55*, 299–303. [CrossRef]
85. Rendina, D.; Abate, V.; Cacace, G.; Elia, L.; De Filippo, G.; Del Vecchio, S.; Galletti, F.; Cuocolo, A.; Strazzullo, P. Tumor induced osteomalacia: A systematic review and individual patient's data analysis. *J. Clin. Endocrinol. Metab.* **2022**, dgac253. [CrossRef]
86. Takeuchi, Y.; Suzuki, H.; Ogura, S.; Imai, R.; Yamazaki, Y.; Yamashita, T.; Miyamoto, Y.; Okazaki, H.; Nakamura, K.; Nakahara, K.; et al. Venous sampling for fibroblast growth factor-23 confirms preoperative diagnosis of tumor-induced osteomalacia. *J. Clin. Endocrinol. Metab.* **2004**, *89*, 3979–3982. [CrossRef] [PubMed]
87. Lee, J.C.; Jeng, Y.M.; Su, S.Y.; Wu, C.T.; Tsai, K.S.; Lee, C.H.; Lin, C.Y.; Carter, J.M.; Huang, J.W.; Chen, S.H.; et al. Identification of a novel FN1-FGFR1 genetic fusion as a frequent event in phosphaturic mesenchymal tumour. *J. Pathol.* **2015**, *235*, 539–545. [CrossRef]
88. Lee, J.C.; Su, S.Y.; Changou, C.A.; Yang, R.S.; Tsai, K.S.; Collins, M.T.; Orwoll, E.S.; Lin, C.Y.; Chen, S.H.; Shih, S.R.; et al. Characterization of FN1-FGFR1 and novel FN1-FGF1 fusion genes in a large series of phosphaturic mesenchymal tumors. *Mod. Pathol.* **2016**, *29*, 1335–1346. [CrossRef]
89. Riminucci, M.; Collins, M.T.; Fedarko, N.S.; Cherman, N.; Corsi, A.; White, K.E.; Waguespack, S.; Gupta, A.; Hannon, T.; Econs, M.J.; et al. FGF-23 in fibrous dysplasia of bone and its relationship to renal phosphate wasting. *J. Clin. Investig.* **2003**, *112*, 683–692. [CrossRef]
90. Bhattacharyya, N.; Wiench, M.; Dumitrescu, C.; Connolly, B.M.; Bugge, T.H.; Patel, H.V.; Gafni, R.I.; Cherman, N.; Cho, M.; Hager, G.L.; et al. Mechanism of FGF23 processing in fibrous dysplasia. *J. Bone Miner. Res.* **2012**, *27*, 1132–1141. [CrossRef]
91. Groesser, L.; Herschberger, E.; Ruetten, A.; Ruivenkamp, C.; Lopriore, E.; Zutt, M.; Langmann, T.; Singer, S.; Klingseisen, L.; Schneider-Brachert, W.; et al. Postzygotic HRAS and KRAS mutations cause nevus sebaceous and Schimmelpenning syndrome. *Nat. Genet.* **2012**, *44*, 783–787. [CrossRef] [PubMed]
92. Lim, Y.H.; Ovejero, D.; Sugarman, J.S.; Deklotz, C.M.; Maruri, A.; Eichenfield, L.F.; Kelley, P.K.; Juppner, H.; Gottschalk, M.; Tifft, C.J.; et al. Multilineage somatic activating mutations in HRAS and NRAS cause mosaic cutaneous and skeletal lesions, elevated FGF23 and hypophosphatemia. *Hum. Mol. Genet.* **2014**, *23*, 397–407. [CrossRef] [PubMed]
93. Zweifler, L.E.; Ao, M.; Yadav, M.; Kuss, P.; Narisawa, S.; Kolli, T.N.; Wimer, H.F.; Farquharson, C.; Somerman, M.J.; Millan, J.L.; et al. Role of PHOSPHO1 in Periodontal Development and Function. *J. Dent. Res.* **2016**, *95*, 742–751. [CrossRef] [PubMed]
94. Schipani, E.; Kruse, K.; Jüppner, H. A constitutively active mutant PTH-PTHrP receptor in Jansen-type metaphyseal chondrodysplasia. *Science* **1995**, *268*, 98–100. [CrossRef]

95. Brown, W.W.; Jüppner, H.; Langman, C.B.; Price, H.; Farrow, E.G.; White, K.E.; McCormick, K.L. Hypophosphatemia with elevations in serum fibroblast growth factor 23 in a child with Jansen's metaphyseal chondrodysplasia. *J. Clin. Endocrinol. Metab.* **2009**, *94*, 17–20. [CrossRef]
96. Lavi-Moshayoff, V.; Wasserman, G.; Meir, T.; Silver, J.; Naveh-Many, T. PTH increases FGF23 gene expression and mediates the high-FGF23 levels of experimental kidney failure: A bone parathyroid feedback loop. *Am. J. Physiol. Renal Physiol.* **2010**, *299*, F882–F889. [CrossRef]
97. Shimizu, Y.; Tada, Y.; Yamauchi, M.; Okamoto, T.; Suzuki, H.; Ito, N.; Fukumoto, S.; Sugimoto, T.; Fujita, T. Hypophosphatemia induced by intravenous administration of saccharated ferric oxide: Another form of FGF23-related hypophosphatemia. *Bone* **2009**, *45*, 814–816. [CrossRef]
98. Schouten, B.J.; Hunt, P.J.; Livesey, J.H.; Frampton, C.M.; Soule, S.G. FGF23 elevation and hypophosphatemia after intravenous iron polymaltose: A prospective study. *J. Clin. Endocrinol. Metab.* **2009**, *94*, 2332–2337. [CrossRef]

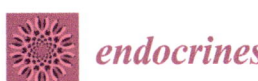

Review

Pathogenic Variants of the *PHEX* Gene

Yasuhisa Ohata [1,*] and Yasuki Ishihara [1,2,3]

1. Department of Pediatrics, Osaka University Graduate School of Medicine, 2-2 Yamadaoka, Suita 565-0871, Osaka, Japan
2. The First Department of Oral and Maxillofacial Surgery, Osaka University Graduate School of Dentistry, 1-8 Yamadaoka, Suita 565-0871, Osaka, Japan
3. Department of Cardiovascular Medicine, Osaka University Graduate School of Medicine, 2-2 Yamadaoka, Suita 565-0871, Osaka, Japan
* Correspondence: yasuhisa1@ped.med.osaka-u.ac.jp; Tel.: +81-6-6879-3932

Abstract: Twenty-five years ago, a pathogenic variant of the phosphate-regulating endopeptidase homolog X-linked (*PHEX*) gene was identified as the cause of X-linked hypophosphatemic rickets (XLH). Subsequently, the overproduction of fibroblast growth factor 23 (FGF23) due to *PHEX* defects has been found to be associated with XLH pathophysiology. However, the mechanism by which PHEX deficiency contributes to the upregulation of FGF23 and the function of PHEX itself remain unclear. To date, over 700 pathogenic variants have been identified in patients with XLH, and functional assays and genotype–phenotype correlation analyses based on pathogenic variant data derived from XLH patients have been reported. Genetic testing for XLH is useful for the diagnosis. Not only have single-nucleotide variants causing missense, nonsense, and splicing variants and small deletion/insertion variants causing frameshift/non-frameshift alterations been observed, but also gross deletion/duplication variants causing copy number variants have been reported as pathogenic variants in *PHEX*. With the development of new technologies including next generation sequencing, it is expected that an increasing number of pathogenic variants will be identified. This chapter aimed to summarize the genotype of *PHEX* and related analyses and discusses the pathophysiology of PHEX defects to seek clues on unsolved questions.

Keywords: X-linked hypophosphatemic rickets; phosphate-regulating endopeptidase homolog X-linked; fibroblast growth factor 23; genotype–phenotype correlation; multiplex ligation-dependent probe amplification; nonsense-mediated decay; cryptic splice site; mosaicism; zinc-binding site; truncating variant

1. Introduction

Previously, genetic linkage analyses have revealed the pathogenic variants of the gene associated with the disorder X-linked hypophosphatemic rickets (XLH) located in Xp22 [1]. In 1995, the HYP consortium defined the XLH locus using a positional cloning approach and identified the phosphate-regulating endopeptidase homolog X-linked (*PHEX*) gene in this region [2]. *Hyp*, *Gy*, and *Ska1* mice have been identified as model mice for studying XLH, and it was later revealed that these mice harbor pathogenic variants in the mouse *Phex* homolog [3–5]. XLH is inherited in an X-linked dominant manner, with complete penetrance. The female-to-male ratio is approximately 2:1, and there is no male-to-male transmission. Genetic testing for XLH is available and can be used for differential diagnosis, especially when the inheritance pattern is unclear [6]. To date, 729 different *PHEX* variants available on the Human Gene Mutation Database (HGMD, http://www.hgmd.cf.ac.uk/ac/index.php, accessed on 7 May 2022) have been reported as a cause of XLH. Recently, a new PHEX variant database (*PHEX* Locus Specific Database [LSDB] sponsored by UltraGenyx Pharmaceutical Inc.: https://www.rarediseasegenes.com/, accessed on 7 May 2022) has been established using four data sources including an old database [7], results from a sponsored genetic testing program [8], unpublished variants identified in previous burosumab clinical studies, and published variant data collected in a literature review [9]. The number of reported *PHEX* pathogenic variants is increasing.

Patients with XLH have hypophosphatemia, phosphaturia, and low or inappropriately normal 1, 25-dihydroxy vitamin D (1,25[OH]$_2$D) levels caused by high levels of fibroblast growth factor 23 (FGF23) [10]. In renal tubules, FGF23 increases phosphate excretion in urine by downregulating type 2a and 2c sodium phosphate cotransporters, which reabsorb phosphate. In vitamin D metabolism, FGF23 downregulates 1-alpha-hydroxylase, which converts 25 hydroxy-vitamin D to 1,25(OH)$_2$D, the active form of vitamin D. FGF23 also upregulates 24-hydroxylase, which converts 1,25(OH)$_2$D to 24, 25-dihydroxy vitamin D, an inactive form of vitamin D. Therefore, excess FGF23 suppresses vitamin D activity and phosphate absorption from the intestine, which also contributes to hypophosphatemia in patients with XLH [11–13]. In addition to *PHEX*, the pathogenic variants of dentin matrix protein 1 (*DMP1*), *FGF23*, ectonucleotide pyrophosphatase phosphodiesterase-1 (*ENPP1*), and *FAM20C* can lead to the overproduction of FGF23 and cause hypophosphatemic rickets [14–19].

Although it has been shown that PHEX deficiency leads to the overproduction of FGF23, which contributes to the pathogenesis of XLH, the mechanism by which an abnormality in PHEX causes an increase in FGF23 levels remains to be elucidated. Rowe et al. showed that PHEX bound to matrix extracellular phophoglycoprotein (MEPE), which belongs to a group of extracellular matrix proteins (small integrin-binding ligand, N-linked glycoproteins [SIBLINGs]) involved in bone mineralization. MEPE contains an acidic serine–aspartate-rich MEPE-associated motif (ASARM) and the ASARM peptide released from MEPE negatively affects mineralization and phosphate uptake [20]. The ASARM motif is also present in other SIBLINGs including DMP1 and osteopontin. Martin et al. reported that the degradation of SIBLINGs and release of ASARM peptides were responsible to the impaired mineralization in XLH [21]. *Hyp* mice harboring deletions in the 3' region of *Phex* have high levels of FGF23 and hypophosphatemia with inappropriately normal 1,25(OH)$_2$D levels similar to that in patients with XLH [22]. *Fgf23* mRNA expression is increased in *Hyp* mouse bones and in osteoblasts and osteocytes isolated from these mice [22,23]. Sitara et al. generated hyperphosphatemic *Fgf23* null mice and crossed them with hypophosphatemic *Hyp* mice and showed the same phenotype [24], which suggested both defects are involved in the same pathway. These findings indicate that FGF23 may function downstream of PHEX; however, the precise mechanism is not fully understood. *PHEX* is predominantly expressed in osteoblasts, osteocytes, and odontoblasts, but not in kidney tubules [25], and it encodes a protein that structurally resembles the M13 family of membrane-binding metalloproteases. Neutral endopeptidase 24.11 or neprilysin (NEP) and endothelin converting enzyme-1 [2] belong to this family of metalloproteases, which are type II integral membrane glycoproteins containing a large extracellular domain that retains catalytic activity [25]. It has been postulated that the large extracellular domain of PHEX contains a zinc-binding motif which is essential for the catalytic activity in NEP [2]. Since the members of this family are known to cleave small peptides, FGF23 was initially considered to serve as a substrate for PHEX and degraded by PHEX [26]. However, several studies have revealed that FGF23 is not a substrate for PHEX [27–29], and the endogenous PHEX protein substrate remains to be verified. To identify any clues to clarify the function of PHEX and the pathogenesis of how PHEX deficiency causes XLH, we reviewed data on the *PHEX* genotype based on published papers.

2. Pathogenic Variants of the *PHEX* Gene

We reviewed 97 papers that were obtained from the HGMD database, including 55 case reports in which pathogenic variants of *PHEX* were described. Among these reports, 252 missense or nonsense, 117 splicing, 155 small deletions, 86 small insertions or duplications, 13 deletion/insertions (delins), 80 gross deletions, 16 gross insertions, 4 regulatory, and 6 complex rearrangement variants have been reported to cause XLH. The analyses of pathogenic variants other than those in case reports are summarized in Table 1.

Table 1. List of studies describing *PHEX* genotypes other than case reports.

Author	Year	Probands	Variant Positive	Variant Positivity Rate (%)	Variants	Reference
Rowe	1997	106	NR	83	NR	[30]
Francis	1997	43	33	77	26	[31]
Holm	1997	22	9	41	9	[32]
Dixon	1998	68	31	46	31	[33]
Filisetti	1999	22	22	100	22	[34]
Tyynismaa	2000	20	19	95	18	[35]
Popowska	2000	35	35	100	29	[36]
Holm	2001	41	22	54	20	[37]
Christie	2001	11 [a]	1	NA	NR	[38]
Cho	2005	17	8	47	7	[39]
Song	2007	15	9	60	8	[40]
Ichikawa	2008	26	26	100	18	[41]
Gaucher	2009	118	93	79	NR	[42]
Clausmeyer	2009	71 [b]	37	52	28	[43]
Morey	2011	36	36	100	34	[44]
Ruppe	2011	46	27	59	27	[45]
Jap	2011	9	5	56	5	[46]
Quinlan	2012	46	38	83	24	[47]
Beck-Nielsen	2012	24	21	88	20	[48]
Kinoshita	2012	27	26	96	17	[49]
Lee	2012	6	6 [c]	NA	4	[50]
Durmaz	2013	6	6	100	6	[51]
Yue	2014	9	9	100	10	[52]
Capelli	2015	26	22	84	19	[53]
Zhang	2015	13	9	69	9	[54]
Rafaelsen	2016	19	15	79	13	[55]
Li	2016	18	18	100	17	[56]
Guven	2017	9	7	78	7	[57]
Acar	2018	15	12	80	12	[58]
Chesher	2018	35	35	100	37	[59]
Gu	2018	86	7	NA	NR	[60]
Marik	2018	32	8	25	NR	[61]
Hernández-Frías	2019	22	22 [c]	NA	NR	[62]
Zhang	2019	216	216 [c]	NA	166	[63]
Lin	2020	76	61	80	51	[64]
Zheng	2020	53	53 [c]	NA	47	[65]
Baroncelli	2021	24	24	100	NR	[66]
Ishihara	2021	28	28 [c]	NA	23	[67]
Jiménez	2021	17	17	100	16	[68]
Lin	2021	105	105 [c]	NA	88	[69]
Park	2021	50	47	94	48	[70]
Rodríguez-Rubio	2021	39	39 [c]	83	NR	[71]

[a] The authors analyzed only probands for which no pathogenic variant was identified in the *PHEX* coding region. [b] All patients were counted. [c] The authors evaluated only probands for which pathogenic variants were confirmed. NA: not applicable. NR: not reported.

From these data, pathogenic variants of *PHEX* has been found to be located across the entire gene [44], which is consistent with data from the *PHEX* LSDB [9]. Sarafrazi et al. described the mapping data of *PHEX* pathogenic variants [9]. After excluding reports in which only genetic variants confirmed probands were analyzed, the median positive rate of genetic analysis was 83% (interquartile range: 59.3, 100). Rush et al. reported that approximately 10% of clinically diagnosed XLH patients had no variant of *PHEX* in a hypophosphatemia genetic testing program [8]. Owing to the high positivity rate, genetic testing for XLH is useful for diagnosis. Not only single nucleotide variants causing missense, nonsense, and splicing variants and small deletion/insertion variants causing frameshift/non-frameshift alteration, but also gross deletion/duplication variants causing copy number variants (CNV) have been reported as pathogenic variants of *PHEX* [43,44,48,49,53,57–59,63,64,67]. The CNV ranges from 3.8–23% in these reports. Sanger sequencing-based entire gene analysis and gene panel tests are performed as a genetic testing tool for *PHEX*. Multiplex ligation-dependent probe amplification (MLPA) often complements these methods to detect CNV [72]. Since a certain number of CNV has been reported in XLH, MLPA should be considered if any variants are not identified by Sanger sequencing or gene panel testing. Advances in next generation sequencing (NGS)-based whole exome or whole genome sequencing are reducing the cost and time taken for sequencing [72]. In *PHEX* analysis, whole exome sequencing has been used in certain studies [68,73,74]. It is expected that NGS-based methods will eventually replace conventional sequencing methods.

2.1. Mosaicism

In some studies, several mosaicism cases have been found only in male patients with XLH [43,63,64,75–77]. In a Chinese cohort study, de novo mosaic variants have been identified in 6.15% of probands [64]. Lin et al. reported the first case of isolated germline mosaicism in which a heterozygous pathogenic variant was initially detected in the *PHEX* gene in a girl with XLH and was not found in her healthy parents based on gDNA from peripheral blood. Since her father had an occasional abnormality in his serum phosphate level, they conducted an additional genetic analysis using gDNA from eight different tissues of the father. They found the same pathogenic variant with the proband only in the sperm, while there was no variant in the hair, oral epithelium, saliva, nail, cuticle, whole blood, or urine [75]. Since the penetrance of XLH is considered to be 100%, the inheritance pattern can be determined from family history. However, the possibility of an isolated germline mosaic should be considered during genetic counseling [64]. Notably, the *PHEX* mosaic variants have been found in male patients alone. Since female patients usually harbor heterozygous pathogenic variants, mosaicism in women may be missed. In contrast, male patients usually have hemizygous variants and the mosaicism is apparent seen in heterozygous variants and can be detected.

2.2. Splice Site Variants

Using the HGMD database, 117 variants affecting mRNA splicing were identified. Almost all of these variants are located at the splicing junctions of the first two or last two nucleotides at the beginning or end of the exon, respectively. These variants result in exon skipping; if the number of nucleotides in the deleted exon is not a multiple of three, this alteration leads to a frameshift and produces a truncated protein owing to a new stop codon [72]. However, several *PHEX* variants have been reported to be located outside the canonical splicing junction. To clarify the effect of these variants on splicing, BinEssa et al. investigated 13 previously reported variants located outside the splicing junction consisting of canonical GT-AG dinucleotide splice donor or acceptor sites. The constructs were transfected into HEK293 cells and pre-mRNA splicing was analyzed using a reverse transcription polymerase chain reaction (RT-PCR) and sequencing. They found that 8 out of 13 variants, including c.1701-16T>A, result in complete exon skipping, and two variants (c.436+6T>C and c.1586+6T>C) cause a partial splicing error (60% exon skipping occurred in both variants). The c.1645+5G>A and c.1645+6 variants lead to 72 bp intron retention by activating the cryptic splice donor site located 70 bp downstream from the canonical splice donor site. Notably, c.437-3C>G resulted in an in-frame deletion due to activation of the adjacent cryptic splice acceptor site. The authors concluded that non-canonical spice site variants should not be missed when they are located within 50 bp from the exon–intron boundary [78]. Zou et al. described the c.633+12del variant of *PHEX* as a pathogenic variant for XLH. They analyzed *PHEX* mRNA extracted from the peripheral blood leukocytes of a patient and revealed that c.633+12del leads to a frameshift resulting from alternative splicing using a cryptic donor splice site. They concluded that the c.633+12del variant activates nearby cryptic 5′ splice sites [79]. Such variants located in deep intron should be evaluated because they can alter mRNA transcription.

2.3. Nonsense Mediated mRNA Decay (NMD)

Many nonsense variants lead to disease by degrading mRNA via NMD [80–82]. Most pathogenic variants of PHEX detected in XLH are nonsense, frame-shift, splice site, and delins variants, which may result in either truncated proteins or degradation of mRNA via NMD [83]. NMD can be activated via several mechanisms. If a premature stop codon is located >50–55 nucleotides upstream from a final exon–exon junction, with an exon junction complex located approximately 24 nucleotides upstream of the junction, it is sufficiently far from the stop codon and cannot be removed by the terminating ribosome and NMD can occur [82]. However, Li et al. identified the p.Trp403* variant of an XLH family member located 939 nucleotides upstream from the last exon–exon junction, and they revealed that the variant does not undergo mRNA decay by showing that mRNA expression level was not reduced [84]. Functional analysis, as discuss later, is needed to determine whether NMD actually occurs in each nonsense variant. It is important to determine whether mRNA-containing pathogenic variants are degraded by NMD when we discuss the phenotype–genotype correlation. Therefore, the accumulation of such data is valuable.

2.4. c.*231A>G Variant

Four variants causing regulatory abnormalities have been reported: c.*231A>G [41,85,86], c.349+11149A>T, c.1482+3997G>A, and c.1646-9276T>G [62]. Ichikawa et al. initially reported six XLH probands harboring c.*231A>G, a novel non-coding single nucleotide substitution variant located in the 3′-untranslated region (UTR) and 3 bp upstream of the putative polyadenylation signal. They also conducted allele-specific PCR in 440 healthy individuals and showed that no controls harbor c.*231A>G. Although this variant has been postulated to affect posttranscriptional transport and translation of mRNA, they did not perform functional analysis to determine whether it can alter the polyadenylation of PHEX mRNA [41]. Mumm et al. reported that all individuals with c.*231A>G have exon 13–15 duplication [87]. Rush et al. suggested that exon 13–15 duplication may contribute to the pathogenesis of XLH in these patients because one patient carried the duplication without *231A>G [8]. However, it is possible that *231A>G may facilitate the duplication of exon 13–15 and indirectly contribute to the pathophysiology of XLH. Further investigations are required to clarify the pathogenicity of *231A>G.

3. Functional Analysis Based on Pathogenic Variants Associated with XLH

Functional analyses of pathogenic variants have been conducted in certain studies. Based on the amino acid sequence of PHEX, it has been hypothesized that PHEX is a transmembrane glycoprotein containing a short N-terminal cytoplasmic region, single N-terminal transmembrane region, and large extracellular C-terminal domain [88]. The PHEX protein is thought to contain multiple glycosylation, enzymatic active, and zinc-binding sites [9]. Although the precise function of PHEX has not been determined, the glycosylation status, endopeptidase activity, and intracellular trafficking have been investigated in mutant PHEX via functional analysis because it is homologous to the M13 zinc metallopeptidases, which function as extramembrane endopeptidases [89]. Sabbagh et al. generated three disease-causing missense variant PHEX cDNAs via PCR mutagenesis, including p.Cys85Arg, p.Gly579Arg, and p.Ser711Arg, identified in patients with XLH. They transfected wild-type and mutant PHEX cDNAs into HEK293 cells and showed that these mutants were not appropriately glycosylated because they were fully sensitive to endoglycosidase H digestion. They also showed that these mutants accumulate in the endoplasmic reticulum (ER) and targeting to the plasma membrane is disrupted [88].

Zheng et al. also analyzed 10 *PHEX* variants in the expression of mutant proteins, cellular trafficking, and endopeptidase activity. They showed that certain nonsense variants, including p.Arg567*, p.Gln714*, and p.Arg747*, are not degraded by NMD and produce mutant proteins with relatively lower molecular weights that have trafficking defects. They also evaluated seven non-truncating variants and revealed that p.Cys77Tyr, p.Cys85Ser, p.Ile281Lys, p.Ile333del, p.Ala514Pro, and p.Gly572Ser mutants accumulate in cells and are not secreted into the medium, whereas the p.Gly553Glu mutant is normally secreted; however, the endopeptidase activity is reduced [65]. Since this variant has been predicted as a pathogenic variant using the American College of Medical Genetics interpretation software [90,91], their results indicated that such defects in endopeptidase activity can result in XLH pathogenesis. Li et al. identified a novel missense variant (p.Phe727Leu) in *PHEX* in patients with XLH and revealed that the mutant is glycosylated inappropriately. They showed that the intracellular transport is blocked and the mutant protein is retained in the ER. Finally, they measured the concentration of FGF23 in the conditioned medium and reported that the level of FGF23 is elevated in the medium with mutant transfected cells when compared to that in the control sample [74]. These findings suggested that those PHEX deficiencies, including abnormalities in glycosylation, can cause an increase of FGF23 expression.

Li et al. reported a p.Trp403* variant in a large Chinese family with XLH. To evaluate the function of this variant, they examined the p38 mitogen-activated protein kinase (MAPK) and extracellular signal-regulated kinase 1/2 (ERK1/2) signaling pathways, because Greenblatt et al. showed that these pathways are involved in osteoblastic differentiation and maintenance of bone structure and function [92]. They overexpressed wild-type or mutant *PHEX* in HEK293 cells and confirmed that phosphorylation of p38 MAPK is significantly decreased in cells transfected with mutant *PHEX*, while the phosphorylation of ERK1/2 is comparable. Based on these data, they concluded that this variant of PHEX causes XLH by downregulating the p38 MAPK signaling pathway [84]. Further studies are needed to confirm whether defects in the p38 MAPK signaling are derived from mutant *PHEX* and cause XLH.

4. Genotype–Phenotype Relationship
4.1. Gene Dosage Effect

Previously, comprehensive clinical studies on untreated adults with XLH suggested that radiographic abnormalities are generally more severe in men than in women, which is explained by X-chromosome inactivation [93]. Theoretically, heterozygous females should have a less severe phenotype because approximately half of the normal alleles remain, whereas males have none [56]. However, it is not clear whether such a gene dosage effect is involved in the XLH phenotype. To analyze the genetic influences on the XLH phenotype, several studies have evaluated the effect of sex on disease severity (Table 2).

Holm et al. tested the skeletal and dental phenotypes and found no significant correlation between these parameters. They then sub-grouped the population into prepuberty and postpuberty and found a trend toward more severe dental disease in males in the postpubertal group (male: 10, female: 15; $p = 0.064$) [37]. Morey et al. compared the clinical features between men and women with XLH independent of the *PHEX* pathogenic variant type and reported that women develop nephrocalcinosis to a lower extent than in men ($p = 0.03$) [44]. However, the gene dosage effect has not been verified, even in a relatively large population [63].

4.2. Location of Pathogenic Variant

To test the hypothesis that patients harboring pathogenic variants located at the N-terminal side have a relatively more severe phenotype, Holm et al. assigned patients into groups with variants at the N-terminal and C-terminal regions, and compared the severity of the phenotype. In this study, the authors found no significant differences in skeletal and dental severities [37]. Several studies performed similar analyses (Table 3).

Table 2. Summary of gene dosage effect analyses.

Author	Year	Subject (Male, Female)	Analyzed Phenotype	p Value	Reference
Whyte	1996	30 (7, 23)	serum Pi	0.34	[94]
			serum ionized Ca	0.89	
			serum Ca	0.99	
			serum $Ca^{2+} \times Pi$	0.30	
			serum ALP	0.075	
			serum iPTH	0.91	
			urinary Ca/Cr	0.65	
			urinary Pi/Cr	0.51	
			% TRP	0.79	
			Tmp/GFR	0.59	
Holm	2001	27 (9, 18)	height z-score	0.11	[37]
		76 (26, 50)	skeletal severity	0.145	
		60 (19, 41)	dental severity	0.272	
Cho	2005	8 (3, 5)	biochemical parameters skeletal severity dental severity	n.s.	[39]
Song	2007	9 (1, 8)	no description	n.s.	[40]
Morey	2011	46 (11, 35)	nephrocalcinosis	**0.03**	[44]
Quinlan	2012	23 (11, 12)	height z-score	n.s.	[47]
Zhang	2019	139 (46, 93)	serum Pi	0.251	[63]
		174 (60, 114)	onset age for any signs	0.284	
		150 (55, 95)	age for first walking	0.844	
		124 (46, 78)	onset age for lower limb deformity	0.817	
		164 (59, 108)	height z-score	0.094	
		47 (19, 28)	RSS	0.850	
		230 (72, 158)	serum i-FGF23	0.696	
Ishihara	2021	26 (5, 21)	RSS	0.11	[67]
		24 (4, 20)	serum iFGF23	0.54	
		29 (6, 23)	height z-score	0.23	
		29 (6, 23)	serum phosphate	0.47	
		28 (5, 23)	serum ALP	**0.048**	
		27 (7, 23)	Tmp/GFR	0.47	
Rodríguez-Rubio	2021	48 (15, 33)	clinical manifestation growth impairment biochemical parameters	n.s.	[71]

Ca, calcium; Pi, phosphate; ALP, alkaline phosphatase; iPTH, intact parathyroid hormone; TRP, tubular reabsorption of phosphorus; Tmp/GFR, tubular maximum phosphate reabsorption per glomerular filtration rate; RSS, rickets severity score; n.s., not significant, FGF23, fibroblast growth factor 23. The value smaller than 0.05 should be highlighted with bold font.

Zhang et al. analyzed the severity of XLH in patients harboring pathogenic variants in the first 649 amino acids (N-terminal) and those with variants located from 650 amino acids to 3′ ends (C-terminal), similar to the study of Holm et al. They found that patients with variants in the N-terminal region showed relatively more severity with any signs at an earlier age (p = 0.015) and had higher serum i-FGF23 levels (p = 0.045) [63]. In contrast, other studies did not show significant differences in any of these parameters. Lin et al. evaluated a large population and stratified them using the same method as that of Holm et al. and Zhang et al.; however, there was no significant difference in onset age and serum i-FGF23 levels [69]. Further studies with relatively larger sample sizes are needed to determine the effect of the location of pathogenic variants on the phenotype.

4.3. Truncating and Non-Truncating Variants

Nonsense, frameshift, and splicing variants result in truncating mutants which may cause more severe functional defects than those caused by non-truncating mutants due to missense variants. To assess the influence of the type of variant on the phenotype, several studies have compared the severity of phenotypes between truncating and non-truncating variants (Table 4).

Table 3. Summary of analyses on *PHEX* variant location.

Author	Year	Subject (N Terminal, C Terminal)	Analyzed Phenotype	p Value	Reference
Holm	2001	23, 6	skeletal severity	1.000	[37]
		22, 5	dental severity	0.621	
Song	2007	2, 7	onset age	n.s.	[40]
			skeletal severity	0.083	
			dental severity	n.s.	
Zhang	2019	113, 26	serum Pi	0.573	[63]
		141, 33	onset age for any signs	**0.015**	
		119, 31	age for first walking	0.478	
		104, 20	onset age for lower limb deformity	0.055	
		132, 25	height z-score	0.692	
		37, 10	RSS	0.711	
		187, 46	serum i-FGF23	0.045	
Baroncelli	2021	24 [a]	dental severity height z-score skeletal severity biochemical parameters	n.s.	[66]
Lin	2021	105, 24	onset age	0.360	[69]
			height z-score	0.759	
			serum Pi	0.286	
			serum ALP	0.077	
			serum i-FGF23	0.485	
			RSS	0.538	

[a] No subject number of subgroup (N-terminal and C-terminal) described. Pi, phosphate; ALP, alkaline phosphatase; RSS, rickets severity score; n.s., not significant; PHEX, phosphate regulating endopeptidase homolog X-linked. The value smaller than 0.05 should be highlighted with bold font.

As predicted from the mutant structure caused by pathogenic variants, Morey et al. reported that truncating variants lead to a relatively more severe phenotype in the percentage of tubular reabsorption of phosphorus (%TRP) and 1,25(OH)$_2$D levels [44]. Jiménez et al. detected the severity of height z-score in patients harboring truncating variants [68]. Nevertheless, other studies that analyzed a relatively larger number of subjects showed no significant difference in phenotypes between truncating and non-truncating variants [63,65,69,70]. Thus, the influence of variant type seems to be limited.

4.4. Preservation of Zinc-Binding Sites in Mutant PHEX

PHEX has a high amino acid sequence homology with NEP. Since NEP is a zinc-dependent metalloprotease, it has been postulated that PHEX also possesses a zinc-binding site and functions as a zinc-dependent metalloprotease [2,30,95–97]. We hypothesized that the preservation of the zinc-binding site structure is effective in improving the severity of XLH; we predicted three-dimensional structures of mutant PHEX and sub-grouped them with and without zinc-binding sites. Notably, the level of serum i-FGF23 was significantly higher in patients with variants that cause defective zinc-binding sites than that in patients with variants which preserve the three-dimensional structure of the zinc-binding site of PHEX [67]. Although a relatively larger sample size should be evaluated, these data may indicate the importance of zinc-binding sites and help clarify the function of PHEX.

Table 4. Summary of analyses on PHEX variants.

Author	Year	Subject (Truncating, Non-Truncating)	Analyzed Phenotype	p Value	Reference
Holm	2001	21, 8 20, 7	skeletal severity dental severity	0.112 1.000	[37]
Cho	2005	5, 3	biochemical parameters skeletal severity dental severity	n.s.	[39]
Song	2007	3, 6	onset age skeletal severity dental severity	n.s.	[40]
Morey	2011	28, 6 24, 6 24, 6 22, 5 16, 6 14, 6 20, 6 22, 6	onset age height z-score serum Pi % TRP 1,25(OH)$_2$D 25(OH)D serum PTH serum ALP	0.08 0.11 0.53 **0.028** **0.013** 0.30 0.06 0.48	[44]
Rafaelsen	2016	21 [a]	height z-score skeletal severity dental severity	n.s.	[55]
Zhang	2019	107, 32 143, 31 121, 29 106, 18 133, 34 42, 5 184, 49	serum Pi onset age for any signs age for first walking onset age for lower limb deformity height z-score RSS serum i-FGF23	0.674 0.641 0.235 0.312 0.379 0.724 0.777	[63]
Zheng	2020	39, 14 39, 14 38, 13 39, 14	height z-score serum Pi Tmp/GFR serum ALP	0.42 0.94 0.42 0.37	[65]
Park	2021	39, 9 [a]	onset age height z-score serum Pi serum Ca serum ALP serum 25(OH)D serum PTH %TRP Tmp/GFR urine Ca/Cr	0.561 0.793 0.672 0.750 0.916 **0.023** 0.235 0.362 0.362 0.644	[70]
Baroncelli	2021	24 [b]	dental severity height z-score skeletal severity biochemical parameters	n.s.	[66]
Jiménez	2021	17 [b]	height z-score onset age serum i-FGF23 skeletal severity	**<0.05** n.s. n.s. n.s.	[68]
Ishihara	2021	21, 4 19, 4 22, 6 22, 6 21, 6 21, 5	RSS serum i-FGF23 height z-score serum Pi serum ALP Tmp/GFR	0.53 0.60 0.29 0.25 0.49 0.35	[67]
Lin	2021	124, 29	onset age height z-score serum Pi serum ALP serum i-FGF23 RSS	0.996 0.510 0.925 0.700 0.695 0.895	[69]

[a] The detailed number of subjects with defects has not been described. [b] No subject number of subgroups (truncating and non-truncating) described. Ca, calcium; Pi, phosphate; ALP, alkaline phosphatase; PTH, parathyroid hormone; Cr, creatinine; TRP, tubular reabsorption of phosphorus; Tmp/GFR, tubular maximum phosphate reabsorption per glomerular filtration rate; RSS, rickets severity score; n.s., not significant; PHEX, phosphate-regulating endopeptidase homolog X-linked. The value smaller than 0.05 should be highlighted with bold font.

5. Conclusions

Twenty-five years have passed since the pathogenic variant of *PHEX* was determined to cause XLH. Subsequently, PHEX impairment has been found to lead to the elevation of FGF23 level, which is involved in the pathogenesis of XLH. To date, a novel treatment to inhibit excessive FGF23 levels has been developed and clinically approved. Although our understanding of the pathophysiology of XLH and the development of therapeutic strategies based on molecular pathology are remarkable, the function of PHEX itself remains unclear. Further investigations associated with the *PHEX* genotype, including functional assays and genotype–phenotype analyses are expected to provide clues to this unsolved problem and lead to further elucidation of the pathophysiology of XLH.

Author Contributions: Conceptualization, writing—original draft preparation, writing—review and editing, Y.O.; Data curation and editing, Y.I. All authors have read and agreed to the published version of the manuscript.

Funding: This research was funded by the Ministry of Health, Labor, and Welfare (grant number 21FC1010 and 22FC1012).

Institutional Review Board Statement: Not applicable.

Informed Consent Statement: Not applicable.

Conflicts of Interest: The authors declare no conflict of interest.

References

1. Read, A.P.; Thakker, R.V.; Davies, K.E.; Mountford, R.C.; Brenton, D.P.; Davies, M.; Glorieux, F.; Harris, R.; Hendy, G.N.; King, A.; et al. Mapping of human X-linked hypophosphataemic rickets by multilocus linkage analysis. *Hum. Genet.* **1986**, *73*, 267–270. [CrossRef]
2. Consortium, T.H. A gene (PEX) with homologies to endopeptidases is mutated in patients with X-linked hypophosphatemic rickets. The HYP Consortium. *Nat. Genet.* **1995**, *11*, 130–136.
3. Carpinelli, M.R.; Wicks, I.P.; Sims, N.A.; O'Donnell, K.; Hanzinikolas, K.; Burt, R.; Foote, S.J.; Bahlo, M.; Alexander, W.S.; Hilton, D.J. An ethyl-nitrosourea-induced point mutation in phex causes exon skipping, x-linked hypophosphatemia, and rickets. *Am. J. Pathol.* **2002**, *161*, 1925–1933. [CrossRef]
4. Eicher, E.M.; Southard, J.L.; Scriver, C.R.; Glorieux, F.H. Hypophosphatemia: Mouse model for human familial hypophosphatemic (vitamin D-resistant) rickets. *Proc. Natl. Acad. Sci. USA* **1976**, *73*, 4667–4671. [CrossRef]
5. Strom, T.M.; Francis, F.; Lorenz, B.; Boddrich, A.; Econs, M.J.; Lehrach, H.; Meitinger, T. Pex gene deletions in Gy and Hyp mice provide mouse models for X-linked hypophosphatemia. *Hum. Mol. Genet.* **1997**, *6*, 165–171. [CrossRef]
6. Carpenter, T.O.; Imel, E.A.; Holm, I.A.; Jan de Beur, S.M.; Insogna, K.L. A clinician's guide to X-linked hypophosphatemia. *J. Bone Miner. Res.* **2011**, *26*, 1381–1388. [CrossRef]
7. Sabbagh, Y.; Jones, A.O.; Tenenhouse, H.S. PHEXdb, a locus-specific database for mutations causing X-linked hypophosphatemia. *Hum. Mutat.* **2000**, *16*, 1–6. [CrossRef]
8. Rush, E.T.; Johnson, B.; Aradhya, S.; Beltran, D.; Bristow, S.L.; Eisenbeis, S.; Guerra, N.E.; Krolczyk, S.; Miller, N.; Morales, A.; et al. Molecular Diagnoses of X-Linked and Other Genetic Hypophosphatemias: Results From a Sponsored Genetic Testing Program. *J. Bone Miner. Res.* **2022**, *37*, 202–214. [CrossRef]
9. Sarafrazi, S.; Daugherty, S.C.; Miller, N.; Boada, P.; Carpenter, T.O.; Chunn, L.; Dill, K.; Econs, M.J.; Eisenbeis, S.; Imel, E.A.; et al. Novel PHEX gene locus-specific database: Comprehensive characterization of vast number of variants associated with X-linked hypophosphatemia (XLH). *Hum. Mutat.* **2022**, *43*, 143–157. [CrossRef]
10. Jonsson, K.B.; Zahradnik, R.; Larsson, T.; White, K.E.; Sugimoto, T.; Imanishi, Y.; Yamamoto, T.; Hampson, G.; Koshiyama, H.; Ljunggren, O.; et al. Fibroblast growth factor 23 in oncogenic osteomalacia and X-linked hypophosphatemia. *N. Engl. J. Med.* **2003**, *348*, 1656–1663. [CrossRef]
11. Shimada, T.; Mizutani, S.; Muto, T.; Yoneya, T.; Hino, R.; Takeda, S.; Takeuchi, Y.; Fujita, T.; Fukumoto, S.; Yamashita, T. Cloning and characterization of FGF23 as a causative factor of tumor-induced osteomalacia. *Proc. Natl. Acad. Sci. USA* **2001**, *98*, 6500–6505. [CrossRef]
12. Fukumoto, S.; Yamashita, T. FGF23 is a hormone-regulating phosphate metabolism–unique biological characteristics of FGF23. *Bone* **2007**, *40*, 1190–1195. [CrossRef]
13. Shimada, T.; Hasegawa, H.; Yamazaki, Y.; Muto, T.; Hino, R.; Takeuchi, Y.; Fujita, T.; Nakahara, K.; Fukumoto, S.; Yamashita, T. FGF-23 is a potent regulator of vitamin D metabolism and phosphate homeostasis. *J. Bone Miner. Res.* **2004**, *19*, 429–435. [CrossRef]
14. Lorenz-Depiereux, B.; Bastepe, M.; Benet-Pages, A.; Amyere, M.; Wagenstaller, J.; Muller-Barth, U.; Badenhoop, K.; Kaiser, S.M.; Rittmaster, R.S.; Shlossberg, A.H.; et al. DMP1 mutations in autosomal recessive hypophosphatemia implicate a bone matrix protein in the regulation of phosphate homeostasis. *Nat. Genet.* **2006**, *38*, 1248–1250. [CrossRef]

15. Feng, J.Q.; Ward, L.M.; Liu, S.; Lu, Y.; Xie, Y.; Yuan, B.; Yu, X.; Rauch, F.; Davis, S.I.; Zhang, S.; et al. Loss of DMP1 causes rickets and osteomalacia and identifies a role for osteocytes in mineral metabolism. *Nat. Genet.* **2006**, *38*, 1310–1315. [CrossRef]
16. Consortium, T.A. Autosomal dominant hypophosphataemic rickets is associated with mutations in FGF23. *Nat. Genet.* **2000**, *26*, 345–348.
17. Lorenz-Depiereux, B.; Schnabel, D.; Tiosano, D.; Hausler, G.; Strom, T.M. Loss-of-function ENPP1 mutations cause both generalized arterial calcification of infancy and autosomal-recessive hypophosphatemic rickets. *Am. J. Hum. Genet.* **2010**, *86*, 267–272. [CrossRef]
18. Levy-Litan, V.; Hershkovitz, E.; Avizov, L.; Leventhal, N.; Bercovich, D.; Chalifa-Caspi, V.; Manor, E.; Buriakovsky, S.; Hadad, Y.; Goding, J.; et al. Autosomal-recessive hypophosphatemic rickets is associated with an inactivation mutation in the ENPP1 gene. *Am. J. Hum. Genet.* **2010**, *86*, 273–278. [CrossRef]
19. Simpson, M.A.; Hsu, R.; Keir, L.S.; Hao, J.; Sivapalan, G.; Ernst, L.M.; Zackai, E.H.; Al-Gazali, L.I.; Hulskamp, G.; Kingston, H.M.; et al. Mutations in FAM20C are associated with lethal osteosclerotic bone dysplasia (Raine syndrome), highlighting a crucial molecule in bone development. *Am. J. Hum. Genet.* **2007**, *81*, 906–912. [CrossRef]
20. Rowe, P.S.; Garrett, I.R.; Schwarz, P.M.; Carnes, D.L.; Lafer, E.M.; Mundy, G.R.; Gutierrez, G.E. Surface plasmon resonance (SPR) confirms that MEPE binds to PHEX via the MEPE-ASARM motif: A model for impaired mineralization in X-linked rickets (HYP). *Bone* **2005**, *36*, 33–46. [CrossRef]
21. Martin, A.; David, V.; Laurence, J.S.; Schwarz, P.M.; Lafer, E.M.; Hedge, A.M.; Rowe, P.S. Degradation of MEPE, DMP1, and release of SIBLING ASARM-peptides (minhibins): ASARM-peptide(s) are directly responsible for defective mineralization in HYP. *Endocrinology* **2008**, *149*, 1757–1772. [CrossRef]
22. Liu, S.; Zhou, J.; Tang, W.; Jiang, X.; Rowe, D.W.; Quarles, L.D. Pathogenic role of Fgf23 in Hyp mice. *Am. J. Physiol. Endocrinol. Metab.* **2006**, *291*, E38–E49. [CrossRef]
23. Miao, D.; Bai, X.; Panda, D.; McKee, M.; Karaplis, A.; Goltzman, D. Osteomalacia in hyp mice is associated with abnormal phex expression and with altered bone matrix protein expression and deposition. *Endocrinology* **2001**, *142*, 926–939. [CrossRef]
24. Sitara, D.; Razzaque, M.S.; Hesse, M.; Yoganathan, S.; Taguchi, T.; Erben, R.G.; Juppner, H.; Lanske, B. Homozygous ablation of fibroblast growth factor-23 results in hyperphosphatemia and impaired skeletogenesis, and reverses hypophosphatemia in Phex-deficient mice. *Matrix Biol.* **2004**, *23*, 421–432. [CrossRef]
25. Beck, L.; Soumounou, Y.; Martel, J.; Krishnamurthy, G.; Gauthier, C.; Goodyer, C.G.; Tenenhouse, H.S. Pex/PEX tissue distribution and evidence for a deletion in the 3′ region of the Pex gene in X-linked hypophosphatemic mice. *J. Clin. Investig.* **1997**, *99*, 1200–1209. [CrossRef]
26. Bowe, A.E.; Finnegan, R.; Jan de Beur, S.M.; Cho, J.; Levine, M.A.; Kumar, R.; Schiavi, S.C. FGF-23 inhibits renal tubular phosphate transport and is a PHEX substrate. *Biochem. Biophys. Res. Commun.* **2001**, *284*, 977–981. [CrossRef]
27. Benet-Pages, A.; Lorenz-Depiereux, B.; Zischka, H.; White, K.E.; Econs, M.J.; Strom, T.M. FGF23 is processed by proprotein convertases but not by PHEX. *Bone* **2004**, *35*, 455–462. [CrossRef]
28. Guo, R.; Liu, S.; Spurney, R.F.; Quarles, L.D. Analysis of recombinant Phex: An endopeptidase in search of a substrate. *Am. J. Physiol. Endocrinol. Metab.* **2001**, *281*, E837–E847. [CrossRef]
29. Liu, S.; Guo, R.; Simpson, L.G.; Xiao, Z.S.; Burnham, C.E.; Quarles, L.D. Regulation of fibroblastic growth factor 23 expression but not degradation by PHEX. *J. Biol. Chem.* **2003**, *278*, 37419–37426. [CrossRef]
30. Rowe, P.S.; Oudet, C.L.; Francis, F.; Sinding, C.; Pannetier, S.; Econs, M.J.; Strom, T.M.; Meitinger, T.; Garabedian, M.; David, A.; et al. Distribution of mutations in the PEX gene in families with X-linked hypophosphataemic rickets (HYP). *Hum. Mol. Genet.* **1997**, *6*, 539–549. [CrossRef]
31. Francis, F.; Strom, T.M.; Hennig, S.; Boddrich, A.; Lorenz, B.; Brandau, O.; Mohnike, K.L.; Cagnoli, M.; Steffens, C.; Klages, S.; et al. Genomic organization of the human PEX gene mutated in X-linked dominant hypophosphatemic rickets. *Genome. Res.* **1997**, *7*, 573–585. [CrossRef] [PubMed]
32. Holm, I.A.; Huang, X.; Kunkel, L.M. Mutational analysis of the PEX gene in patients with X-linked hypophosphatemic rickets. *Am. J. Hum. Genet.* **1997**, *60*, 790–797. [PubMed]
33. Dixon, P.H.; Christie, P.T.; Wooding, C.; Trump, D.; Grieff, M.; Holm, I.; Gertner, J.M.; Schmidtke, J.; Shah, B.; Shaw, N.; et al. Mutational analysis of PHEX gene in X-linked hypophosphatemia. *J. Clin. Endocrinol. Metab.* **1998**, *83*, 3615–3623. [CrossRef]
34. Filisetti, D.; Ostermann, G.; von Bredow, M.; Strom, T.; Filler, G.; Ehrich, J.; Pannetier, S.; Garnier, J.M.; Rowe, P.; Francis, F.; et al. Non-random distribution of mutations in the PHEX gene, and under-detected missense mutations at non-conserved residues. *Eur. J. Hum. Genet.* **1999**, *7*, 615–619. [CrossRef]
35. Tyynismaa, H.; Kaitila, I.; Nanto-Salonen, K.; Ala-Houhala, M.; Alitalo, T. Identification of fifteen novel PHEX gene mutations in Finnish patients with hypophosphatemic rickets. *Hum. Mutat.* **2000**, *15*, 383–384. [CrossRef]
36. Popowska, E.; Pronicka, E.; Sulek, A.; Jurkiewicz, D.; Rowe, P.; Rowinska, E.; Krajewska-Walasek, M. X-linked hypophosphatemia in Polish patients. 1. Mutations in the PHEX gene. *J. Appl. Genet.* **2000**, *41*, 293–302.
37. Holm, I.A.; Nelson, A.E.; Robinson, B.G.; Mason, R.S.; Marsh, D.J.; Cowell, C.T.; Carpenter, T.O. Mutational analysis and genotype-phenotype correlation of the PHEX gene in X-linked hypophosphatemic rickets. *J. Clin. Endocrinol. Metab.* **2001**, *86*, 3889–3899. [CrossRef]
38. Christie, P.T.; Harding, B.; Nesbit, M.A.; Whyte, M.P.; Thakker, R.V. X-linked hypophosphatemia attributable to pseudoexons of the PHEX gene. *J. Clin. Endocrinol. Metab.* **2001**, *86*, 3840–3844. [CrossRef]

39. Cho, H.Y.; Lee, B.H.; Kang, J.H.; Ha, I.S.; Cheong, H.I.; Choi, Y. A clinical and molecular genetic study of hypophosphatemic rickets in children. *Pediatr. Res.* **2005**, *58*, 329–333. [CrossRef]
40. Song, H.R.; Park, J.W.; Cho, D.Y.; Yang, J.H.; Yoon, H.R.; Jung, S.C. PHEX gene mutations and genotype-phenotype analysis of Korean patients with hypophosphatemic rickets. *J. Korean Med. Sci.* **2007**, *22*, 981–986. [CrossRef]
41. Ichikawa, S.; Traxler, E.A.; Estwick, S.A.; Curry, L.R.; Johnson, M.L.; Sorenson, A.H.; Imel, E.A.; Econs, M.J. Mutational survey of the PHEX gene in patients with X-linked hypophosphatemic rickets. *Bone* **2008**, *43*, 663–666. [CrossRef] [PubMed]
42. Gaucher, C.; Walrant-Debray, O.; Nguyen, T.M.; Esterle, L.; Garabedian, M.; Jehan, F. PHEX analysis in 118 pedigrees reveals new genetic clues in hypophosphatemic rickets. *Hum. Genet.* **2009**, *125*, 401–411. [CrossRef] [PubMed]
43. Clausmeyer, S.; Hesse, V.; Clemens, P.C.; Engelbach, M.; Kreuzer, M.; Becker-Rose, P.; Spital, H.; Schulze, E.; Raue, F. Mutational analysis of the PHEX gene: Novel point mutations and detection of large deletions by MLPA in patients with X-linked hypophosphatemic rickets. *Calcif. Tissue Int.* **2009**, *85*, 211–220. [CrossRef] [PubMed]
44. Morey, M.; Castro-Feijoo, L.; Barreiro, J.; Cabanas, P.; Pombo, M.; Gil, M.; Bernabeu, I.; Diaz-Grande, J.M.; Rey-Cordo, L.; Ariceta, G.; et al. Genetic diagnosis of X-linked dominant Hypophosphatemic Rickets in a cohort study: Tubular reabsorption of phosphate and 1,25(OH)2D serum levels are associated with PHEX mutation type. *BMC Med. Genet.* **2011**, *12*, 116. [CrossRef]
45. Ruppe, M.D.; Brosnan, P.G.; Au, K.S.; Tran, P.X.; Dominguez, B.W.; Northrup, H. Mutational analysis of PHEX, FGF23 and DMP1 in a cohort of patients with hypophosphatemic rickets. *Clin. Endocrinol.* **2011**, *74*, 312–318. [CrossRef] [PubMed]
46. Jap, T.S.; Chiu, C.Y.; Niu, D.M.; Levine, M.A. Three novel mutations in the PHEX gene in Chinese subjects with hypophosphatemic rickets extends genotypic variability. *Calcif. Tissue Int.* **2011**, *88*, 370–377. [CrossRef]
47. Quinlan, C.; Guegan, K.; Offiah, A.; Neill, R.O.; Hiorns, M.P.; Ellard, S.; Bockenhauer, D.; Hoff, W.V.; Waters, A.M. Growth in PHEX-associated X-linked hypophosphatemic rickets: The importance of early treatment. *Pediatr. Nephrol.* **2012**, *27*, 581–588. [CrossRef]
48. Beck-Nielsen, S.S.; Brixen, K.; Gram, J.; Brusgaard, K. Mutational analysis of PHEX, FGF23, DMP1, SLC34A3 and CLCN5 in patients with hypophosphatemic rickets. *J. Hum. Genet.* **2012**, *57*, 453–458. [CrossRef]
49. Kinoshita, Y.; Saito, T.; Shimizu, Y.; Hori, M.; Taguchi, M.; Igarashi, T.; Fukumoto, S.; Fujita, T. Mutational analysis of patients with FGF23-related hypophosphatemic rickets. *Eur. J. Endocrinol.* **2012**, *167*, 165–172. [CrossRef]
50. Lee, S.H.; Agashe, M.V.; Suh, S.W.; Yoon, Y.C.; Song, S.H.; Yang, J.H.; Lee, H.; Song, H.R. Paravertebral ligament ossification in vitamin D-resistant rickets: Incidence, clinical significance, and genetic evaluation. *Spine* **2012**, *37*, E792–E796. [CrossRef]
51. Durmaz, E.; Zou, M.; Al-Rijjal, R.A.; Baitei, E.Y.; Hammami, S.; Bircan, I.; Akcurin, S.; Meyer, B.; Shi, Y. Novel and de novo PHEX mutations in patients with hypophosphatemic rickets. *Bone* **2013**, *52*, 286–291. [CrossRef] [PubMed]
52. Yue, H.; Yu, J.B.; He, J.W.; Zhang, Z.; Fu, W.Z.; Zhang, H.; Wang, C.; Hu, W.W.; Gu, J.M.; Hu, Y.Q.; et al. Identification of two novel mutations in the PHEX gene in Chinese patients with hypophosphatemic rickets/osteomalacia. *PLoS ONE* **2014**, *9*, e97830. [CrossRef] [PubMed]
53. Capelli, S.; Donghi, V.; Maruca, K.; Vezzoli, G.; Corbetta, S.; Brandi, M.L.; Mora, S.; Weber, G. Clinical and molecular heterogeneity in a large series of patients with hypophosphatemic rickets. *Bone* **2015**, *79*, 143–149. [CrossRef] [PubMed]
54. Zhang, H.; Yang, R.; Wang, Y.; Ye, J.; Han, L.; Qiu, W.; Gu, X. A pilot study of gene testing of genetic bone dysplasia using targeted next-generation sequencing. *J. Hum. Genet.* **2015**, *60*, 769–776. [CrossRef] [PubMed]
55. Rafaelsen, S.; Johansson, S.; Raeder, H.; Bjerknes, R. Hereditary hypophosphatemia in Norway: A retrospective population-based study of genotypes, phenotypes, and treatment complications. *Eur. J. Endocrinol.* **2016**, *174*, 125–136. [CrossRef]
56. Li, S.S.; Gu, J.M.; Yu, W.J.; He, J.W.; Fu, W.Z.; Zhang, Z.L. Seven novel and six de novo PHEX gene mutations in patients with hypophosphatemic rickets. *Int. J. Mol. Med.* **2016**, *38*, 1703–1714. [CrossRef]
57. Guven, A.; Al-Rijjal, R.A.; BinEssa, H.A.; Dogan, D.; Kor, Y.; Zou, M.; Kaya, N.; Alenezi, A.F.; Hancili, S.; Tarim, O.; et al. Mutational analysis of PHEX, FGF23 and CLCN5 in patients with hypophosphataemic rickets. *Clin. Endocrinol.* **2017**, *87*, 103–112. [CrossRef]
58. Acar, S.; BinEssa, H.A.; Demir, K.; Al-Rijjal, R.A.; Zou, M.; Catli, G.; Anik, A.; Al-Enezi, A.F.; Ozisik, S.; Al-Faham, M.S.A.; et al. Clinical and genetic characteristics of 15 families with hereditary hypophosphatemia: Novel Mutations in PHEX and SLC34A3. *PLoS ONE* **2018**, *13*, e0193388. [CrossRef]
59. Chesher, D.; Oddy, M.; Darbar, U.; Sayal, P.; Casey, A.; Ryan, A.; Sechi, A.; Simister, C.; Waters, A.; Wedatilake, Y.; et al. Outcome of adult patients with X-linked hypophosphatemia caused by PHEX gene mutations. *J. Inherit. Metab. Dis.* **2018**, *41*, 865–876. [CrossRef]
60. Gu, J.; Wang, C.; Zhang, H.; Yue, H.; Hu, W.; He, J.; Fu, W.; Zhang, Z. Targeted resequencing of phosphorus metabolismrelated genes in 86 patients with hypophosphatemic rickets/osteomalacia. *Int. J. Mol. Med.* **2018**, *42*, 1603–1614.
61. Marik, B.; Bagga, A.; Sinha, A.; Hari, P.; Sharma, A. Genetics of Refractory Rickets: Identification of Novel PHEX Mutations in Indian Patients and a Literature Update. *J. Pediatr. Genet.* **2018**, *7*, 47–59. [CrossRef]
62. Hernandez-Frias, O.; Gil-Pena, H.; Perez-Roldan, J.M.; Gonzalez-Sanchez, S.; Ariceta, G.; Chocron, S.; Loza, R.; de la Cerda Ojeda, F.; Madariaga, L.; Vergara, I.; et al. Risk of cardiovascular involvement in pediatric patients with X-linked hypophosphatemia. *Pediatr. Nephrol.* **2019**, *34*, 1077–1086. [CrossRef] [PubMed]
63. Zhang, C.; Zhao, Z.; Sun, Y.; Xu, L.; JiaJue, R.; Cui, L.; Pang, Q.; Jiang, Y.; Li, M.; Wang, O.; et al. Clinical and genetic analysis in a large Chinese cohort of patients with X-linked hypophosphatemia. *Bone* **2019**, *121*, 212–220. [CrossRef] [PubMed]

64. Lin, Y.; Xu, J.; Li, X.; Sheng, H.; Su, L.; Wu, M.; Cheng, J.; Huang, Y.; Mao, X.; Zhou, Z.; et al. Novel variants and uncommon cases among southern Chinese children with X-linked hypophosphatemia. *J. Endocrinol. Investig.* **2020**, *43*, 1577–1590. [CrossRef] [PubMed]
65. Zheng, B.; Wang, C.; Chen, Q.; Che, R.; Sha, Y.; Zhao, F.; Ding, G.; Zhou, W.; Jia, Z.; Huang, S.; et al. Functional Characterization of PHEX Gene Variants in Children With X-Linked Hypophosphatemic Rickets Shows No Evidence of Genotype-Phenotype Correlation. *J. Bone Miner. Res.* **2020**, *35*, 1718–1725. [CrossRef] [PubMed]
66. Baroncelli, G.I.; Zampollo, E.; Manca, M.; Toschi, B.; Bertelloni, S.; Michelucci, A.; Isola, A.; Bulleri, A.; Peroni, D.; Giuca, M.R. Pulp chamber features, prevalence of abscesses, disease severity, and PHEX mutation in X-linked hypophosphatemic rickets. *J. Bone Miner. Metab.* **2021**, *39*, 212–223. [CrossRef]
67. Ishihara, Y.; Ohata, Y.; Takeyari, S.; Kitaoka, T.; Fujiwara, M.; Nakano, Y.; Yamamoto, K.; Yamada, C.; Yamamoto, K.; Michigami, T.; et al. Genotype-phenotype analysis, and assessment of the importance of the zinc-binding site in PHEX in Japanese patients with X-linked hypophosphatemic rickets using 3D structure modeling. *Bone* **2021**, *153*, 116135. [CrossRef]
68. Jimenez, M.; Ivanovic-Zuvic, D.; Loureiro, C.; Carvajal, C.A.; Cavada, G.; Schneider, P.; Gallardo, E.; Garcia, C.; Gonzalez, G.; Contreras, O.; et al. Clinical and molecular characterization of Chilean patients with X-linked hypophosphatemia. *Osteoporos. Int.* **2021**, *32*, 1825–1836. [CrossRef]
69. Lin, X.; Li, S.; Zhang, Z.; Yue, H. Clinical and Genetic Characteristics of 153 Chinese Patients With X-Linked Hypophosphatemia. *Front. Cell Dev. Biol.* **2021**, *9*, 617738. [CrossRef]
70. Park, P.G.; Lim, S.H.; Lee, H.; Ahn, Y.H.; Cheong, H.I.; Kang, H.G. Genotype and Phenotype Analysis in X-Linked Hypophosphatemia. *Front Pediatr.* **2021**, *9*, 699767. [CrossRef]
71. Rodriguez-Rubio, E.; Gil-Pena, H.; Chocron, S.; Madariaga, L.; de la Cerda-Ojeda, F.; Fernandez-Fernandez, M.; de Lucas-Collantes, C.; Gil, M.; Luis-Yanes, M.I.; Vergara, I.; et al. Correction to: Phenotypic characterization of X-linked hypophosphatemia in pediatric Spanish population. *Orphanet J Rare. Dis.* **2021**, *16*, 154. [CrossRef]
72. Jacobsen, C.; Shen, Y.; Holm, I. *Approaches to Genetic Testing*, 9th ed.; Bilezikian, J.P., American Society for Bone and Mineral Research, Eds.; Wiley Blackwell: New York, NY, USA, 2019.
73. Ma, S.L.; Vega-Warner, V.; Gillies, C.; Sampson, M.G.; Kher, V.; Sethi, S.K.; Otto, E.A. Whole Exome Sequencing Reveals Novel PHEX Splice Site Mutations in Patients with Hypophosphatemic Rickets. *PLoS ONE* **2015**, *10*, e0130729. [CrossRef]
74. Li, B.; Wang, X.; Hao, X.; Liu, Y.; Wang, Y.; Shan, C.; Ao, X.; Liu, Y.; Bao, H.; Li, P. A novel c.2179T>C mutation blocked the intracellular transport of PHEX protein and caused X-linked hypophosphatemic rickets in a Chinese family. *Mol. Genet. Genom. Med.* **2020**, *8*, e1262. [CrossRef] [PubMed]
75. Lin, Y.; Cai, Y.; Xu, J.; Zeng, C.; Sheng, H.; Yu, Y.; Li, X.; Liu, L. 'Isolated' germline mosaicism in the phenotypically normal father of a girl with X-linked hypophosphatemic rickets. *Eur. J. Endocrinol.* **2020**, *182*, K1–K6. [CrossRef]
76. Weng, C.; Chen, J.; Sun, L.; Zhou, Z.W.; Feng, X.; Sun, J.H.; Lu, L.P.; Yu, P.; Qi, M. A de novo mosaic mutation of PHEX in a boy with hypophosphatemic rickets. *J. Hum. Genet.* **2016**, *61*, 223–227. [CrossRef]
77. Goji, K.; Ozaki, K.; Sadewa, A.H.; Nishio, H.; Matsuo, M. Somatic and germline mosaicism for a mutation of the PHEX gene can lead to genetic transmission of X-linked hypophosphatemic rickets that mimics an autosomal dominant trait. *J. Clin. Endocrinol. Metab.* **2006**, *91*, 365–370. [CrossRef] [PubMed]
78. BinEssa, H.A.; Zou, M.; Al-Enezi, A.F.; Alomrani, B.; Al-Faham, M.S.A.; Al-Rijjal, R.A.; Meyer, B.F.; Shi, Y. Functional analysis of 22 splice-site mutations in the PHEX, the causative gene in X-linked dominant hypophosphatemic rickets. *Bone* **2019**, *125*, 186–193. [CrossRef]
79. Zou, M.; Bulus, D.; Al-Rijjal, R.A.; Andiran, N.; BinEssa, H.; Kattan, W.E.; Meyer, B.; Shi, Y. Hypophosphatemic rickets caused by a novel splice donor site mutation and activation of two cryptic splice donor sites in the PHEX gene. *J. Pediatr. Endocrinol. Metab.* **2015**, *28*, 211–216. [CrossRef] [PubMed]
80. Frischmeyer, P.A.; Dietz, H.C. Nonsense-mediated mRNA decay in health and disease. *Hum. Mol. Genet.* **1999**, *8*, 1893–1900. [CrossRef] [PubMed]
81. Mort, M.; Ivanov, D.; Cooper, D.N.; Chuzhanova, N.A. A meta-analysis of nonsense mutations causing human genetic disease. *Hum. Mutat.* **2008**, *29*, 1037–1047. [CrossRef] [PubMed]
82. Kurosaki, T.; Popp, M.W.; Maquat, L.E. Quality and quantity control of gene expression by nonsense-mediated mRNA decay. *Nat. Rev. Mol. Cell Biol.* **2019**, *20*, 406–420. [CrossRef] [PubMed]
83. Chang, Y.F.; Imam, J.S.; Wilkinson, M.F. The nonsense-mediated decay RNA surveillance pathway. *Annu. Rev. Biochem.* **2007**, *76*, 51–74. [CrossRef] [PubMed]
84. Li, W.; Tan, L.; Li, X.; Zhang, X.; Wu, X.; Chen, H.; Hu, L.; Wang, X.; Luo, X.; Wang, F.; et al. Identification of a p.Trp403* nonsense variant in PHEX causing X-linked hypophosphatemia by inhibiting p38 MAPK signaling. *Hum. Mutat.* **2019**, *40*, 879–885. [CrossRef]
85. Mumm, S.; Huskey, M.; Cajic, A.; Wollberg, V.; Zhang, F.; Madson, K.L.; Wenkert, D.; McAlister, W.H.; Gottesman, G.S.; Whyte, M.P. PHEX 3'-UTR c.*231A>G near the polyadenylation signal is a relatively common, mild, American mutation that masquerades as sporadic or X-linked recessive hypophosphatemic rickets. *J. Bone Miner. Res.* **2015**, *30*, 137–143. [CrossRef]
86. Smith, P.S.; Gottesman, G.S.; Zhang, F.; Cook, F.; Ramirez, B.; Wenkert, D.; Wollberg, V.; Huskey, M.; Mumm, S.; Whyte, M.P. X-Linked Hypophosphatemia: Uniquely Mild Disease Associated With PHEX 3'-UTR Mutation c.*231A>G (A Retrospective Case-Control Study). *J. Bone Miner. Res.* **2020**, *35*, 920–931. [CrossRef]

87. Mumm, S.; Huskey, M.; Duan, S.; Wollberg, V.; Bijanki, V.; Gottesman, G.S.; Whyte, M.P.; Smith, P. (Eds.) X-Linked Hypophosphatemia: All Eight Individuals Representing Separate American Families Carrying the PHEX 3'UTR Mutation c.* 231A> G Tested Positive for an Exon 13-15 Duplication. In *Journal of Bone and Mineral Research*; Wiley: Hoboken, NJ, USA, 2019.
88. Sabbagh, Y.; Boileau, G.; DesGroseillers, L.; Tenenhouse, H.S. Disease-causing missense mutations in the PHEX gene interfere with membrane targeting of the recombinant protein. *Hum. Mol. Genet.* **2001**, *10*, 1539–1546. [CrossRef]
89. Lipman, M.L.; Panda, D.; Bennett, H.P.; Henderson, J.E.; Shane, E.; Shen, Y.; Goltzman, D.; Karaplis, A.C. Cloning of human PEX cDNA. Expression, subcellular localization, and endopeptidase activity. *J. Biol. Chem.* **1998**, *273*, 13729–13737. [CrossRef] [PubMed]
90. Richards, S.; Aziz, N.; Bale, S.; Bick, D.; Das, S.; Gastier-Foster, J.; Grody, W.W.; Hegde, M.; Lyon, E.; Spector, E.; et al. Standards and guidelines for the interpretation of sequence variants: A joint consensus recommendation of the American College of Medical Genetics and Genomics and the Association for Molecular Pathology. *Genet. Med.* **2015**, *17*, 405–424. [CrossRef]
91. Nykamp, K.; Anderson, M.; Powers, M.; Garcia, J.; Herrera, B.; Ho, Y.Y.; Kobayashi, Y.; Patil, N.; Thusberg, J.; Westbrook, M.; et al. Sherloc: A comprehensive refinement of the ACMG-AMP variant classification criteria. *Genet. Med.* **2017**, *19*, 1105–1117. [CrossRef] [PubMed]
92. Greenblatt, M.B.; Shim, J.H.; Glimcher, L.H. Mitogen-activated protein kinase pathways in osteoblasts. *Annu. Rev. Cell Dev. Biol.* **2013**, *29*, 63–79. [CrossRef] [PubMed]
93. Hardy, D.C.; Murphy, W.A.; Siegel, B.A.; Reid, I.R.; Whyte, M.P. X-linked hypophosphatemia in adults: Prevalence of skeletal radiographic and scintigraphic features. *Radiology* **1989**, *171*, 403–414. [CrossRef]
94. Whyte, M.P.; Schranck, F.W.; Armamento-Villareal, R. X-linked hypophosphatemia: A search for gender, race, anticipation, or parent of origin effects on disease expression in children. *J. Clin. Endocrinol. Metab.* **1996**, *81*, 4075–4080.
95. Bianchetti, L.; Oudet, C.; Poch, O. M13 endopeptidases: New conserved motifs correlated with structure, and simultaneous phylogenetic occurrence of PHEX and the bony fish. *Proteins* **2002**, *47*, 481–488. [CrossRef]
96. Turner, A.J.; Isaac, R.E.; Coates, D. The neprilysin (NEP) family of zinc metalloendopeptidases: Genomics and function. *Bioessays* **2001**, *23*, 261–269. [CrossRef]
97. Schiering, N.; D'Arcy, A.; Villard, F.; Ramage, P.; Logel, C.; Cumin, F.; Ksander, G.M.; Wiesmann, C.; Karki, R.G.; Mogi, M. Structure of neprilysin in complex with the active metabolite of sacubitril. *Sci. Rep.* **2016**, *6*, 27909. [CrossRef]

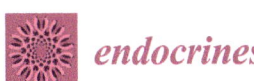

Communication

Presentation and Diagnosis of Pediatric X-Linked Hypophosphatemia

Kento Ikegawa [1,2,*] and Yukihiro Hasegawa [1]

1. Division of Endocrinology and Metabolism, Tokyo Metropolitan Children's Medical Center, Fuchu 183-8561, Japan
2. Clinical Research Support Center, Tokyo Metropolitan Children's Medical Center, Fuchu 183-8561, Japan
* Correspondence: ikegawakento721@gmail.com; Tel.: +81-42-300-5111

Abstract: X-linked hypophosphatemia (XLH) is a rare type of hereditary hypophosphatemic rickets. Patients with XLH have various symptoms that lower their QOL as defined by HAQ, RAPID3, SF36-PCS, and SF36-MCS in adult patients and SF-10 and PDCOI in pediatric patients. Early diagnosis and treatment are needed to reduce the burden, but the condition is often diagnosed late in childhood. The present review aims to summarize the symptoms, radiological and biological characteristics, and long-term prognosis of pediatric XLH. Typical symptoms of XLH are lower leg deformities (age six months or later), growth impairment (first year of life or later), and delayed gross motor development with progressive lower limb deformities (second year of life or later). Other symptoms include dental abscess, bone pain, hearing impairment, and Chiari type 1 malformation. Critical, radiological findings of rickets are metaphyseal widening, cupping, and fraying, which tend to occur in the load-bearing bones. The Rickets Severity Score, validated for XLH, is useful for assessing the severity of rickets. The biochemical features of XLH include elevated FGF23, hypophosphatemia, low 1,25(OH)2D, and elevated urine phosphate. Renal phosphate wasting can be assessed using the tubular maximum reabsorption of phosphate per glomerular filtration rate (TmP/GFR), which yields low values in patients with XLH. XLH should be diagnosed early because the multisystem symptoms often worsen over time. The present review aims to help physicians diagnose XLH at an early stage.

Keywords: X-linked hypophosphatemia; PHEX; QOL; lower leg deformities; growth impairment; TmP/GFR; FGF23; Rickets Severity Score

1. Introduction

X-linked hypophosphatemia (XLH) is a rare form of renal phosphate wasting and the most common type of hereditary hypophosphatemic rickets [1,2]. Its prevalence is estimated to be 1.7 per 100,000 in Norway and 5.0 per 100,000 in Japan [3,4]. These numbers are similar to those in North America, suggesting that there is little racial difference in the prevalence of this disease [4,5]. XLH is caused by a variant of the phosphate-regulating endopeptidase homolog X-linked (*PHEX*) gene, which regulates the expression of fibroblast growth factor 23 (FGF23) [6]. However, it remains unclear how *PHEX* mutations cause FGF23 elevation [2], which leads to phosphate wasting from the proximal tubule and decreased intestinal phosphate absorption owing to reduced 1,25-hydroxyvitamin D [1,25(OH)2D] [7]. The low phosphate level gives rise to various symptoms, such as short stature, wrist enlargement, bowed legs, frontal bossing, and dental abscess [8].

The conventional therapy of oral vitamin D and phosphate is normally used to treat short stature, one of the most common symptoms of hereditary XLH [9]. The mean final/adult height in Danish patients with XLH, more than 70% of whom did not receive the conventional treatment continuously, was 166.4 cm for males and 156.4 cm for females while that of the general population was 179.0 cm for males and 166.6 cm for females, indicating that patients with XLH can have a final height 10 cm lower than that of the general population [10]. Another study reported that the standard deviation score (SDS) of final height in patients with XLH receiving oral vitamin D and phosphate was −2.8 [11]. Yet another study demonstrated that the SDS of height in patients receiving the conventional treatment was −2.38 ± 0.88 at diagnosis and −1.69 ± 1.11 at the final/adult height [12].

As with short stature, reduced quality of life (QOL) is a major problem for patients with XLH. Several reports demonstrated that adults with XLH had a lower QOL than the general population [13,14]. A previous study reported that 55.8%, 76.9%, 50%, and 50% of adult patients with XLH had a low QOL on the Health Assessment Questionnaire (HAQ), Routine Assessment of Patient Index 3 (RAPID3), Short Form 36-Physical Component Score (SF36-PCS), and Short Form 36-Mental Component Score (SF36-MCS), respectively [14]. Dental defects and enthesopathies were associated with poor QOL on HAQ and RAPID3 [14]. Treatment with oral vitamin D and phosphate improved the SF36-MCS score [14].

Low QOL was also reported in children with the disease [15]. Health-related QOL as defined by the SF-10 Physical Health Summary score in children with XLH was nearly 1.5 SDs below the score of 50 reported for the general population in the US [15]. Similarly, Pediatrics Outcomes Data Collection Instrument (PODCI) scores for the transfers/basic mobility, sports/physical function, and pain/comfort domains in children with XLH were 1 to 2 SDs below those of the general population in the US [15].

Early diagnosis and treatment with oral vitamin D and phosphate are needed to reduce the burden on patients with XLH. Early diagnosis is necessary to enable early treatment, which can improve the final height, biochemical parameters, radiographic outcome, and dental health of patients [16–18]. A previous study reported that the median (interquartile range) z-score for height after treatment was higher in patients who began treatment before one year old than in those who began treatment later (−0.7 [−1.5, 0.3], −2.0 [−2.3, −1.0], p = 0.009) [19]. Another study divided 17 patients with XLH into two groups based on their age at treatment onset (group 1: <1.0 years old; group 2: >1.0 years old) and demonstrated that the radiographic score at treatment onset, at the end of the first treatment year, and at prepuberty was higher in group 2 [17]. Another study demonstrated that the mean number of teeth in adulthood was higher in patients treated continuously during childhood than those treated after the age of five years [18]. To the best of our knowledge, there are no reports of early treatment improving future QOL in patients with XLH, but this outcome is likely, considering that dental complications, which negatively affect QOL, can be improved by early treatment [14].

Burosumab, an anti-FGF23 antibody recently introduced as a treatment for XLH [20], was shown to improve patient-reported outcomes in children with XLH, which were assessed using the Brief Pain Inventory (BPI) Worst Pain Score and the full Western Ontario and McMaster Universities Osteoarthritis Index (WOMAC) score [20]. However, its efficacy, like that of the other treatments, may depends on early initiation [21].

XLH is diagnosed in childhood on the basis of a family history, symptoms, radiological findings, laboratory findings, and genetic analysis. A previous study reported that XLH is readily diagnosed in most patients with a family history of the disease [17]. Similarly, the condition may be readily diagnosed in the presence of severe symptoms, even without a family history. In contrast, the disease is more challenging to diagnose in patients with no family history and only mild symptoms. A survey of experts in Italy demonstrated that 16% of patients with XLH received their diagnosis at the age of 12 years or older [9]. Another study reported that the mean age at diagnosis in children with XLH stemming from a de novo *PHEX* mutation was 3.9 ± 3.1 years (range: 0.9–13.1 years) [22]. Diagnosis may be further delayed in developing countries where vitamin D deficiency is common [7].

To diagnose XLH early, it is important that pediatricians and orthopedic surgeons be familiar with the characteristics of this disease. While several recent reviews have summarized the clinical characteristics of XLH [1,6,7,22–24], only a few reports have discussed the frequency and timing of the symptoms. The present review aims to summarize the symptoms of pediatric XLH by focusing on their frequency, timing, and related radiological and biological findings.

2. Clinical Features

Patients with XLH have a variety of symptoms associated with low serum phosphate. The clinician should be aware of the typical age at the onset of each symptom and its frequency. Table 1 summarizes the timing of XLH symptoms.

Table 1. Clinical features for diagnosing XLH presented in recent reviews.

Age	Clinical Features	Haffner, 2019 [23]	Lambert, 2019 [24]	Rothenbuhler, 2020 [22]	Juraibah, 2021 [7]	Laurent, 2021 [1]	Baroncelli, 2021 [6]
From age 6 months to 1 year	Lower leg deformities	O	O ‡	O ‡	O ‡	O ‡	O ‡
	Craniosynostosis	O	O ‡	O ‡	O ‡	O ‡	O
	Growth impairment †	O ‡	O ‡	O ‡	O ‡	O ¶	O ‡
From age 1 year to 2 years	Waddling gait	O	O ‡	O ‡	O ‡	O ‡	O ‡
	Progressive lower limb deformities	O	O §	ND	ND	ND	O ‡
	Delayed gross motor development	O	O ‡	O ‡	O ‡	ND	O ‡
	Delayed standing	ND	ND	O ‡	ND	ND	ND
	Delayed walking	O	O ‡	O ‡	ND	ND	O ‡
	Torsional components	O	ND	ND	O ‡	ND	ND
	Widening of the distal metaphysis at the wrists and ankles	O	O ‡	O ‡	O ‡	ND	O ‡
Age 3 years or older	Dental abscess	O	O ‡	O ‡	O ‡	O ‡	O ‡
	Dental malposition	ND	ND	ND	ND	ND	O ‡
Older children	Bone pain	O	O ‡	O ‡	O ‡	O	O ‡
	Hearing loss	O	O ‡	O ‡	O ‡	O ‡	O

Abbreviations: XLH, X-linked hypophosphatemia; ND, not described. † Also appears at later ages. ‡ No mention of when they appeared. § Varus deformity develops in younger children, and valgus deformity develops in children approaching puberty. ¶ Growth impairment becomes evident from 9 to 12 months of age.

Lower leg deformities begin to materialize as early as six months of age [23]. However, many parents of patients become aware of the symptoms as these deteriorate when the patient begins walking [23]. A previous study reported that most patients (94.8%) had leg deformities, which were severe, moderate, and mild in 28%, 47%, and 25% of the cohort, respectively [9]. Delayed tooth emergence and premature craniosynostosis may begin at this age or a little later [6]. The latter symptom, which was found to occur in 60% of children with XLH, is usually caused by abnormal fusion of the sagittal suture and results in a dolichocehalic head conformation [23,25]. Because both these symptoms also occur in other diseases, diagnosing XLH on the basis of these symptoms alone is challenging, and careful monitoring and testing are necessary in children who have them.

Growth impairment is another major symptom of pediatric XLH. Children with XLH are of average height at birth and begin to exhibit growth impairment during the first year of life [17,26]. A survey of 175 Italian patients found stature lower than −2 SD in 67% of patients with XLH [9]. One study reported that growth of the legs was uncoupled from that of the trunk, with the leg length SDS decreasing progressively during childhood and adolescence while sitting height SDS increased during late childhood [27].

Delayed gross motor development, waddling gait, and progressive lower limb deformities become apparent during the second year of life [6,23]. Blood tests and X-rays should be performed if patients present with any of these symptoms. In addition to delayed gross motor development, such as delayed standing or walking, XLH patients have weaker muscle strength than controls [28]. One researcher mechanographically compared the muscle force of thirty XLH patients to that of age- and gender-matched controls and found that muscle strength was significantly weaker in the former [28]. Torsional components and distal metaphyseal widening in the wrists and ankles were also documented at a similar age [23].

Dental abscesses, especially in the canine teeth, are highly prevalent in patients aged >3 years [23,29]. Approximately one third of patients with XLH have at least one dental abscess [9]. Poor mineralization leading to dentin defects is one of the causes of these abscesses [6]. Other dental symptoms, such as dental malposition, are also observed [9].

Bone pain, which becomes more prevalent with age, is also a common symptom [1,9]. Data from pediatric hospitals in Italy demonstrated that two thirds of patients with XLH experienced bone pain [9]. A study in East Asia demonstrated the frequency of patients with XLH with bone pain to be 5/14 (35.7%) among children and 19/32 (59.4%) among adults [30].

Bone pain in young adults is classified into spontaneous fracture-related and osteomalacia-related types [2,23]. Fractures occur in the femur or tibia and usually present as localized pain [2]. Osteomalacia-related bone pain, the mechanism of which is unknown, should be considered if fractures are absent [1,2]. Oral vitamin D and phosphate therapy improve the bone pain but are insufficient for a cure [2]. Many pediatric and young adult patients with XLH receiving conventional treatment experience bone pain, which negatively affects their QOL [14,30]. The survey in East Asia cited above demonstrated that patients with XLH had a physical component summary score of 41.2 on their 36-item Short Form health survey version 2 (SF-36v2), which was lower than the normal score of 50 [30].

Other symptoms of XLH include hearing impairment and Chiari type 1 malformation, which occurred in five and 25% of cases, respectively, in previous studies [9,31]. Most patients with Chiari type 1 malformation are asymptomatic, but central apnea and lower cranial nerve dysfunction may be present [23]. Although hearing loss is infrequent, it becomes more evident with age and therefore, hearing tests are recommended for children aged eight years or older if symptoms of hearing difficulty begin to appear [23].

A previous study described the long-term consequences of this disorder when no treatment was administered. A study of the natural history of 22 adults with XLH demonstrated that 8, 17, and 19 had bone pain, genu varum, and significant dental problems, respectively [10], indicating that patients without treatment were more likely to experience these symptoms.

3. Radiological Findings

Patients with XLH have hypophosphatemia, which in children impairs bone and growth plate mineralization or causes rickets. Critical radiological findings of rickets include metaphyseal widening, cupping, and fraying [1,7], which tend to occur in the load-bearing bones, such as the femur and tibia [32]. Radiography of the left hand, lower femur, and upper tibia is an easy, non-invasive method of detecting these findings [32,33]. Metaphyseal enlargement in these bones can be detectable on the medial side [33]. Another radiological finding of rickets is long bone deformities, such as genu varum or genu valgum [32]. Bone-within-a-bone, which is caused by differences in bone growth and the periosteal reaction and indicates new bone formation in response to abnormal stimulation, is also a crucial radiological finding of rickets [32], although it is also observed in other disorders.

X-rays are also useful for assessing the severity of rickets. The Rickets Severity Score (RSS) is based on the degree of metaphyseal fraying and concavity and the proportion of affected growth plates in the wrists, knees, and ankles [1,33]. The RSS is a ten-point scale, with a score of ten indicating the highest severity, as described in Table 2 [34]. The RSS, which has been validated for XLH [35], correlates with the serum ALP value [34,35]. In recent years, the Radiographic Global Impression of Change (RGI-C) score, a seven-point, subjective scale assessing changes between X-ray findings at two time points, has come to be used when evaluating the severity of rickets [35]. The RGI-C score correlates with the serum phosphate, serum ALP, RSS, and comfort/pain functioning values and is considered a reliable, valid, and sensitive tool for assessing pediatric XLH [36].

Table 2. Rickets Severity Score [a] [34].

Evaluation Site	Grade or Multiplier	Radiographic Features
Radius and ulna [b]	Grade	
	0	Normal
	1	Widened growth plate, irregularity of metaphyseal margins, no concave cupping
	2	Metaphyseal concavity with fraying of margins
Femur and tibia [b]	Grade	
	0	Normal
	1	Partial lucency, smooth metaphyseal margin visible
	2	Partial lucency, smooth metaphyseal margin not visible
	3	Complete lucency, epiphysis appears widely separated from distal metaphysis
	Multiplier	
	0.5	≤1 condyle or plateau
	1	2 condyles or plateaus

[a] Rickets Severity Score = grade of radius + grade of ulna + grade of femur × Multiplier + grade of tibia × Multiplier, [b] Scored separately.

The radiological findings of osteomalacia in older children include insufficiency fractures, a coarse trabecular pattern, and Loozer zones. The latter, also known as Milkman lines or pseudofractures, are radiolucent lines composed of non-mineralized osteoid [32,37]. These findings occur in high-stress areas, such as the femoral neck and tibial shaft [32,37].

4. Biochemical Findings

The biochemical features of XLH include elevated FGF23, hypophosphatemia, low 1,25(OH)2D, and elevated urine phosphate [6] (Table 3). If XLH is suspected on the basis of a family history, clinical symptoms, or radiological findings, the patients should receive blood and urine tests.

Table 3. Summary of test findings for diagnosing XLH.

Radiologic Findings	Biochemical Findings	Genetic Findings
Widening of the metaphysis	*Blood test*	*Sanger sequencing*
Cupping of the metaphysis	Decreased P	MLPA
Fraying of the metaphysis	Increased ALP	*Next-generation sequencing*
Enlarged metaphysis	Normal or increased PTH	Deletion
Long bone deformities	Low or normal 1,25(OH)$_2$D	Missense variant
Bone-within-a-bone	Increased FGF23	Nonsense variant
	Urine test	Splicing variant
	Low TmP/GFR	Frameshift variant

Abbreviations: XLH, X-linked hypophosphatemia; P, phosphate; ALP, alkaline phosphatase; PTH, parathyroid hormone; 1,25(OH)$_2$D, 1,25-hydroxyvitamin D; FGF23, fibroblast growth factor 23; TmP/GFR, tubular maximum reabsorption of phosphate per glomerular filtration rate; MLPA, multiple ligation-dependent probe amplification.

The simplest screening test for XLH involves assessing for a decreased serum phosphate concentration, increased alkaline phosphatase (ALP), normal or slightly elevated parathyroid hormone (PTH), and low or normal 1,25(OH)2D in blood [6,23]. However, there are several pitfalls. First, the serum phosphate level might be normal in the first three to four months of life [23,38]. Frequent breastfeeding may compensate for renal phosphate wasting, and several months are usually required for the phosphate level to fall below the lower limit of the age-appropriate reference value [7]. Second, the normal range of serum phosphate and ALP differ by age group. The Pathology Harmony Group (UK) demonstrated that the serum phosphate reference interval in neonates and adolescents was 1.3–2.6 mmol/L (4.0–8.1 mg/dL) and 0.9–1.8 mmol/L (2.8–5.6 mg/dL), respectively, suggesting that serum phosphate decreases with age [39]. Similarly, serum ALP is high in early childhood and adolescence, when bone formation is at its height [40].

Tubular maximum reabsorption of phosphate per glomerular filtration rate (TmP/GFR), a marker of renal phosphate wasting, was found in one study to be lower in patients with XLH than in control subjects [23]; the same was found to be the case in patients with secondary hyperparathyroidism, such as nutritional vitamin D deficiency or vitamin D-dependent rickets [7]. The serum PTH level is helpful in differentiating XLH from other conditions; for instance, it is normal or mildly elevated in XLH and high in secondary hyperparathyroidism [7]. Moreover, in patients with rickets caused by impaired dietary phosphate absorption, TmP/GFR is normal or high [7]. As with serum phosphate and ALP, the normal TmP/GFR value varies by age. Previous reports demonstrated that the mean TmP/GFR level was highest at the age of 0–6 months at approximately 1.5–1.6 μmol/mL (4.6–5.0 mg/dL) and decreased to 0.9–1.0 μmol/mL (2.8–3.1 mg/dL) by adulthood [41,42].

Last but not least, serum FGF23 is helpful in the differential diagnosis of XLH [43,44]. For example, FGF23 is a useful marker for distinguishing patients with XLH from those with vitamin D deficiency rickets [43]. However, these two conditions sometimes demonstrate similar 25-hydroxyvitamin D (25[OH]D) and PTH values. Chemiluminescent enzyme immunoassays for FGF23 are available in some developed countries [44,45].

5. Genetic Findings

Genetic testing is useful for diagnosing XLH and is often employed when clinical features, radiological findings, and biological features are insufficient for diagnosis. Furthermore, genetic testing can differentiate XLH from other forms of hypophosphatemic rickets, such as autosomal recessive hypophosphatemic rickets (ARHR). Patients with ARHR with loss-of-function mutations in *ENPP1* [46] have widespread arterial calcification in early life or symptoms associated with hypophosphatemic rickets in later life [47]. Since the clinical course and inheritance pattern of ARHR differ from those of XLH, it is important to differentiate between these two conditions.

The genetic tests most often performed are Sanger sequencing, multiple ligation-dependent probe amplification (MLPA), and next-generation sequencing [48–51]. Approximately 80–90% of clinically diagnosed XLH cases involve a *PHEX* variant [1,52,53]. Although some studies have reported a genotype–phenotype correlation in XLH [54,55], other reports have not reported this correlation [1,56]. While genetic testing is useful, it should be performed in a facility that can also provide genetic counseling.

6. Treatment

A brief summary of treatments for rickets in XLH is in order. The classical therapy for XLH is oral vitamin D and phosphate. This therapy improves short stature and QOL [11,12,14], as described in the Introduction. However, it is difficult completely to normalize the serum ALP value, Tmp/GFR, and RSS [2,57], and the treatment cannot resolve dental complications or improve the patient's QOL [57,58].

Another treatment for short stature is growth hormone (GH), which improves the height SDS of patients with XLH [11,59,60]. A previous study reported that the height SDS in patients with XLH increased from −3.5 SD to −2.4 SD after three years of GH administration [16]. Baroncelli et al. demonstrated that the final height SDS in patients with XLH receiving GH and classical therapy improved from −3.4 SD to −2.1 SD, while patients receiving conventional therapy alone failed to demonstrate an increase [11].

Burosumab, an anti-FGF23 antibody recently introduced as a treatment for XLH [20], improves biochemical markers, such as serum phosphorus, TmP/GFR, and 1, 25(OH)2D; osteoid volume/bone volume as assessed by transiliac bone biopsies; fracture healing; and RSS, RGI-C, and height Z scores [61–65]. Burosumab, which targets increased FGF23, is expected to improve various symptoms as a radical treatment, although data on the long-term outcomes are not yet available.

7. Conclusions

The present review summarized the clinical, radiological, and biochemical features and genetic analysis of patients with XLH. This multisystem disorder is rare and challenging to diagnose. However, early diagnosis is of paramount importance because the multisystem symptoms deteriorate over time, negatively impacting the patients' QOL.

Author Contributions: Conceptualization, K.I. and Y.H.; writing—original draft preparation, K.I.; writing—review and editing, Y.H.; visualization, K.I.; supervision, Y.H. All authors have read and agreed to the published version of the manuscript.

Funding: This research received no external funding.

Institutional Review Board Statement: Ethical review and approval were waived for this study because it is a review article.

Informed Consent Statement: Not applicable.

Data Availability Statement: Not applicable.

Acknowledgments: We are indebted to James R. Valera for his assistance with editing this manuscript.

Conflicts of Interest: The authors declare no conflict of interest.

References

1. Laurent, M.R.; De Schepper, J.; Trouet, D.; Godefroid, N.; Boros, E.; Heinrichs, C.; Bravenboer, B.; Velkeniers, B.; Lammens, J.; Harvengt, P.; et al. Consensus Recommendations for the Diagnosis and Management of X-Linked Hypophosphatemia in Belgium. *Front. Endocrinol.* **2021**, *12*, 641543. [CrossRef]
2. Carpenter, T.O.; Imel, E.A.; Holm, I.A.; Jan de Beur, S.M.; Insogna, K.L. A clinician's guide to X-linked hypophosphatemia. *J. Bone Miner. Res.* **2011**, *26*, 1381–1388. [CrossRef]
3. Rafaelsen, S.; Johansson, S.; Raeder, H.; Bjerknes, R. Hereditary hypophosphatemia in Norway: A retrospective population-based study of genotypes, phenotypes, and treatment complications. *Eur. J. Endocrinol.* **2016**, *174*, 125–136. [CrossRef]
4. Endo, I.; Fukumoto, S.; Ozono, K.; Namba, N.; Inoue, D.; Okazaki, R.; Yamauchi, M.; Sugimoto, T.; Minagawa, M.; Michigami, T.; et al. Nationwide survey of fibroblast growth factor 23 (FGF23)-related hypophosphatemic diseases in Japan: Prevalence, biochemical data and treatment. *Endocr. J.* **2015**, *62*, 811–816. [CrossRef]
5. Carpenter, T.O. New perspectives on the biology and treatment of X-linked hypophosphatemic rickets. *Pediatr. Clin. N. Am.* **1997**, *44*, 443–466. [CrossRef]
6. Baroncelli, G.I.; Mora, S. X-Linked Hypophosphatemic Rickets: Multisystemic Disorder in Children Requiring Multidisciplinary Management. *Front. Endocrinol.* **2021**, *12*, 688309. [CrossRef]
7. Al Juraibah, F.; Al Amiri, E.; Al Dubayee, M.; Al Jubeh, J.; Al Kandari, H.; Al Sagheir, A.; Al Shaikh, A.; Beshyah, S.A.; Deeb, A.; Habeb, A.; et al. Diagnosis and management of X-linked hypophosphatemia in children and adolescent in the Gulf Cooperation Council countries. *Arch. Osteoporos.* **2021**, *16*, 52. [CrossRef]
8. Acar, S.; Demir, K.; Shi, Y. Genetic Causes of Rickets. *J. Clin. Res. Pediatr. Endocrinol.* **2017**, *9* (Suppl. 2), 88–105. [CrossRef]
9. Emma, F.; Cappa, M.; Antoniazzi, F.; Bianchi, M.L.; Chiodini, I.; Eller Vainicher, C.; Di Iorgi, N.; Maghnie, M.; Cassio, A.; Balsamo, A.; et al. X-linked hypophosphatemic rickets: An Italian experts' opinion survey. *Ital. J. Pediatr.* **2019**, *45*, 67. [CrossRef]
10. Beck-Nielsen, S.S.; Brusgaard, K.; Rasmussen, L.M.; Brixen, K.; Brock-Jacobsen, B.; Poulsen, M.R.; Vestergaard, P.; Ralston, S.H.; Albagha, O.M.; Poulsen, S.; et al. Phenotype presentation of hypophosphatemic rickets in adults. *Calcif. Tissue Int.* **2010**, *87*, 108–119. [CrossRef]
11. Baroncelli, G.I.; Bertelloni, S.; Ceccarelli, C.; Saggese, G. Effect of growth hormone treatment on final height, phosphate metabolism, and bone mineral density in children with X-linked hypophosphatemic rickets. *J. Pediatr.* **2001**, *138*, 236–243. [CrossRef]
12. Miyamoto, J.; Koto, S.; Hasegawa, Y. Final height of Japanese patients with X-linked hypophosphatemic rickets: Effect of vitamin D and phosphate therapy. *Endocr. J.* **2000**, *47*, 163–167. [CrossRef]
13. Padidela, R.; Nilsson, O.; Makitie, O.; Beck-Nielsen, S.; Ariceta, G.; Schnabel, D.; Brandi, M.L.; Boot, A.; Levtchenko, E.; Smyth, M.; et al. The international X-linked hypophosphataemia (XLH) registry (NCT03193476): Rationale for and description of an international, observational study. *Orphanet J. Rare Dis.* **2020**, *15*, 172. [CrossRef]
14. Che, H.; Roux, C.; Etcheto, A.; Rothenbuhler, A.; Kamenicky, P.; Linglart, A.; Briot, K. Impaired quality of life in adults with X-linked hypophosphatemia and skeletal symptoms. *Eur. J. Endocrinol.* **2016**, *174*, 325–333. [CrossRef]
15. Skrinar, A.; Dvorak-Ewell, M.; Evins, A.; Macica, C.; Linglart, A.; Imel, E.A.; Theodore-Oklota, C.; San Martin, J. The Lifelong Impact of X-Linked Hypophosphatemia: Results From a Burden of Disease Survey. *J. Endocr. Soc.* **2019**, *3*, 1321–1334. [CrossRef]

64. Insogna, K.L.; Rauch, F.; Kamenický, P.; Ito, N.; Kubota, T.; Nakamura, A.; Zhang, L.; Mealiffe, M.; San Martin, J.; Portale, A.A. Burosumab Improved Histomorphometric Measures of Osteomalacia in Adults with X-Linked Hypophosphatemia: A Phase 3, Single-Arm, International Trial. *J. Bone Miner. Res.* **2019**, *34*, 2183–2191. [CrossRef]
65. Carpenter, T.O.; Imel, E.A.; Ruppe, M.D.; Weber, T.J.; Klausner, M.A.; Wooddell, M.M.; Kawakami, T.; Ito, T.; Zhang, X.; Humphrey, J.; et al. Randomized trial of the anti-FGF23 antibody KRN23 in X-linked hypophosphatemia. *J. Clin. Investig.* **2014**, *124*, 1587–1597. [CrossRef]

Disclaimer/Publisher's Note: The statements, opinions and data contained in all publications are solely those of the individual author(s) and contributor(s) and not of MDPI and/or the editor(s). MDPI and/or the editor(s) disclaim responsibility for any injury to people or property resulting from any ideas, methods, instructions or products referred to in the content.

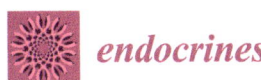

Review

Adult Presentation of X-Linked Hypophosphatemia

Nobuaki Ito [1,2]

1. Division of Nephrology and Endocrinology, The University of Tokyo Hospital, Tokyo 113-8655, Japan; nobitotky@gmail.com
2. Osteoporosis Center, The University of Tokyo Hospital, Tokyo 113-8655, Japan

Abstract: Adult X-linked hypophosphatemia (XLH) patients present with specific symptoms, including enthesopathies (e.g., ossification of longitudinal ligaments (OPLL), osteophytes around large joints, and enthesopathy in the Achilles tendons), early osteoarthritis, the development of severe secondary and tertiary hyperparathyroidism (SHPT/THPT), and the subsequent progression of chronic kidney disease (CKD). In addition, these patients exhibit the typical phenotypes of osteomalacia, such as pseudofracture and fracture in weight-bearing bones, odontitis, and tooth abscesses. The mechanism underlying enthesopathy development is unknown; however, a common underlying mechanism among XLH and autosomal recessive hypophosphatemic rickets (ARHR1/2) due to mutations in *PHEX*, *DMP1*, and *ENPP1* is assumed. Clarification of the pathogenesis and drug discovery for this complication is an urgent issue, as many adult XLH patients suffer subsequent debilitating nervous symptoms or impingement syndrome, and existing treatments are ineffective. Severe SHPT and THPT are associated with conventional therapy, including active vitamin D and phosphate supplementation, and complicated and careful adjustment of dosages by experienced clinicians is required to avoid SHPT/THPT. Burosumab is a very effective therapy without risk for the development of SHPT/THPT. However, indications for this drug should be carefully considered, along with cost-effectiveness, guidelines or recommendations, and the health care system of each country.

Keywords: X-linked hypophosphatemia; fibroblast growth factor 23; osteomalacia; enthesopathy; secondary hyperparathyroidism; tertiary hyperparathyroidism; chronic kidney disease; oral disease; quality of life; burosumab

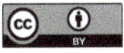

1. Introduction

X-linked hypophosphatemia (XLH) is a genetic disease caused by inactivating mutations of the phosphate-regulating endopeptidase gene (*PHEX*). Symptoms that develop during childhood are typical rachitic phenotypes, including leg deformity, short stature, odontitis, tooth abscesses, and craniosynostosis. In contrast, adult XLH patients present variable symptoms, including complications resulting from its treatment, such as enthesopathy, early osteoarthritis, secondary/tertiary hyperparathyroidism (SHPT/THPT), and chronic kidney disease (CKD), in addition to characteristic phenotypes for osteomalacia, such as pseudofracture and fracture in weight-bearing bones [1,2]. Some clinicians believe that treatment could be terminated after epiphyseal closure even among patients with severe XLH; however, adult XLH patients are currently recognized to be at risk of pseudofractures and fractures in weight-bearing bones due to low turnover even with normal to high bone mineral density (BMD) [3,4]. The mechanism for the development of enthesopathy in adults with XLH is unknown, and even among adult XLH patients treated with active vitamin D and phosphate supplementation or burosumab, remarkable enthesopathies sometimes develop, and these patients experience significant difficulty in activities of daily life (ADL) and lower quality of life (QOL) with nervous symptoms due to ossification of the posterior longitudinal ligament (OPLL), ossification of the ligamentum flavum (OLF), and other ossification-related nerve entrapment, or impingement syndromes in the hip, and the development of osteoarthritis [4].

Treatment for adult XLH with active vitamin D and inorganic phosphate is very difficult, as well as for child patients with XLH, because excess of this treatment is associated with the development of SHPT/THPT and subsequent nephrotic diabetes insipidus, prerenal renal failure, postrenal renal failure, and the progression of CKD [5]. Therefore, the transition of XLH patients to specialized clinicians is vital, especially when patients are treated with conventional therapy, although there are a limited number of specialists for bone and mineral disorders in adults. Burosumab is an anti-fibroblast growth factor (FGF) 23 humanized monoclonal antibody developed by a pharmaceutical company in collaboration with our laboratory, which led to the improvement of phosphate metabolism in children with XLH and adults with XLH up to 96 weeks in clinical studies [6–11]. A beneficial effect of burosumab on pseudofracture and fracture healing was confirmed in the clinical studies, and, theoretically, it is protective against the progression of CKD, as burosumab enables patients to withdraw phosphate preparation, although its effect on the prevention or improvement of enthesopathy and early osteoarthritis is unknown.

In this review article about the adult presentation of XLH, the estimated underlying mechanisms for the development of adult XLH-specific problems, including enthesopathy, early osteoarthritis, SHPT/THPT, and CKD, are illustrated, and the recommended indication and selection of pharmaceuticals and detailed adjustment procedure of dosage according to previous publications and personal experience are introduced.

2. Diagnosis of Adult XLH

Mild cases of undiagnosed XLH are infrequently suspected among adults with pseudofractures and fractures in weight-bearing bones or remarkable enthesopathies in the spinal ligament, around the hip joints, and in the Achilles tendons, with concomitant chronic hypophosphatemia. To accelerate an accurate diagnosis, appropriate treatment and prevention of additional pseudofracture, fracture, and dental disorders, clinicians should suspect low turnover disorders such as FGF23-related hypophosphatemia, including XLH and tumor-induced osteomalacia, Fanconi syndrome, vitamin D deficient osteomalacia, mild vitamin D dependent rickets (e.g., heterozygous mutation in *CYP3A4*), mild hypophosphatasia (e.g., heterozygous mutation in *ALPL*), mild osteogenesis imperfecta (e.g., Sillence type I), and mild osteopetrosis (e.g., dominant negative type of heterozygous mutation in *CLCN7*). These ailments should be suspected among adult patients who develop pseudofractures and fractures in weight-bearing bones (costa, pelvis, femoral head subchondral fragility fracture, diaphyses of femur/tibia/fibula, calcaneus, and metatarsal) spontaneously, with low-power trauma, with relatively short-term use of anti-resorptive reagents for osteoporosis (e.g., ≤5 years), among adult patients who develop odontitis, tooth abscesses, necrosis of the jaw spontaneously, or with relatively short-term use of anti-resorptive reagents for osteoporosis.

In Japan, once chronic hypophosphatemia with the relevant symptoms of rickets/osteomalacia is recognized, measurement of serum intact fibroblast growth factor (FGF) 23 (Determinar CL FGF23; Minaris Medical, Tokyo, Japan) is encouraged to determine the etiology of hypophosphatemia, with a cutoff value of 30 pg/mL to discriminate FGF23-related hypophosphatemic rickets/osteomalacia and others, which was revealed to possess high sensitivity and specificity [12–14]. Among adult patients with osteomalacia accompanied by FGF23 values of 30 pg/mL or more, diagnosis of XLH is strongly supported by the presence of one or more of the following symptoms: mildly short stature, leg deformity (genu varum, genu vulgus), enthesopathy, or X-linked inheritance of rickets/osteomalacia. However, even among these cases, genetic diagnosis of *PHEX* mutation is recommended, if available, in an effort to make an accurate diagnosis [15]. In the cases of adult-onset FGF23-related hypophosphatemic osteomalacia without any of the symptoms above, the possibilities of tumor-induced osteomalacia, intravenous infusion of iron preparation-induced osteomalacia, and alcohol-induced FGF23-related hypophosphatemic osteomalacia should be explored [16–18].

3. Symptoms of Adult XLH

3.1. Pseudofracture and Fracture

As stated above, some clinicians used to believe that treatment could be terminated after epiphyseal closure, probably due to the normal or relatively high bone mineral density detected in the majority of adults with mild XLH [3,4]. Normal-to-high BMD observed in patients with mild XLH might stem from suppressed osteoclastic function and is probably due to the excessive ossification caused for the same reason XLH patients tend to develop enthesopathy [4]. However, the risk of pseudofractures and fractures in weight-bearing bones (costa, pelvis, femoral head subchondral fragility fracture, diaphyses of femur/tibia/fibula, calcaneus, and metatarsal) is usually not correlated with BMD and is strongly associated with low turnover of bone (e.g., also shown in other hypophosphatemic rickets/otsteomalacia, hypophosphatasia, osteogenesis imperfecta, osteopetrosis, and long-term use of anti-osteoclastic reagents), as accumulated micro bone cracks with delayed healing in weight-bearing bones eventually lead to pseudofracture and fracture. Therefore, the treatment for hypophosphatemia should be continued among adult XLH patients with typical rachitic phenotypes, including short stature, leg deformity, or a past history of surgical correction of leg deformity, with continuously elevated bone-specific alkaline phosphatase (BAP) in the absence of treatment [1,2]. Figure 1a,b show typical femoral pseudofractures developed after years of treatment cessation and surgically treated fractures in the diaphysis of the femur and bilateral tibiae developed under conventional therapy (Figure 1). To detect tiny pseudofractures, X-rays in multiple directions, bone scintigraphy (^{99m}Tc-methylene diphosphonate/hydroxymethylene diphosphonate), and T2-weighted fat-suppressed magnetic resonance imaging (MRI) are beneficial.

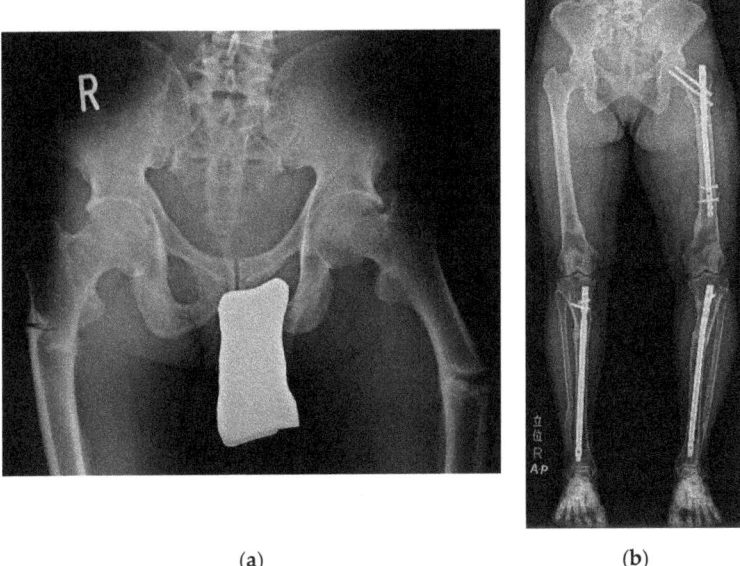

(a)   (b)

Figure 1. Pseudofracture and fracture in the femurs and tibiae in adult XLH patients. (**a**) Pseudofractures developed spontaneously in both femurs in an adult XLH patient after years of conventional therapy cessation. (**b**) Fractures developed spontaneously in the left femur and both tibiae in an adult XLH patient with conventional therapy.

To prevent the development of pseudofracture and fracture, long periods of strenuous exercise and labor (e.g., long period of walking, stomping exercise for osteoporosis, or weightbearing exercise/labor) should be avoided in adult XLH patients with uncontrolled chronic hypophosphatemia manifested by elevated BAP, and patients should be encouraged to visit their attending clinician immediately when warning pain is recognized in the diaphysis of the femur/tibia/fibula. Adult XLH patients with new pseudofracture or fracture should be treated with conventional therapy or burosumab. It is recommended that patients who developed pseudofracture or fracture under treatment with conventional therapy consider changing the treatment to burosumab. When a surgical procedure is unavoidable for the developed pseudofracture/fracture, medical treatment should be provided for 1 to 3 months before surgery to prevent the loosening of prosthesis or the development of additional pseudofracture/fracture around prosthesis, unless urgent surgery is required [2].

Please note that anti-resorptive reagents (bisphosphonates and denosumab) are contraindicated for patients with uncontrolled low bone turnover disorders, including adult XLH, as these reagents aggravate low bone turnover and increase the risk of developing pseudofracture and fracture in weight-bearing bones, tooth abscesses, and necrosis of the jaw. If coexisting osteoporosis is suspected in postmenopausal females with XLH or older patients with XLH, anti-osteoporotic treatment should not be initiated until osteomalacia improvement by normalization of BAP with conventional therapy or burosumab is confirmed.

Based on retrospective case reviews, conventional therapy with active vitamin D and phosphate preparation is suggested to be beneficial to prevent and heal pseudofractures and fractures in weight-bearing bones; however, this speculation has not been proven, as there are no prospective trials. On the other hand, burosumab treatment improved pseudofractures and fractures in adult XLH patients in clinical trials [7,9,19].

3.2. Muscle Weakness

In 2013, Veilleux et al. reported that muscle force in the lower extremities in 13 XLH patients (6 to 60 years old) was significantly decreased despite normal muscle size in comparison with age- and sex-matched control participants [20]. Clinicians tend to ascribe this muscle weakness in XLH patients to the direct effect of hypophosphatemia on myocytes. However, the observed muscle weakness was also explained by bone pain due to osteomalacia and inefficient transduction of muscle contraction due to leg deformity or impingement syndrome stemming from enthesopathy. Of note, rapidly induced hypophosphatemia is not associated with muscle weakness [21]. The effect of conventional therapy on muscle weakness is inconclusive as there is no prospective trial, and burosumab was associated with an increased distance of 6 min in walk tests, although this might be associated with the improvement of pseudofractures and fractures [11]. Further clinical studies are warranted to clarify whether there is a direct effect of hypophosphatemia on myocytes.

3.3. Dental Health

Uncontrolled rickets/osteomalacia is evidently associated with a high risk of periodontitis, odontitis, and tooth abscesses in children and adults [22,23]. The underlying mechanism for this might be the accumulation of microcracks with delayed healing in the enamel and dentin that penetrate from the pit on the surface to the pulp, similar to how pseudofractures and fractures develop in weight-bearing bones. Orthodontic treatment sometimes results in the loss of permanent teeth in XLH patients with uncontrolled osteomalacia. Early intervention with conventional treatment was reported to have a prophylactic effect on the development of these dental diseases, although this finding was not discovered in a prospective trial [24,25]. In the post hoc analysis of a 64-week, open-label, randomized controlled study with 61 children aged 1 to 12 years with XLH, dental abscesses occurred in 3 of 12 (25%) younger (<5 years) children with conventional therapy, while 0 of 20 (0%) younger children from the burosumab group developed dental abscesses. However, in older (5–12 years) children with XLH, dental abscesses presented more frequently with burosumab than with conventional therapy (9/29 (31%) vs. 2/32 (6%)) [26]. Based on the results of this study, burosumab seems to possess weaker protective effects or, at least, not more intense protective effects, against the development of dental abscesses compared to conventional therapy; however, a longer duration study is needed.

The effect of burosumab on dental health in XLH patients has not yet been reported.

3.4. Enthesopathy

We examined the prevalence of enthesopathies in 25 adult XLH patients (18 to 72 y) and revealed a high prevalence of OPLL (32%), osteophytes around the hip joints equivalent to a Kellgren–Lawrence grade of 2 and more (96%), and enthesopathies in the Achilles tendon (72%), which explained that XLH is an obvious genetic condition in which patients are prone to developing enthesopathies [4]. Normal to high BMD in adult XLH patients was also reported in the same article and was attributed to the same osteogenic nature of XLH [4]. In some adult XLH patients, neurological symptoms due to OPLL and limited range of motion (ROM) in the hip and intervertebral joints severely lowered ADL and QOL [27]. Figure 2a–c are typical images of OPLL, osteophytes around the hip joint, and enthesopathy in the Achilles tendon present in adult XLH patients (Figure 2).

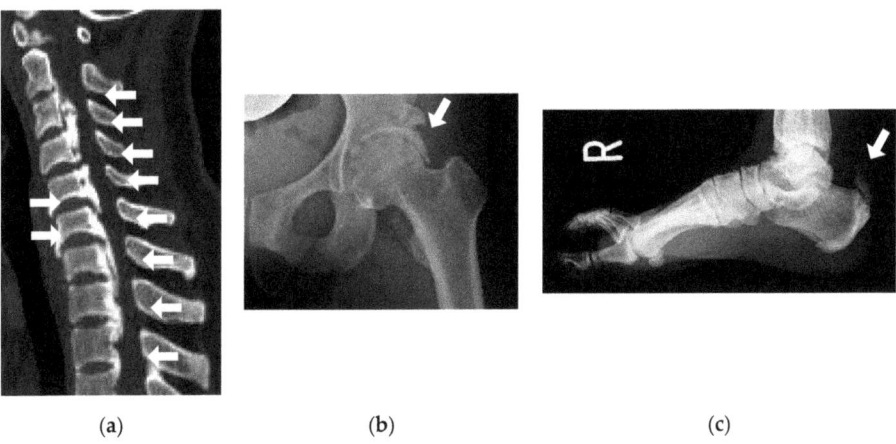

Figure 2. Enthesopathies in adult XLH patients. (**a**) Severe ossification of the posterior longitudinal ligament and ossification of the anterior longitudinal ligament presented in an adult XLH patient. (**b**) A large osteophyte developed around the left hip joint in an adult XLH patient, causing severe impingement syndrome. (**c**) Enthesopathy developed in the right Achilles tendon in an adult XLH patient.

Currently, the precise mechanism for the development of enthesopathy in adult XLH patients (typically over 30 years old) is unknown. It has been recognized that enthesopathy is also frequently present in patients with other inherited FGF23-related hypophosphatemic rickets, including autosomal recessive hypophosphatemic rickets 1 and 2 caused by homozygous mutations in *DMP1* and *ENPP1*, respectively, although other types of inherited or acquired FGF23-related hypophosphatemia are not associated with the development of enthesopathy [28,29]. Recently, we reported that haploinsufficiency of ectonucleotide pyrophosphatase/phosphodiesterase (ENPP1) with heterozygous or compound heterozygous mutations of *ENPP1* is also associated with milder phenotypes of enthesopathy, manifested by OPLL and diffuse idiopathic skeletal hyperostosis (DISH) [30]. This means that the enthesopathy present in patients with XLH and ARHR1/2 is not a consequence of chronic hypophosphatemia or high levels of serum FGF23, and there is a common mechanism to develop enthesopathy among XLH and ARHR1/2. Therefore, unfortunately, conventional treatment did not exert a prophylactic effect on the development of enthesopathy or improve enthesopathy [25]. In my view, burosumab is suspected to be ineffective in the prevention or improvement of enthesopathy, as other conditions with highly elevated FGF23, such as advanced CKD patients on renal replacement therapy, are not associated with increased risk for enthesopathy, although this finding will not be conclusive until the results of a long-term study with burosumab are reported. Severe neurologic symptoms, such as paraparesis due to OPLL, are an indication for surgical decompression of the spinal cord.

ENPP1 is a membranous enzyme that metabolizes adenosine triphosphate (ATP) into adenosine monophosphate (AMP) and inorganic pyrophosphate (PPi). PPi was identified to antagonize the formation of hydroxyapatite. Thus, lowering plasma PPi is the candidate mechanism for the development of enthesopathy in patients with homozygous, compound heterozygous, or heterozygous ENPP1 mutations [31,32]. Furthermore, Maulding et al. reported that low plasma PPi levels were identified in Hyp mice, the model mouse for XLH [33]. Therefore, one possible explanation for this tendency to develop enthesopathy in adult XLH patients is the involvement of lowered PPi, albeit the PPi levels in XLH patients have not been reported.

3.5. Osteoarthritis

Early osteoarthritis is the other debilitating symptom commonly recognized among adult XLH patients. Development of early osteoarthritis is partly due to abnormal mechanical loading stemming from leg deformity, although it is not fully explained by this [34]. Existence of enthesopathy and excessive ossification in adults with XLH might be associated with the development of early osteoarthritis. We reported the prevalence of hip osteoarthritis (Kellgren–Lawrence grade ≥2, 3) to be 96% and 88%, respectively, and the prevalence of knee osteoarthritis (Kellgren–Lawrence grade ≥2, 3) to be 68% and 36%, which is markedly higher than the general population [4]. Figure 3a,b are typical images of osteoarthritis in the hip and knee joints presented in a 29-year-old male and 30-year-old female with XLH, respectively (Figure 3). As in the case with enthesopathy, conventional therapy did not improve or prevent the development of osteoarthritis in the adults with XLH, while the effect of burosumab on this complication is indecisive.

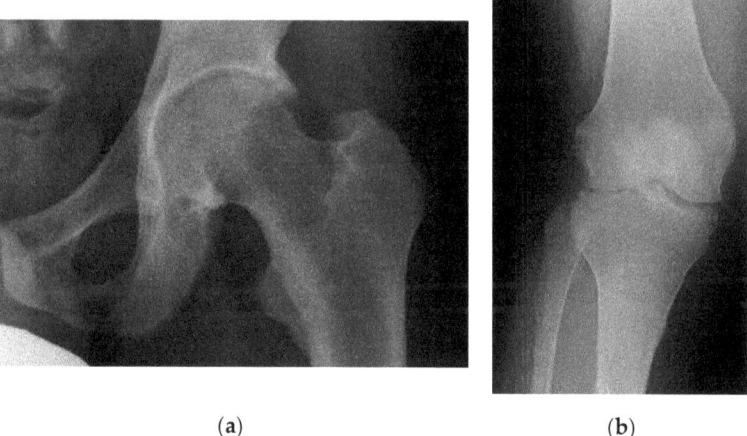

Figure 3. Early osteoarthritis in adult XLH patients. (**a**) Osteoarthritis with a Kellgren–Lawrence grade of 3 in the left hip joint of a 29-year-old male XLH patient. (**b**) Osteoarthritis with a Kellgren–Lawrence grade of 3 in the right knee joint of a 30-year-old female XLH patient.

3.6. SHPT/THPT

XLH patients tend to develop SHPT (hyperparathyroidism with the value of calcium less than the middle of the reference range) due to low 1,25(OH)$_2$D stemming from excessive action of FGF23 and exogenous supplementation of inorganic phosphate. SHPT is an undesired phenotype in XLH patients because hyperparathyroidism stimulates osteoclastic activity, leading to bone loss in addition to rickets/osteomalacia, and accelerates hypophosphatemia as parathyroid hormone (PTH) decreases the expression of sodium–phosphate cotransporter independent of FGF23. Additionally, we recently reported that PTH directly stimulates the transcription of FGF23 in an osteocytic cell line [35]. Furthermore, a handful of XLH patients who already suffer from SHPT develop THPT (hyperparathyroidism with the value of calcium greater than or equal to the middle of the reference range), which is an equivalent clinical condition to primary hyperparathyroidism (PHPT) that causes hypercalciuria and nephrotic diabetes insipidus, leading to repetitive episodic prerenal and postrenal renal failure and progression of CKD.

In 2019, DeLacey et al. reported that among 84 patients with XLH (40 adults, 44 children), 83.3% had SHPT or THPT, and THPT developed in 16.7% of patients [5]. Seventy-five percent (6/8) of the patients who underwent parathyroidectomy for THPT experienced persistent or recurrent THPT, which explains why other parathyroid cells are also ready to convert into autonomous PTH-producing cells in XLH patients who once developed THPT [5]. We are now analyzing the relationship between the highest or cumulative dose of phosphate supplementation and the development of SHPT or THPT in a large cohort of XLH patients in Japan and Korea [36]. To prevent the development of severe SHPT and THPT, the dosage of conventional treatment with active vitamin D and phosphate supplementation should be adjusted with great care by experienced clinicians, and the change in treatment to burosumab should be considered for XLH patients who develop severe SHPT or THPT, as burosumab is not supposed to be associated with the development of severe SHPT and THPT as it enables patients to be freed from phosphate preparation. Once THPT is developed, immediate cessation of conventional therapy and initiation of an allosteric modulator of the calcium sensing receptor should be considered until parathyroidectomy conduction occurs, and treatment for hypophosphatemia should be resumed with burosumab afterward. Detailed guidance for conventional therapy recommended by the author is described in "Section 6.2. Conventional therapy (active vitamin D and phosphate supplementation)."

3.7. CKD

Some adult XLH patients with conventional treatment experience CKD progression uncommon for their age or for those with other medical conditions, and very rarely, patients need renal replacement therapy. The main reason for the progression of CKD in patients with adult XLH is described in "Section 3.5. SHPT/THPT" above; that is, the main reason is hypercalciuria and nephrotic diabetes insipidus due to conventional therapy, leading to repetitive episodic prerenal and postrenal renal failure, which often follows development of THPT. In fact, in the article by DeLacey et al. introduced in the previous section and including 84 XLH patients, nephrocalcinosis and CKD G3 and over (eGFR < 60 mL/min/1.73 m^2) were more prevalent in patients with THPT than in patients without THPT (60% vs. 18.6% and 35.7% vs. 1.5%, respectively) [5]. Therefore, to prevent the progression of CKD, adequate handling of severe SHPT and THPT by experienced clinicians is necessary, and appropriate water consumption and intake of salt should be recommended among XLH patients treated with conventional therapy, especially in those with febrile and gastrointestinal disorders or who labor and spend leisure time in the hot sun over a long period. Please note that the dosage of active vitamin D and phosphate supplementation needs to be decreased as CKD progresses; otherwise, a persistent excessive dose of conventional therapy might be associated with the development of THPT and further progression of CKD. The correlation between the highest or cumulative dose of phosphate supplementation and active vitamin D and the progression of CKD to stage

G3 and over is also under examination in a large cohort of XLH patients in Japan and Korea [37]. The use of burosumab is thought to be protective against the progression of CKD, as patients can disregard phosphate preparations; however, its protectiveness remains unclear until the result of a long-term study is reported.

3.8. Hypertension and Left Ventricular Hypertrophy

A high prevalence of elevated blood pressure (27.3%, 6/22) unmatched to age has been reported in a small cohort of adult XLH patients, and this characteristic could be the consequence of the progression of CKD. A cohort study with a larger number of adult XLH patients is necessary to address this issue [38]. The effects of conventional therapy and burosumab on the prevention of development and progression of hypertension and left ventricular hypertrophy are unknown.

3.9. Hearing Loss

The prevalence of hearing loss among XLH patients varies from 16% to 76% depending on the population or method of evaluation [39]. In 25 adult XLH patients with a median age of 39 (range 18–60) years from our hospital, 8 (32%) patients presented with hearing impairment. Seven cases had a sensorineural pattern, and one case had both sensorineural and conductive patterns [4]. The precise mechanism of hearing loss in XLH patients has not been clarified; however, temporal bone malformation due to osteomalacia and endolymphatic hydrops stemming from hypophosphatemia have been suggested to be the causes [38]. There has been no report suggesting a beneficial effect of conventional therapy or burosumab to prevent or improve hearing impairment in adults with XLH.

4. QOL of Adult XLH

There are several reports about the QOL of adult XLH patients [39–41]. In 2019, Skrinar et al. reported that among 232 adult patients with XLH, 97% had bone or joint pain/stiffness, 44% had a history of fractures, 46% had osteophytes, 27% had enthesopathy in the Achilles tendon, and 19% had spinal stenosis. In addition, the mean scores for age-specific patient-reported outcomes (PROs) evaluating pain, stiffness, and physical function were worse than those of the control population [39]. In 2020, Seefried et al. conducted a systematic literature review including 91 articles and 44 congress abstracts, revealing that XLH had a substantial and wide-ranging negative impact on health-related quality of life (HRQOL), particularly relating to physical function and pain measured by the 36-item Short-Form Health Survey (SF-36), Western Ontario and McMaster Universities Osteoarthritis Index (WOMAC), and Brief Pain Inventory (BPI) [40]. We evaluated the HRQOL in Japanese and Korean patients with XLH, including 32 adult patients; this investigation revealed that among adult XLH patients, 59.4% had bone pain, 65.6% had joint pain, 9.5% had CKD G3 or higher, 15.6% had nephrocalcinosis, 15.6% had SHPT or THPT, and 6.3% underwent parathyroidectomy [41]. In our study, the SF-36, WOMAC, and BPI also revealed lower QOL in adult XLH patients [41]. In fact, it is hard to distinguish if musculoskeletal pain is due to enthesopathy, osteoarthritis, bone pain, or pain from myalgias among adult patients with XLH. However, given the higher prevalence of reported joint pain (65.6%) than that of bone pain (59.4%) observed in our study, (1) early initiation of pharmaceutical intervention to prevent leg deformity and (2) exploration of the mechanism for the development of enthesopathy and early osteoarthritis to develop new treatment options to conquer these debilitating complications are important to further improve the QOL among adult XLH patients.

5. Transition of XLH Patients

Clinical follow-up of XLH patients should be transferred from pediatricians to adult endocrinologists or rheumatologists when patients are approximately 18 to 20 years of age to encourage independence from their caregivers and facilitate the care of other adult-specific medical problems. At the time of transition, patients need to be educated or re-educated about XLH, including the genetic information. XLH patients should be followed by experienced clinicians, as stated above, in the institutions where multidisciplinary care, which involves physical and occupational therapy, dental care, pain clinics, etc., can be offered. For more information about the transition of XLH, please refer to the well-organized mini-review by Dahir et al. [42]. Most importantly, XLH patients should be referred to experienced clinicians, although there are too few endocrinologists, rheumatologists, and medical geneticists worldwide specializing in bone metabolic disorders and skeletal dysplasia to meet demand. Therefore, the need for an increased number of endocrinologists, rheumatologists, and medical geneticists who are educated about bone metabolic disorders and skeletal dysplasia is one of the urgent issues to resolve in this field.

6. Treatment of Adult XLH

6.1. Indication and Selection of Treatment

The indication and selection of conventional treatment and burosumab among adult XLH patients might be influenced by the health care system of each nation. In Japan, I suggest the indication and selection of pharmaceutical treatment in adult XLH patients as described in Table 1; this information reflects my personal opinion based on my own experience with adult XLH patients (Table 1). The severity of the symptoms among adult XLH patients varies widely even between family members sharing the same mutation, and treatment for hypophosphatemia is not necessarily required among patients with mild symptoms defined by a normal value of BAP, stature ≥ -1.0 SD, lack of genu varum and genu valgus, and no history of pseudofracture/bone pain, fracture in weight-bearing bones, or odontitis/tooth abscesses without treatment. In contrast, adult XLH patients with severe phenotypes should be treated with burosumab, which is more effective than conventional therapy. In my opinion, severe phenotypes are defined by short stature (< -2.0 SD), deviation of mechanical axis of the leg into zone 3 or greater [43], history of corrective surgery on the leg, history of pseudofracture/bone pain in weight-bearing bones, odontitis, tooth abscesses more than twice without any treatment, more than once under conventional therapy, or more than once but requiring surgery, and history of fracture in weight-bearing bone. The indication for conventional treatment is between the indications for observation and burosumab. Additionally, I recommend changing the treatment approach to include burosumab for adult XLH patients who develop uncontrolled SHPT or THPT with conventional treatment and patients with moderate symptoms (between mild and severe symptoms) and eGFR < 45 mL/min/1.73 m^2 to prevent further progression of CKD.

Table 1. Suggested indication and selection of therapy for adult XLH patients.

Observation	Conventional Therapy	Burosumab
BAP ($\leq$ upper limit of the reference range)	BAP (>upper limit of reference range) with eGFR ≥ 45 mL/min/1.73 m^2	BAP (>upper limit of the reference range) with conventional treatment
Stature (≥ -1.0 SD)	Short stature ($-2.0 \leq -1.0$ SD) with eGFR ≥ 45 mL/min/1.73 m^2	Short stature (< -2.0 SD)
Mechanical axis of the leg within zone 1 [43]	Deviation of the mechanical axis of the leg into zone 2 [43] with eGFR ≥ 45 L/min/1.73 m^2	Deviation of the mechanical axis of the leg into zone 3 or greater [43] or history of corrective surgery for leg deformity
No history of pseudofracture/bone pain/fracture in weight-bearing bone or odontitis/tooth abscesses	Pseudofracture/bone pain in weight-bearing bone or odontitis/tooth abscess once with eGFR ≥ 45 mL/min/1.73 m^2	Pseudofracture/bone pain in weight-bearing bone or odontitis/tooth abscesses more than two times or more than once with conventional treatment or once requiring impending surgery
	No response or trivial response to burosumab	Fracture in weight-bearing bone

Table 1. *Cont.*

Observation	Conventional Therapy	Burosumab
	Severe adverse event with burosumab	Uncontrolled severe SHPT with conventional treatment (e.g., peak intact PTH ≥ twice the upper limit of the reference range);
		THPT;
		Patients with symptoms described in the "conventional therapy" and eGFR < 45 mL/min/1.73 m^2;
		Severe adverse event with conventional therapy

Please note that enthesopathy cannot be improved by therapeutically targeting the increase in serum phosphate. Supplementation of natural vitamin D preparation (ergocalciferol, cholecalciferol) or encouraged intake of natural vitamin D from diet targeting serum 25OHD of 30 ng/mL and higher is recommended in XLH patients to avoid detriment to the bone due to vitamin D deficiency.

6.2. Conventional Therapy (Active Vitamin D and Phosphate Supplementation)

Treatment of XLH patients with conventional therapy is the tricky part of patient management, as inadequate and careless dosage adjustment results in the development of SHPT/THPT and consequent irreversible progression of CKD. Thus, clinicians should always prioritize prevention of the development of severe SHPT and THPT as long as patients are treated with conventional therapy.

In Japan, a powdered preparation is used, containing 330 mg of monobasic sodium phosphate monohydrate (NaH_2PO_4/H_2O) and 119 mg of dibasic sodium phosphate anhydrous (Na_2HPO_4) in a packet, which is equivalent to 100 mg of inorganic phosphate. Other formulae of phosphate preparations (e.g., K-Phos, neutraphos) are also used to treat XLH patients [1]. Relatively frequent adverse events associated with phosphate preparation include nephrocalcinosis, abdominal pain, nausea, vomiting, and diarrhea, among others, in addition to the aforementioned SHPT, THPT, acute kidney injury, and progression of CKD. Active vitamin D-associated adverse events include nephrocalcinosis, hypercalciuria, thirst, appetite loss, abdominal pain, nausea, vomiting, diarrhea, and constipation, among others, in addition to acute kidney injury and progression of CKD.

The range of daily dosages of conventional therapy described in the consensus statement introduced by specialists from European countries (calcitriol: 0.50 to 0.75 μg, alfacalcidol: 0.75 to 1.5 μg, phosphate supplementation: 750 to 1600 mg) appears very appropriate from the viewpoint of preventing severe SHPT and THPT [2]. Calcitriol should be taken twice daily due to its shorter half-life compared to alfacalcidol, which is taken once daily. Active vitamin D should precede phosphate supplementation by approximately one week, and treatment with phosphate supplementation should always be accompanied by active vitamin D to prevent the development of severe SHPT and THPT [1,2]. Importantly, the serum phosphate level peaks approximately 1.5 h after the intake of phosphate supplementation and goes back to the trough value 2 to 3 h after intake [44]. Thus, phosphate supplementation should be taken four or more times daily to maximize the antihypophosphatemic effect and minimize the risk of developing SHPT/THPT.

I propose laboratory tests, including serum phosphate, calcium, albumin, intact PTH, creatinine, and BAP, with blood samples drawn 1 to 2 h after the intake of phosphate supplementation to detect the peak value of serum phosphate and intact PTH because these values are associated with bone mineralization and risk for the development of severe SHPT/THPT. These effects and risks cannot be inferred from the trough value of serum phosphate and intact PTH.

In our facility, conventional therapy usually starts with 1.0 µg of alfacalcidol, and 1 to 2 weeks later, phosphate supplementation is initiated with 200 mg four times daily. In the dose-adjusting phase, laboratory data are followed every one to four weeks, and phosphate supplementation is adjusted by 100 mg increments until the peak phosphate level stably settles within the lower 50% of the reference range. Most importantly, we do not attempt to adjust conventional therapy to increase trough phosphate levels within the reference range, as this is strongly associated with the development of SHPT/THPT and consequent progression of CKD [1]. Additionally, in adult XLH patients with eGFR < 45 mL/min/1.73 m^2, lower dosages of active vitamin D and phosphate are required to maintain the peak serum phosphate level in the target range, and often only a small dose of active vitamin D (e.g., 0.25 to 0.50 µg of alfacalcidol) or no medication is required among adult XLH patients with eGFR < 30 mL/min/1.73 m^2, although the change in treatment to burosumab should be recommended to prevent the further progression of CKD in case phosphate supplementation is still required (e.g., uncontrolled BAP) in patients with eGFR < 45 mL/min/1.73 m^2. In the maintenance phase, laboratory data are followed every 3 to 6 months, and normalization of BAP is the ideal goal of treatment, as it directly reflects the ossification status of the bone. However, in treatment-naive XLH patients with active osteomalacia, BAP initially increases in response to treatment up to 3 to 6 months, indicating the recommencement of mineralization, and then decreases to the basal value approximately 6 to 12 months after the initiation of treatment. Thus, dose adjustment of conventional therapy targeting normalization of BAP should be considered after 12 to 18 months. Changing treatment to burosumab should be considered in patients with uncontrolled BAP.

Once again, the prioritized agenda alongside conventional treatment is the prevention of severe SHPT and THPT; therefore, the dosage of phosphate should be immediately decreased by 100 mg or more for a period of time once overadjustment of peak phosphate (e.g., within the upper 25% of the reference range or more) or severe SHPT (e.g., peak intact PTH $\geq$ double the upper limit of the reference range) is observed. Then, if an increase in phosphate supplementation is required in patients who have developed severe SHPT, escalation of active vitamin D by 0.25 µg for calcitriol and 0.25 to 0.5 µg for alfacalcidol should precede an increase in phosphate supplementation by 1 to 2 weeks. In patients who develop THPT (hyperparathyroidism with the value of calcium > the middle of the reference range), conventional therapy should immediately be terminated to prevent the progression of CKD; in addition, patients should try their best to avoid dehydration, and immediate initiation of an allosteric modulator of calcium sensing receptors (e.g., cinacalcet, evocalcet) is recommended until parathyroidectomy is performed after examination with ultrasound and ^{99m}Tc-sestamibi (MIBI) scintigraphy. In cases with THPT, all recognizable parathyroid glands by ultrasound and MIBI scintigraphy should be removed, as persistenting THPT and recurrence of THPT after parathyroidectomy occur very frequently (75%) among XLH patients [5]. In patients who developed THPT with contraindication for surgery (e.g., severe cardiopulmonary disorder, oldest-old patients), allosteric modulation of calcium sensing receptors should be continued, and in these patients, additional anti-osteoporotic treatment should be considered after the surrogate marker of osteomalacia (e.g., BAP) is well-controlled, because increased intact PTH persists with allosteric modulation of the calcium sensing receptor [45]. It is recommended to change treatment to burosumab in XLH patients with uncontrolled severe SHPT undergoing conventional therapy or who have developed THPT. Supplementation of active vitamin D or replacement therapy with recombinant 1-84 PTH is required in addition to treatment of hypophosphatemia in patients in whom all parathyroid glands have been removed due to THPT. Please refer to Table 2 for guidance for conventional treatment for adults with XLH (Table 2).

Table 2. Suggested guidance of conventional therapy for adult XLH patients.

Priority	Event	Action
	Initiation of treatment	Start with active vitamin D (0.50 µg b.i.d. for calcitriol or 1.0 µg s.i.d. for alfacalcidol) After 1 to 2 weeks, start phosphate supplementation (800 mg q.i.d.)
	Range of dosage	Calcitriol: 0.50 to 0.75 µg b.i.d., alfacalcidol: 0.75 to 1.5 µg s.i.d. Phosphate supplementation: 750 to 1600 mg q.i.d.
	Initial phase	Adjust phosphate supplementation for a period of time by 100 mg Goal: peak phosphate [1] within lower 50% of the reference range; laboratory test: every one to four weeks
	Maintenance phase (after 12 to 18 months)	Adjust phosphate supplementation for a period of time by 100 mg Goal: BAP within the reference range Laboratory test: every 3 months Uncontrolled BAP: change the treatment to burosumab
High	Severe SHPT (peak intact PTH $\geq 2 \times$ upper limit of the reference range)	Immediately decrease phosphate supplementation by 100 mg or more Increase active vitamin D (0.25 µg daily for calcitriol and 0.25 to 0.5 µg daily for alfacalcidol) After 1 to 2 weeks, increase phosphate supplementation Uncontrolled severe SHPT: change the treatment to burosumab
High	Development of THPT (hyperparathyroidism with the value of calcium $\geq$ the middle of the reference range)	Immediately quit conventional therapy Initiate allosteric modulation of calcium sensing receptor Try to prevent dehydration Conduct parathyroidectomy for all recognizable glands, otherwise continue allosteric modulation of the calcium sensing receptor in patients with contraindication for surgery Change the treatment to burosumab afterward
High	Overadjustment of peak phosphate within upper 25% of the reference range or over	Immediately decrease phosphate supplementation by 100 mg or more
High	Progression of CKD to eGFR < 45 mL/min/1.73 m^2	Decrease conventional therapy Change the treatment to burosumab in patients who still need phosphate supplementation (uncontrolled BAP with active vitamin D).

[1] Peak phosphate: phosphate level 1 to 2 h after phosphate supplementation.

6.3. Burosumab

Burosumab has been reported to be associated with improvement in persistent pseudofractures and fractures; the results of PROs in adult XLH patients show that most of them were treated with conventional treatment beforehand [7,9,11,19]. Consequently, the initiation of or change to burosumab should be considered among adult XLH patients with severe symptoms (Table 1). In addition, given that burosumab repairs dysfunctional phosphate metabolism in patients with XLH to a physiologically corrected state by counteracting excess action of FGF23, burosumab should not be associated with the development of SHPT/THPT and subsequent progression of CKD. Therefore, initiation of burosumab should also be considered in patients with CKD (e.g., eGFR < 45 mL/min/1.73 m^2), and a change in treatment from conventional therapy to burosumab should be considered among adult XLH patients with uncontrolled severe SHPT or a history of the development of THPT (Table 1). However, medical economic efficacy should always be considered independently for this kind of expensive orphan drug according to the guidelines/recommendations or the health care system of each country [2].

The initial dosage of burosumab for adult XLH patients is decided worldwide to be 1.0 mg/kg body weight (maximum dose of 90 mg) by subcutaneous injection every four weeks, and concomitant use of active vitamin D and phosphate supplementation are not recommended or are prohibited unless other coexisting medical conditions require active vitamin D (e.g., hypoparathyroidism after parathyroidectomy of all parathyroid glands). In the initial phase, the response to burosumab should be confirmed 1 to 2 weeks after the injection (peak phosphate), as the phosphate level returns to baseline four weeks after the last injection (trough phosphate) in a considerable number of patients. Trough phosphate level should be controlled within the lower half of the reference range, and dosage of burosumab should be decreased by 0.2 to 0.3 mg/kg in patients with trough phosphate levels within the higher half of the reference range. Burosumab should be suspended until phosphate values fall below the normal range in the case of phosphate levels over the reference range; treatment may be restarted at approximately half the initial starting dose. Adverse effects tightly associated with the use of burosumab are injection site reactions, and there are no reports of the development of antagonizing antibodies [7,9,11,19].

When no response or only a trivial response is observed at 1 to 2 weeks after injection (peak phosphate), coexisting vitamin D deficiency should be examined by measuring 25OHD. If the patient develops uncontrolled severe SHPT with conventional therapy, and the treatment is changed to burosumab, the response to burosumab (peak phosphate) might improve after 3 to 6 injections, as intact PTH decreases because stimulation of *FGF23* transcription by PTH is alleviated [35]. THPT is also associated with a diminished response to burosumab, and immediate initiation of allosteric modulators of calcium sensing receptors (e.g., cinacalcet, evocalcet) and subsequent parathyroidectomy are recommended along with careful prevention of dehydration. If no response or trivial response to burosumab continues after these problems are ruled out or adequately addressed, changing the treatment to conventional therapy should be considered. Please refer to Table 3 for guidance for burosumab treatment for adults with XLH (Table 3).

Table 3. Suggested guidance for the use of burosumab for adult XLH patients.

Priority	Event	Action
	Initiation of treatment	1.0 mg/kg body weight (up to 90 mg) subcutaneous injection every four weeks Response to burosumab should be confirmed by peak phosphate [1]; Concomitant use of active vitamin D and phosphate supplementation is not recommended or is prohibited unless another medical condition requires it
High	Trough phosphate [2] within the higher half of the reference range	Decrease burosumab dose by 0.2 to 0.3 mg/kg Subsequently, fine tune burosumab dose by 0.1 mg/kg to target trough phosphate within lower half of the reference range
	Trough phosphate over the reference range	Suspend burosumab until phosphate values fall below the normal range Restarted burosumab at approximately half the initial starting dose
	No or trivial response at peak phosphate	Rule out vitamin D deficiency by measuring 25OHD Severe SHPT: continue burosumab 3 to 6 times and confirm improvement in peak phosphate Continuing no response or trivial response after problems above are ruled out or addressed; change treatment to conventional therapy

Table 3. *Cont.*

Priority	Event	Action
High	THPT	Initiate allosteric modulation of the calcium sensing receptor Try to prevent dehydration Conduct parathyroidectomy for all recognizable glands, otherwise continue allosteric modulation of the calcium sensing receptor in patients with contraindication for surgery

[1] Peak phosphate: phosphate level 1 to 2 weeks after the last injection of burosumab. [2] Trough phosphate: phosphate level 4 weeks after the last injection of burosumab.

7. Remaining Problems and Future Research Topics in Adult XLH Patients

The etiology for the development of enthesopathy and early osteoarthritis needs to be elucidated to develop treatment options, as these complications remarkably debilitate ADL and QOL in a large number of adult XLH patients. Associations between the development of severe SHPT or THPT, progression of CKD, the highest dosage, cumulative dosage of phosphate supplementation, and dosage of active vitamin D needs to be elucidated to create more detailed guidelines for conventional therapy. The mode of administration and dosage of burosumab should be reconsidered, as some of adult XLH patients are obviously undertreated with the current dosage (maximum 1.0 mg/kg body weight) and mode of administration (once every four weeks). The effects of burosumab on oral health and the development or progression of osteoarthritis and enthesopathy have been inconclusive, and we are awaiting the results of long-term observational studies. The impact of burosumab on pregnancy and fetal development must also be clarified.

8. Conclusions

The development of burosumab has been a game changer in the treatment of adult XLH patients, as conventional therapy is associated with undertreatment of osteomalacia, the risk of the developing severe SHPT or THPT, and the progression of CKD. However, there are problems remaining to be addressed, specifically among adults with XLH; of these, the complications of debilitating enthesopathy and early osteoarthritis warrant special attention and must be addressed urgently.

Funding: This research received no external funding.

Institutional Review Board Statement: Not applicable.

Informed Consent Statement: Not applicable.

Data Availability Statement: Not applicable.

Conflicts of Interest: N.I. receives research support from Kyowa Kirin Co. Ltd. (Tokyo, Japan).

References

1. Carpenter, T.O.; Imel, E.A.; Holm, I.A.; Jan de Beur, S.M.; Insogna, K.L. A clinician's guide to X-linked hypophosphatemia. *J. Bone Miner. Res.* **2011**, *26*, 1381–1388. [CrossRef] [PubMed]
2. Haffner, D.; Emma, F.; Eastwood, D.M.; Duplan, M.B.; Bacchetta, J.; Schnabel, D.; Wicart, P.; Bockenhauer, D.; Santos, F.; Levtchenko, E.; et al. Clinical practice recommendations for the diagnosis and management of X-linked hypophosphataemia. *Nat. Rev. Nephrol.* **2019**, *15*, 435–455. [CrossRef] [PubMed]
3. Cheung, M.; Roschger, P.; Klaushofer, K.; Veilleux, L.N.; Roughley, P.; Glorieux, F.H.; Rauch, F. Cortical and trabecular bone density in X-linked hypophosphatemic rickets. *J. Clin. Endocrinol. Metab.* **2013**, *98*, E954–E961. [CrossRef] [PubMed]
4. Kato, H.; Koga, M.; Kinoshita, Y.; Taniguchi, Y.; Kobayashi, H.; Fukumoto, S.; Nangaku, M.; Makita, N.; Ito, N. Incidence of Complications in 25 Adult Patients with X-linked Hypophosphatemia. *J. Clin. Endocrinol. Metab.* **2021**, *106*, e3682–e3692. [CrossRef]
5. DeLacey, S.; Liu, Z.; Broyles, A.; El-Azab, S.A.; Guandique, C.F.; James, B.C.; Imel, E.A. Hyperparathyroidism and parathyroidectomy in X-linked hypophosphatemia patients. *Bone* **2019**, *127*, 386–392. [CrossRef] [PubMed]

6. Aono, Y.; Yamazaki, Y.; Yasutake, J.; Kawata, T.; Hasegawa, H.; Urakawa, I.; Fujita, T.; Wada, M.; Yamashita, T.; Fukumoto, S.; et al. Therapeutic effects of anti-FGF23 antibodies in hypophosphatemic rickets/osteomalacia. *J. Bone Miner. Res.* **2009**, *24*, 1879–1888. [CrossRef] [PubMed]
7. Insogna, K.L.; Briot, K.; Imel, E.A.; Kamenický, P.; Ruppe, M.D.; Portale, A.A.; Weber, T.; Pitukcheewanont, P.; Cheong, H.I.; Jan de Beur, S.; et al. A Randomized, Double-Blind, Placebo-Controlled, Phase 3 Trial Evaluating the Efficacy of Burosumab, an Anti-FGF23 Antibody, in Adults with X-Linked Hypophosphatemia: Week 24 Primary Analysis. *J. Bone Miner. Res.* **2018**, *33*, 1383–1393. [CrossRef]
8. Carpenter, T.O.; Whyte, M.P.; Imel, E.A.; Boot, A.M.; Högler, W.; Linglart, A.; Padidela, R.; Van't Hoff, W.; Mao, M.; Chen, C.Y.; et al. Burosumab Therapy in Children with X-Linked Hypophosphatemia. *N. Engl. J. Med.* **2018**, *378*, 1987–1998. [CrossRef]
9. Portale, A.A.; Carpenter, T.O.; Brandi, M.L.; Briot, K.; Cheong, H.I.; Cohen-Solal, M.; Crowley, R.; Jan De Beur, S.; Eastell, R.; Imanishi, Y.; et al. Continued Beneficial Effects of Burosumab in Adults with X-Linked Hypophosphatemia: Results from a 24-Week Treatment Continuation Period after a 24-Week Double-Blind Placebo-Controlled Period. *Calcif. Tissue Res.* **2019**, *105*, 271–284. [CrossRef]
10. Imel, E.A.; Glorieux, F.H.; Whyte, M.P.; Munns, C.F.; Ward, L.M.; Nilsson, O.; Simmons, J.H.; Padidela, R.; Namba, N.; Cheong, H.I.; et al. Burosumab versus conventional therapy in children with X-linked hypophosphataemia: A randomised, active-controlled, open-label, phase 3 trial. *Lancet* **2019**, *393*, 2416–2427. [CrossRef]
11. Briot, K.; Portale, A.A.; Brandi, M.L.; Carpenter, T.O.; Cheong, H.I.; Cohen-Solal, M.; Crowley, R.K.; Eastell, R.; Imanishi, Y.; Ing, S.; et al. Burosumab treatment in adults with X-linked hypophosphataemia: 96-week patient-reported outcomes and ambulatory function from a randomised phase 3 trial and open-label extension. *RMD Open* **2021**, *7*, e001714. [CrossRef] [PubMed]
12. Fukumoto, S.; Ozono, K.; Michigami, T.; Minagawa, M.; Okazaki, R.; Sugimoto, T.; Takeuchi, Y.; Matsumoto, T. Pathogenesis and diagnostic criteria for rickets and osteomalacia—Proposal by an expert panel supported by the Ministry of Health, Labour and Welfare, Japan, the Japanese Society for Bone and Mineral Research, and the Japan Endocrine Society. *J. Bone Miner. Metab.* **2015**, *33*, 467–473. [CrossRef] [PubMed]
13. Ito, N.; Kubota, T.; Kitanaka, S.; Fujiwara, I.; Adachi, M.; Takeuchi, Y.; Yamagami, H.; Kimura, T.; Shinoda, T.; Minagawa, M.; et al. Clinical performance of a novel chemiluminescent enzyme immunoassay for FGF23. *J. Bone Miner. Metab.* **2021**, *39*, 1066–1075. [CrossRef] [PubMed]
14. Kato, H.; Hidaka, N.; Koga, M.; Ogawa, N.; Takahashi, S.; Miyazaki, H.; Nangaku, M.; Makita, N.; Ito, N. Performance evaluation of the new chemiluminescent intact FGF23 assay relative to the existing assay system. *J. Bone Miner. Metab.* **2022**, *40*, 101–108. [CrossRef] [PubMed]
15. Kinoshita, Y.; Saito, T.; Shimizu, Y.; Hori, M.; Taguchi, M.; Igarashi, T.; Fukumoto, S.; Fujita, T. Mutational analysis of patients with FGF23-related hypophosphatemic rickets. *Eur. J. Endocrinol.* **2012**, *167*, 165–172. [CrossRef]
16. Minisola, S.; Peacock, M.; Fukumoto, S.; Cipriani, C.; Pepe, J.; Tella, S.H.; Collins, M.T. Tumour-induced osteomalacia. *Nat. Rev. Dis. Prim.* **2017**, *3*, 17044. [CrossRef]
17. Shimizu, Y.; Tada, Y.; Yamauchi, M.; Okamoto, T.; Suzuki, H.; Ito, N.; Fukumoto, S.; Sugimoto, T.; Fujita, T. Hypophosphatemia induced by intravenous administration of saccharated ferric oxide: Another form of FGF23-related hypophosphatemia. *Bone* **2009**, *45*, 814–816. [CrossRef]
18. Hidaka, N.; Kato, H.; Koga, M.; Katsura, M.; Oyama, Y.; Kinoshita, Y.; Fukumoto, S.; Makita, N.; Nangaku, M.; Ito, N. Induction of FGF23-related hypophosphatemic osteomalacia by alcohol consumption. *Bone Rep.* **2021**, *15*, 101144. [CrossRef]
19. Insogna, K.L.; Rauch, F.; Kamenický, P.; Ito, N.; Kubota, T.; Nakamura, A.; Zhang, L.; Mealiffe, M.; San Martin, J.; Portale, A.A. Burosumab Improved Histomorphometric Measures of Osteomalacia in Adults with X-Linked Hypophosphatemia: A Phase 3, Single-Arm, International Trial. *J. Bone Miner. Res.* **2019**, *34*, 2183–2191. [CrossRef]
20. Veilleux, L.N.; Cheung, M.S.; Glorieux, F.H.; Rauch, F. The muscle-bone relationship in X-linked hypophosphatemic rickets. *J. Clin. Endocrinol. Metab.* **2013**, *98*, E990–E995. [CrossRef]
21. Ito, N.; Fukumoto, S.; Takeuchi, Y.; Takeda, S.; Suzuki, H.; Yamashita, T.; Fujita, T. Effect of acute changes of serum phosphate on fibroblast growth factor (FGF)23 levels in humans. *J. Bone Miner. Metab.* **2007**, *25*, 419–422. [CrossRef] [PubMed]
22. Beck-Nielsen, S.S.; Brusgaard, K.; Rasmussen, L.M.; Brixen, K.; Brock-Jacobsen, B.; Poulsen, M.R.; Vestergaard, P.; Ralston, S.H.; Albagha, O.M.; Poulsen, S.; et al. Phenotype presentation of hypophosphatemic rickets in adults. *Calcif. Tissue Res.* **2010**, *87*, 108–119. [CrossRef] [PubMed]
23. Ye, L.; Liu, R.; White, N.; Alon, U.S.; Cobb, C.M. Periodontal status of patients with hypophosphatemic rickets: A case series. *J. Periodontol.* **2011**, *82*, 1530–1535. [CrossRef] [PubMed]
24. Biosse Duplan, M.; Coyac, B.R.; Bardet, C.; Zadikian, C.; Rothenbuhler, A.; Kamenicky, P.; Briot, K.; Linglart, A.; Chaussain, C. Phosphate and Vitamin D Prevent Periodontitis in X-Linked Hypophosphatemia. *J. Dent. Res.* **2016**, *96*, 388–395. [CrossRef] [PubMed]
25. Connor, J.; Olear, E.A.; Insogna, K.L.; Katz, L.; Baker, S.; Kaur, R.; Simpson, C.A.; Sterpka, J.; Dubrow, R.; Zhang, J.H.; et al. Conventional Therapy in Adults with X-Linked Hypophosphatemia: Effects on Enthesopathy and Dental Disease. *J. Clin. Endocrinol. Metab.* **2015**, *100*, 3625–3632. [CrossRef] [PubMed]
26. Ward, L.M.; Glorieux, F.H.; Whyte, M.P.; Munns, C.F.; Portale, A.A.; Högler, W.; Simmons, J.H.; Gottesman, G.S.; Padidela, R.; Namba, N.; et al. Impact of Burosumab Compared with Conventional Therapy in Younger versus Older Children with X-Linked Hypophosphatemia. *J. Clin. Endocrinol. Metab.* **2022**, dgac296. [CrossRef]

27. Steele, A.; Gonzalez, R.; Garbalosa, J.C.; Steigbigel, K.; Grgurich, T.; Parisi, E.J.; Feinn, R.S.; Tommasini, S.M.; Macica, C.M. Osteoarthritis, Osteophytes, and Enthesophytes Affect Biomechanical Function in Adults with X-linked Hypophosphatemia. *J. Clin. Endocrinol. Metab.* **2020**, *105*, e1798–e1814. [CrossRef]
28. Karaplis, A.C.; Bai, X.; Falet, J.P.; Macica, C.M. Mineralizing enthesopathy is a common feature of renal phosphate-wasting disorders attributed to FGF23 and is exacerbated by standard therapy in hyp mice. *Endocrinology* **2012**, *153*, 5906–5917. [CrossRef]
29. Saito, T.; Shimizu, Y.; Hori, M.; Taguchi, T.; Igarashi, T.; Fukumoto, S.; Fujita, T. A patient with hypophosphatemic rickets and ossification of posterior longitudinal ligament caused by a novel homozygous mutation in ENPP1 gene. *Bone* **2011**, *49*, 913–916. [CrossRef]
30. Kato, H.; Ansh, A.J.; Lester, E.R.; Kinoshita, Y.; Hidaka, N.; Hoshino, Y.; Koga, M.; Taniguchi, Y.; Uchida, T.; Yamaguchi, H.; et al. Identification of ENPP1 Haploinsufficiency in Patients with Diffuse Idiopathic Skeletal Hyperostosis and Early-Onset Osteoporosis. *J. Bone Miner. Res.* **2022**, *37*, 1125–1135. [CrossRef]
31. Ferreira, C.R.; Kintzinger, K.; Hackbarth, M.E.; Botschen, U.; Nitschke, Y.; Mughal, M.Z.; Baujat, G.; Schnabel, D.; Yuen, E.; Gahl, W.A.; et al. Ectopic Calcification and Hypophosphatemic Rickets: Natural History of ENPP1 and ABCC6 Deficiencies. *J. Bone Miner. Res.* **2021**, *36*, 2193–2202. [CrossRef]
32. Bernhard, E.; Nitschke, Y.; Khursigara, G.; Sabbagh, Y.; Wang, Y.; Rutsch, F. A Reference Range for Plasma Levels of Inorganic Pyrophosphate in Children Using the ATP Sulfurylase Method. *J. Clin. Endocrinol. Metab.* **2021**, *107*, 109–118. [CrossRef] [PubMed]
33. Maulding, N.D.; Kavanagh, D.; Zimmerman, K.; Coppola, G.; Carpenter, T.O.; Jue, N.K.; Braddock, D.T. Genetic pathways disrupted by ENPP1 deficiency provide insight into mechanisms of osteoporosis, osteomalacia, and paradoxical mineralization. *Bone* **2020**, *142*, 115656. [CrossRef]
34. Trombetti, A.; Al-Daghri, N.; Brandi, M.L.; Cannata-Andía, J.B.; Cavalier, E.; Chandran, M.; Chaussain, C.; Cipullo, L.; Cooper, C.; Haffner, D.; et al. Interdisciplinary management of FGF23-related phosphate wasting syndromes: A Consensus Statement on the evaluation, diagnosis and care of patients with X-linked hypophosphataemia. *Nat. Rev. Endocrinol.* **2022**, *18*, 366–384. [CrossRef] [PubMed]
35. Ito, N.; Prideaux, M.; Wijenayaka, A.R.; Yang, D.; Ormsby, R.T.; Bonewald, L.F.; Atkins, G.J. Sclerostin Directly Stimulates Osteocyte Synthesis of Fibroblast Growth Factor-23. *Calcif. Tissue Res.* **2021**, *109*, 66–76. [CrossRef] [PubMed]
36. Kubota, T.; Fukumoto, S.; Cheong, H.I.; Michigami, T.; Namba, N.; Ito, N.; Tokunaga, S.; Gibbs, Y.; Ozono, K. Long-term outcomes for Asian patients with X-linked hypophosphataemia: Rationale and design of the SUNFLOWER longitudinal, observational cohort study. *BMJ Open* **2020**, *10*, e036367. [CrossRef] [PubMed]
37. Nakamura, Y.; Takagi, M.; Takeda, R.; Miyai, K.; Hasegawa, Y. Hypertension is a characteristic complication of X-linked hypophosphatemia. *Endocr. J.* **2017**, *64*, 283–289. [CrossRef]
38. Beck-Nielsen, S.S.; Mughal, Z.; Haffner, D.; Nilsson, O.; Levtchenko, E.; Ariceta, G.; de Lucas Collantes, C.; Schnabel, D.; Jandhyala, R.; Mäkitie, O. FGF23 and its role in X-linked hypophosphatemia-related morbidity. *Orphanet J. Rare Dis.* **2019**, *14*, 58. [CrossRef]
39. Skrinar, A.; Dvorak-Ewell, M.; Evins, A.; Macica, C.; Linglart, A.; Imel, E.A.; Theodore-Oklota, C.; San Martin, J. The Lifelong Impact of X-Linked Hypophosphatemia: Results from a Burden of Disease Survey. *J. Endocr. Soc.* **2019**, *3*, 1321–1334. [CrossRef]
40. Seefried, L.; Smyth, M.; Keen, R.; Harvengt, P. Burden of disease associated with X-linked hypophosphataemia in adults: A systematic literature review. *Osteoporos. Int.* **2020**, *32*, 7–22. [CrossRef]
41. Ito, N.; Kang, H.G.; Nishida, Y.; Evins, A.; Skrinar, A.; Cheong, H.I. Burden of disease of X-linked hypophosphatemia in Japanese and Korean patients: A cross-sectional survey. *Endocr. J.* **2022**, *69*, 373–383. [CrossRef] [PubMed]
42. Dahir, K.; Dhaliwal, R.; Simmons, J.; Imel, E.A.; Gottesman, G.S.; Mahan, J.D.; Prakasam, G.; Hoch, A.I.; Ramesan, P.; Díaz-González de Ferris, M. Health Care Transition from Pediatric- to Adult-Focused Care in X-linked Hypophosphatemia: Expert Consensus. *J. Clin. Endocrinol. Metab.* **2021**, *107*, 599–613. [CrossRef]
43. Horn, A.; Wright, J.; Bockenhauer, D.; Van't Hoff, W.; Eastwood, D.M. The orthopaedic management of lower limb deformity in hypophosphataemic rickets. *J. Child. Orthop.* **2017**, *11*, 298–305. [CrossRef] [PubMed]
44. Bettinelli, A.; Bianchi, M.L.; Mazzucchi, E.; Gandolini, G.; Appiani, A.C. Acute effects of calcitriol and phosphate salts on mineral metabolism in children with hypophosphatemic rickets. *J. Pediatr.* **1991**, *118*, 372–376. [CrossRef]
45. Peacock, M.; Bolognese, M.A.; Borofsky, M.; Scumpia, S.; Sterling, L.R.; Cheng, S.; Shoback, D. Cinacalcet treatment of primary hyperparathyroidism: Biochemical and bone densitometric outcomes in a five-year study. *J. Clin. Endocrinol. Metab.* **2009**, *94*, 4860–4867. [CrossRef] [PubMed]

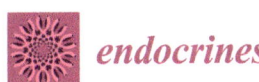

Review

Dental Manifestations and Oral Management of X-Linked Hypophosphatemia

Rena Okawa * and Kazuhiko Nakano

Department of Pediatric Dentistry, Osaka University Graduate School of Dentistry, 1-8 Yamada-oka, Suita 565-0871, Osaka, Japan
* Correspondence: okawa.rena.dent@osaka-u.ac.jp

Abstract: X-linked hypophosphatemia (XLH) is the most common genetic form of rickets and osteomalacia and is characterized by growth retardation, deformities of the lower limbs, and bone and muscular pain. Spontaneous dental abscesses caused by endodontic infections due to dentin dysplasia are well-known dental manifestations. When dentin affected by microcracks or attrition of the enamel is exposed to oral fluids, oral bacteria are able to invade the hypomineralized dentin and pulp space, leading to pulp necrosis, followed by the formation of a periapical gingival abscess. Without appropriate dental management, this dental manifestation results in early loss of teeth and deterioration in the patient's quality of life. Early specific dental intervention and oral management in collaboration with medical personnel are strongly recommended for XLH patients. Importantly, dental manifestations sometimes appear before the diagnosis of XLH. Dentists should be alert for this first sign of XLH and refer affected children to a pediatrician for early diagnosis. A humanized monoclonal antibody for FGF23 (burosumab) is a promising new treatment for XLH; however, the effects on the dental manifestations remain to be elucidated. The establishment of fundamental dental therapy to solve dental problems is still underway and is eagerly anticipated.

Keywords: X-linked hypophosphatemia; dentin dysplasia; pulp infection; periapical abscess; medical and dental collaboration

1. Introduction

X-linked hypophosphatemia (XLH; OMIM# 307800) is the most common genetic form of rickets and osteomalacia and is characterized by growth retardation, deformities of the lower limbs, and bone and muscular pain [1–3]. Sequence variations in the phosphate regulating endopeptidase homolog X-linked (*PHEX*) gene lead to overproduction of fibroblast growth factor 23 (FGF23), resulting in renal phosphate wasting and impaired skeletal mineralization [4]. The incidence of XLH is estimated to be approximately 1 in 20,000 [5].

Spontaneous dental abscesses caused by endodontic infections due to dentin dysplasia are well-known dental manifestations [6–8]. Without appropriate dental management, this dental manifestation of XLH finally results in early loss of teeth and reduced quality of life [9,10]. Early specific dental intervention and ongoing oral management in collaboration with medical professionals are strongly recommended for XLH patients [9,11]. Moreover, this dental manifestation sometimes appears before the diagnosis of XLH [12–14]; dentists should be aware of this first sign of XLH and refer affected children to a pediatrician for early diagnosis.

A combination of active vitamin D and phosphate salts is the conventional medical therapy for patients with XLH [15,16]. A humanized monoclonal antibody for FGF23 (burosumab) is a new and promising treatment for XLH [15–17].

This review summarizes the manifestations and management of XLH from a dental perspective.

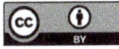

2. Dental Manifestations of XLH

Harris and Sullivan first described dental findings in 1960, after XLH was first reported in 1930 [18]. XLH is caused by loss-of-function sequence variations in *PHEX* [1–3]. *PHEX* sequence variations cause hypophosphatemia indirectly, through the increased expression of FGF23 [4]. A high serum FGF23 concentration impairs renal phosphate reabsorption, thereby increasing phosphate excretion. FGF23 also decreases phosphate absorption in the intestine by suppressing serum 1,25-dyhydroxyvitamin D [1,25(OH)$_2$D] levels. The lack of phosphate leads to a mineralization defect of bone and teeth [7,8,19,20]. *PHEX* protein is also expressed in osteoblasts, osteocytes, and odontoblasts in addition to the kidney [19]. *PHEX* has been proposed to dynamically regulate FGF-23 expression in bone and teeth [20]. The hard mineralized tissue of teeth is composed of enamel, dentin, and cementum [21], and is supported by alveolar bone. Dentin is produced by the mineralization of the organic matrix synthesized and secreted by odontoblasts [22]. Inorganic phosphate and calcium are essential for the mineralization of teeth and bone. Abnormal mineralization of dentin is the main cause of dental problems in XLH patients [23–28].

A spontaneous formation of a periapical gingival abscess or fistula around a visibly healthy tooth with no evidence of dental caries or trauma is a typical dental manifestation of XLH (Figure 1) [6–8]. Owing to microcracks or attrition of the enamel, dentin is exposed to the bacteria abundant in the oral cavity, which invade the hypomineralized dentin and pulp space leading to pulp necrosis and periapical gingival abscess formation (Figure 2) [6–8]. Abscess formation is more commonly found in primary teeth than in permanent teeth [6], possibly because the enamel of primary teeth is half as thick as that of permanent teeth, and less hard, so the dentin is more easily exposed [29,30]. The frequency of occurrence of dental abscesses in children with XLH is reported to range from 25% to 70% [6,19,31–33]. Primary incisors are affected more often than canines, and first and second molars are occasionally involved [6,9]. Teeth in the mandible and maxilla are equally likely to develop an abscess [31]. For XLH, the different expression in the two sexes is not as well-established. The features of XLH are the same in males and females [34]. On the other hand, some reports indicate that XLH is an X-linked dominant disorder and symptoms are mediated by lyonization, and dental manifestations are more severe in male than female individuals, as they also are in bone [7,31]. The dental phenotype is associated with the severity of the disease [35]. The younger the patient when the first abscess appears, the more severe the dental manifestations [13]. An abscess on one tooth indicates that at least one other tooth is likely to be affected [31].

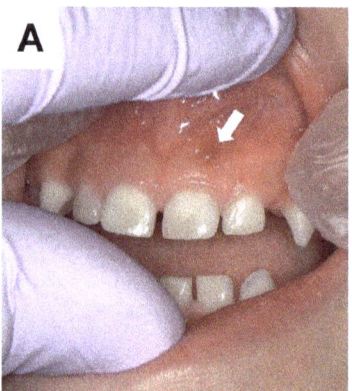 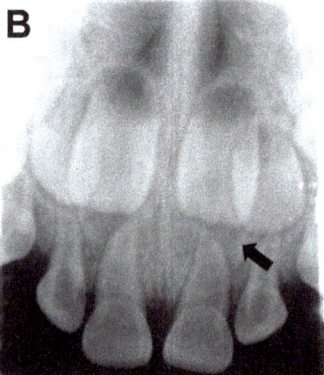

Figure 1. Clinical and radiographic dental manifestations of X-linked hypophosphatemia (XLH). (**A**) Oral photograph of male patient aged 4 years 4 months showing a periapical gingival abscess (white arrow) corresponding to the primary maxillary left central incisor. (**B**) Periapical radiograph showing radiolucency (black arrow) around the periapical region of the primary maxillary left central incisor.

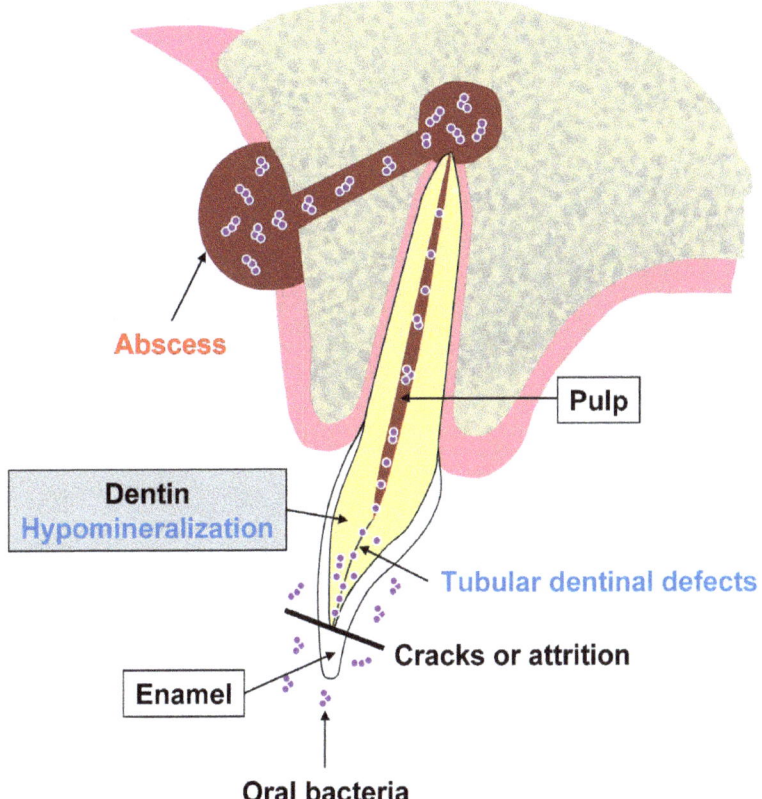

Figure 2. Illustration of the mechanism of gingival abscess formation in a tooth of an X-linked hypophosphatemia (XLH) patient.

The principal dental defects are seen in dentin both radiographically and histologically. Prominent pulp horns, a large pulp chamber suggesting taurodontism, and thin dentin are recognized radiographically (Figure 3) [6–8,13]. A wide predentin layer (the first layer of the non-mineralized matrix), interglobular dentin, and tubular dentinal defects extending from the pulp to the enamel are detected histologically (Figure 4) [6,23–25]. The pulp color can sometimes be observed on the lingual side of the primary incisors due to the thin dentin (Figure 5) [14]. Additionally, an absence of secondary dentin formation in the wall of the pulp chamber after root formation has been reported [36].

The dentin defects found in XLH patients are sometimes accompanied by a thinner layer of enamel [8], although the structure of enamel is normal [7,26]. The thin enamel tends to wear faster and expose the poorly mineralized dentin, leading to pulpal infection [7]. Additionally, delayed eruption, short roots, root resorption, a poorly defined lamina dura, and a hypoplastic alveolar ridge were recognized in a patient with XLH [7]. Whether caries activity is higher in children with XLH compared with healthy subjects is unknown; however, caries progresses easily via the thin enamel and poorly mineralized dentin [7]. Children with XLH often present with delayed dental development, abnormal eruption patterns, and increased frequency of specific malocclusions (Figure 6). An open bite or impacted or ectopic eruption of maxillary canines due to delayed maxillary growth in relation to mandibular growth has been reported [37–39].

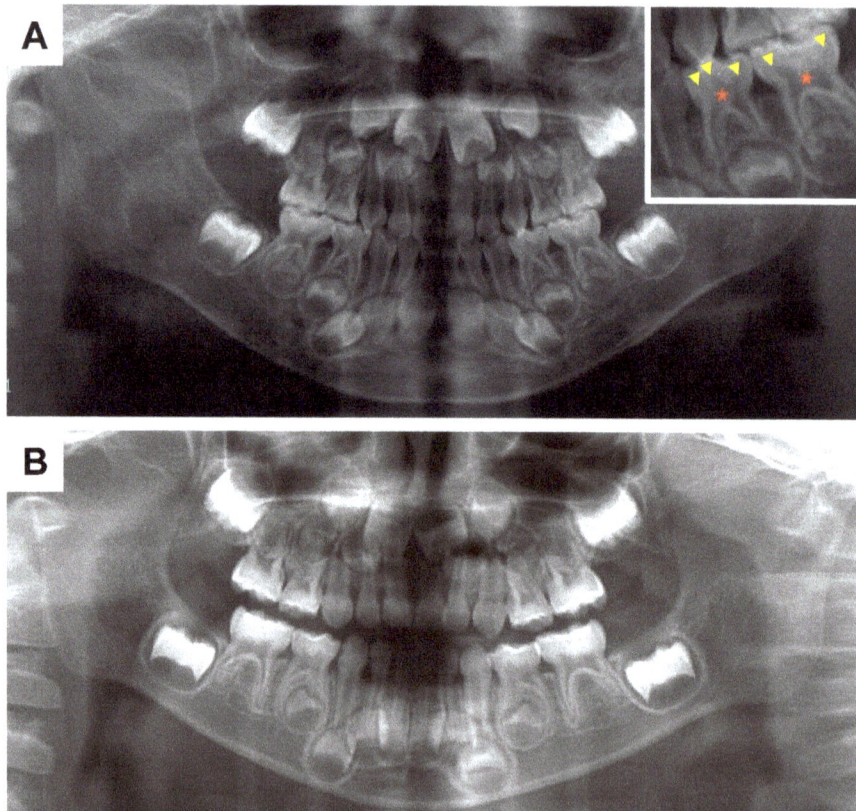

Figure 3. Panoramic radiographs. (**A**) Female X-linked hypophosphatemia (XLH) patient aged 3 years 11 months. The square on the upper right is an enlargement of the primary mandibular left molar region. Wide pulp chambers (asterisks) and prominent pulp horns (arrowheads) can be seen. (**B**) Healthy age-matched female.

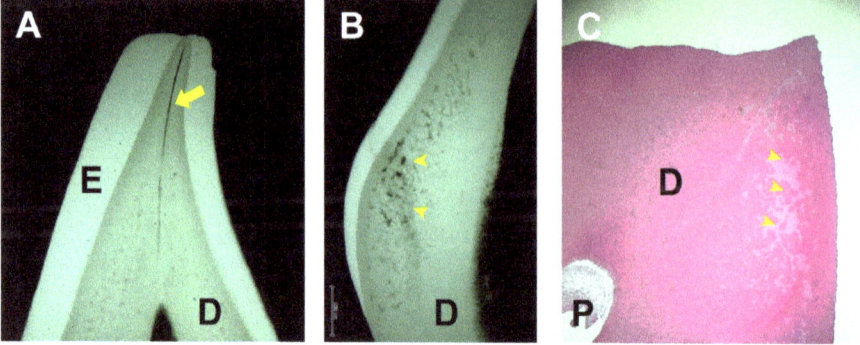

Figure 4. (**A**) Contact microradiograph of a ground section of a primary tooth of a patient with X-linked hypophosphatemia (XLH) showing a tubular defect from the enamel–dentin junction to the pulp (arrow). (**B**) Contact microradiograph of a ground section of a primary tooth of a patient with XLH showing interglobular dentin (arrowheads). (**C**) Histopathological image of a decalcified section of a permanent tooth of a patient with XLH aged 20 years (H-E staining) showing interglobular dentin (arrowheads). E: enamel; D: dentin; P: pulp.

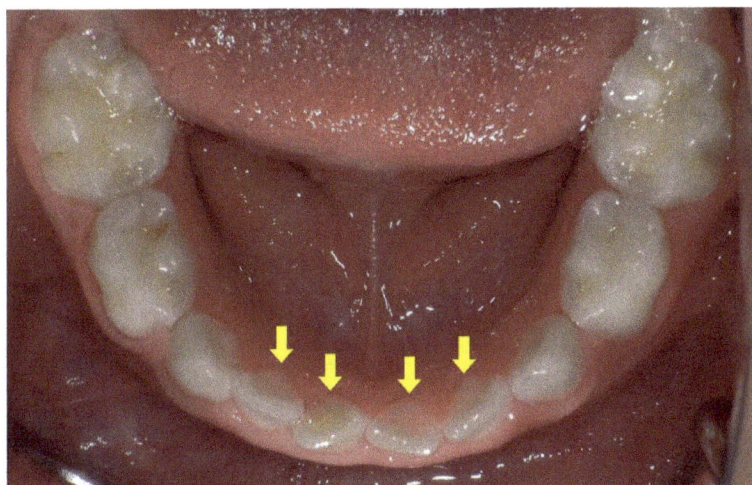

Figure 5. Intraoral photograph of the mandibular arch of a male X-linked hypophosphatemia (XLH) patient aged 3 years 3 months. The pink color of the pulp can be seen through the enamel on the lingual side of the primary mandibular incisors (arrows).

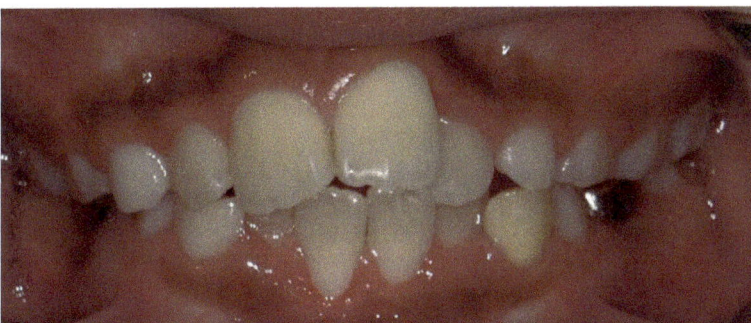

Figure 6. Crowding in the anterior region of a male X-linked hypophosphatemia (XLH) patient aged 10 years 1 month.

Endodontic infections due to poor dentin mineralization are also recognized in permanent teeth [40] (Figure 7). However, maxillofacial cellulitis is rare in adults with XLH [8]. Endodontically affected teeth are common in XLH patients, and the number of affected teeth increases significantly with age [41]. More than 60% of adults with XLH have experienced more than five dental abscesses [42]. The most commonly affected teeth are incisors and canines, followed by molars and premolars [41]. The order in which teeth are affected is determined not only by the time of eruption but also by the rate of natural attrition as a result of mastication [7]. High prevalence and severity of periodontitis are often recognized in adult patients with XLH [43]. Nearly 80% of adult XLH patients are reported to have moderate or severe periodontitis [44]. Periodontitis is a major cause of tooth loss in adults with XLH [8].

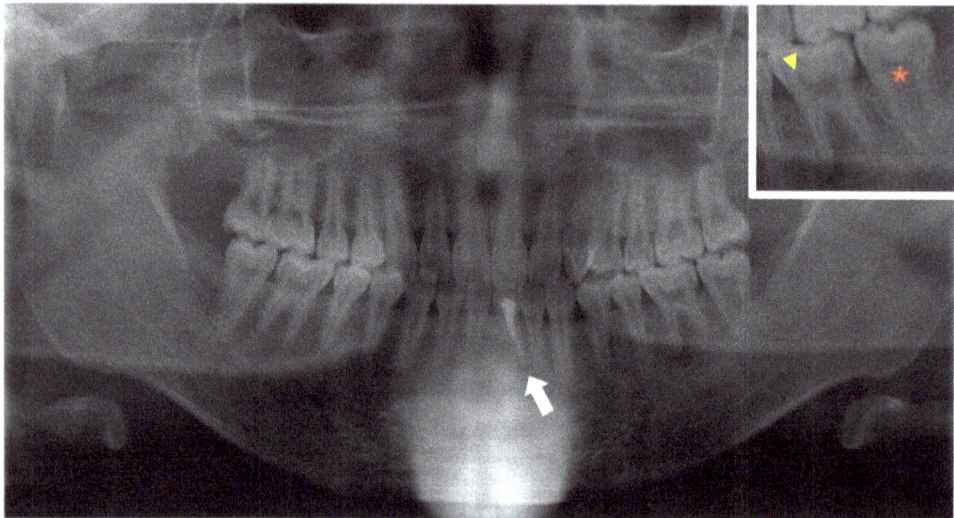

Figure 7. Panoramic radiograph of the permanent dentition of a male X-linked hypophosphatemia (XLH) patient aged 21 years who underwent root canal treatment of the mandibular left central incisor associated with a cystic swelling (arrow). The square on the upper right is an enlargement of the primary mandibular left molar region. Wide pulp chambers (asterisks) and prominent pulp horns (arrowheads) can be seen.

3. Oral Management of XLH

There is no fundamental treatment for dentin dysplasia in XLH. Early detection and management of pulp infection improve the prognosis of the tooth [7,8]. Short-term periodical dental check-ups are required for XLH patients [19,45–47]. The consensus statement of XLH recommends twice-yearly dentist visits [2]. The principle of dental management in XLH patients is to preserve pulp vitality [7]. Professional tooth cleaning, application of topical fluoride, and fissure sealing are recommended [7,13,19,33,45]. Pit and fissure sealing of the enamel is effective in preventing the invasion of oral bacteria [7,8,13,19,45]. Exposed dentin due to attrition or cracking of the enamel should be repaired as soon as possible [14]. The bonding strength of adhesive composite restorations is assumed to be reduced due to mineralization defects in the dentin. Prolonged etching times or a total etch system increases the risk of pulp irritation; therefore, a self-etch system is recommended [13,45].

The crucial purpose of oral management of XLH is to protect vital pulp from being infected by oral bacteria. The vitality of the tooth should be carefully monitored [7]. Early coronal restoration of teeth at high risk is strongly recommended, especially in patients who are diagnosed early with many abscesses [35]. Composite resin crowns in the anterior region, stainless steel crowns for primary teeth and immature permanent teeth, and permanent crowns for permanent teeth in the posterior region are recommended [35,48,49]. Full ceramic crowns should be avoided because of the extensive tooth reduction required when compared with metal crowns [7]. Large pulp chambers and prominent pulp horns should be considered during the preparation of the tooth to prevent exposure or irritation of the pulp [7,13].

When apical periodontitis is detected, a periapical radiograph is taken, and the dentist must decide whether to perform endodontic treatment or extract the tooth. Systemic antibiotics are used in cases of acute abscess [8]. Primary teeth play an important role as space maintainers for permanent successors, and dentists should preserve them for as long as possible until replacement [50]. Early extraction before replacement leads to loss of space for the eruption of permanent teeth [50]. Space maintenance is necessary after the extraction of primary teeth before replacement [50]. Obturation of the root canal system in XLH patients should aim to fill any voids to achieve maximal density, due to the increased risk of reinfection of the root canal because of dentin dysplasia [7]. The use of thermoplasticized techniques using a virtually insoluble sealer is recommended for permanent teeth [7]. Working length should be determined accurately, taking into account the short roots commonly found in XLH patients [7]. In contrast, for primary teeth, the use of calcium hydroxide and iodoform ($Ca(OH)_2$/iodoform), which are absorbed during root resorption, is recommended [51]. Additionally, for permanent teeth undergoing root formation, $Ca(OH)_2$ or mineral trioxide aggregate (MTA) is recommended before obturation to promote apexification [7,52,53].

Once the pulp starts to become necrotic, the blood supply stops, and the devitalized tooth tends to break down [54]. Teeth with broken roots are indicated for extraction [55]. Prosthetic crowns are necessary for teeth that have undergone root canal treatment (Figure 8). The thin dentin perforates easily and does not support restorative posts for prosthetic crowns in permanent teeth [7,13]. The application of posts in the roots should be avoided to prevent root fracture [7,13].

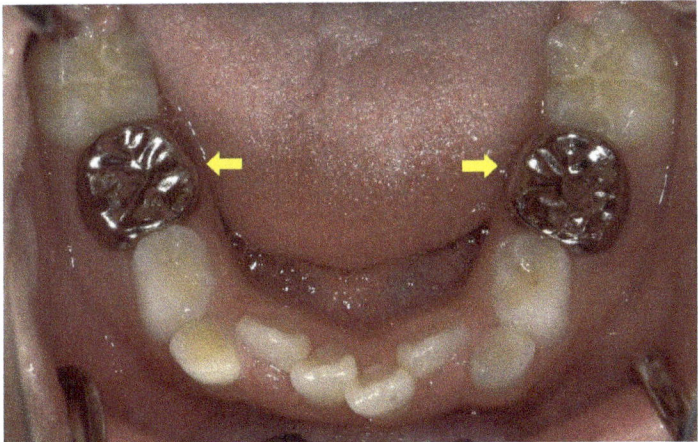

Figure 8. Treatment of a male X-linked hypophosphatemia (XLH) patient aged 8 years 3 months involved full coverage of the primary mandibular second molars with stainless steel crowns (arrows) after root canal treatment associated with a cystic swelling.

There is no established orthodontic treatment for XLH patients [56]. Traumatic orthodontic forces sometimes cause pulp necrosis [46]. It is important to prevent traumatic forces during orthodontic treatment of XLH patients. Orthodontic treatment involves the movement of teeth and extensive remodeling of the alveolar bone [8]. This treatment sometimes results in the loss of permanent teeth in XLH patients with uncontrolled rickets of the jaw [57]. Optimizing conventional medical treatment of XLH is considered mandatory before the initiation of orthodontic treatment [2,8]. A longer period of retention and observation is necessary in cases with abnormal bone remodeling to confirm the stability of the resulting occlusion [58]. The high frequency of permanent tooth loss secondary to endodontic infections or periodontitis often leads to the need for dental implants [2]. Several reports have described cases of XLH patients who have had dental implants [46,59]. Standard surgical protocols in adults with XLH who are not receiving conventional therapy resulted in a decreased success rate compared with healthy control individuals [2]. Some studies reported that the interruption of conventional therapy in XLH may have a negative influence on bone healing around implants [8]. Dental implant surgery should be performed after 3–6 months of medical treatment, which should be continued for 6 months following the implant surgery [2]. The healing time should be extended up to 6 months [2].

4. Dental Effects of Conventional Therapy or Burosumab in XLH

The conventional medical therapy of XLH has consisted of oral phosphate and active vitamin D supplementation [15,16]. However, this therapy has certain limitations related to efficacy and safety [15]. A humanized monoclonal antibody for FGF23 (burosumab) was recently approved as a promising treatment for XLH [15–17].

Early intervention with conventional therapy is reported to have a beneficial effect on dental status [60–66]. The missing and filled teeth index of patients treated since early childhood is similar to that of the healthy, age-matched controls [62]. This therapy improves dentin mineralization and formation, reducing the size of the dental pulp canal and chamber in both the primary and permanent dentitions [8,62]. Dentin mineralization of permanent teeth especially, which mineralize after birth, can be restored by the treatment [65]. The primary dentition usually shows more severe symptoms than the permanent dentition [64]. This can also be explained by the low levels of calcium and phosphorus during odontogenesis of the primary dentition [64]. However, this therapy cannot completely eliminate dentin dysplasia [67]. Remaining defects may result from the early exposure of odontoblasts and the surrounding osteoblasts to hypophosphatemia before the commencement of conventional therapy, and from intrinsic cell disturbances linked to the genetic alteration [62]. Additionally, unlike bone, dentin is not remodeled and is not involved in the regulation of calcium and phosphate metabolism [22]. The effects of burosumab on the dentition of XLH patients has not yet been reported. A post hoc analysis of a 64-week, open-label, randomized controlled study of 61 children with XLH aged 1–12 years revealed that dental abscesses occurred in 3 of 12 (25%) younger (<5 years) children in the conventional therapy group, while 0 of 20 (0%) younger children from the burosumab group developed dental abscesses [68]. However, in older children (5–12 years) with XLH, dental abscesses presented more frequently with burosumab (8/15, 53%) than with conventional therapy (0/20, 0%). Dental caries, which were reported more frequently in the burosumab group (9/29, 31%) than the conventional therapy group (2/32, 6%), occurred slightly more often in older than younger children who received conventional therapy (2/20, 10% vs. 0/12, 0%), and slightly more often in younger than older children who received burosumab (5/14, 36% vs. 4/15, 27%). On the basis of the results of this study, the protective effects of burosumab seem to be weaker, or at least not more intense, against the development of dental abscesses compared with conventional therapy; however, a longer duration study is needed.

5. Importance of Medical and Dental Collaboration in XLH

Without appropriate dental management, spontaneous periapical gingival abscess formation in XLH patients finally leads to early loss of teeth and a reduced quality of life [10,32]. Early oral management soon after diagnosis and follow-up throughout life by dentists are recommended for XLH patients [19,45–47]. There is a need for a system in which medical doctors explain the importance of oral care to parents of children with XLH and ensure they find appropriate dental care [2]. The alveolar bone status is particularly important when XLH patients receive orthodontic treatment or dental implants [2]. Dentists should consult with the patient's medical doctor about the status of rickets control with medical treatment [2,8].

Primary incisors emerge into the oral cavity at around 6 months of age, and the primary dentition is complete by the age of 2 years [69]. Most XLH patients are diagnosed at approximately 1–2 years of age when their delayed walking or bowed legs are observed by pediatricians [3,70]. Spontaneous periapical abscesses sometimes lead to an XLH diagnosis [12–14]. Pediatric dentists must never overlook dental abscesses in teeth that appear to be intact. A system should be established by which dentists can immediately refer patients to pediatricians when this first dental sign of XLH is observed.

6. Conclusions

Renal phosphate wasting in XLH leads to a mineralization defect of teeth, but not bone [1–3]. The main dental manifestations are periapical gingival abscesses, which are derived from endodontic infections caused by poorly mineralized dentin [6–8]. Medical and dental collaboration is important in the treatment of XLH, and dental symptoms should be followed-up as the patient ages [1–3,8,9]. The establishment of fundamental dental therapy to treat dental manifestations is still underway and is eagerly anticipated.

Funding: This research received no external funding.

Institutional Review Board Statement: Not applicable.

Informed Consent Statement: Written informed consent has been obtained from the parents of patients or patients to publish the accompanying images.

Data Availability Statement: Not applicable.

Conflicts of Interest: The authors declare no conflict of interest.

References

1. Carpenter, T.O.; Imel, E.A.; Holm, I.A.; Jan de Beur, S.M.; Insogna, K.L. A clinician's guide to X-linked hypophosphatemia. *J. Bone Miner. Res.* **2011**, *26*, 1381–1388. [CrossRef] [PubMed]
2. Haffner, D.; Emma, F.; Eastwood, D.M.; Duplan, M.B.; Bacchetta, J.; Schnabel, D.; Wicart, P.; Bockenhauer, D.; Santos, F.; Levtchenko, E.; et al. Clinical practice recommendations for the diagnosis and management of X-linked hypophosphataemia. *Nat. Rev. Nephrol.* **2019**, *15*, 435–455. [CrossRef] [PubMed]
3. Dahir, K.; Roberts, M.S.; Krolczyk, S.; Simmons, J.H. X-Linked Hypophosphatemia: A New Era in Management. *J. Endocr. Soc.* **2020**, *4*, bvaa151. [CrossRef] [PubMed]
4. Nakanishi, T.; Michigami, T. Pathogenesis of FGF23-Related Hypophosphatemic Diseases Including X-linked Hypophosphatemia. *Endocrines* **2022**, *3*, 303–316. [CrossRef]
5. Endo, I.; Fukumoto, S.; Ozono, K.; Namba, N.; Inoue, D.; Okazaki, R.; Yamauchi, M.; Sugimoto, T.; Minagawa, M.; Michigami, T.; et al. Nationwide survey of fibroblast growth factor 23 (FGF23)-related hypophosphatemic diseases in Japan: Prevalence, biochemical data and treatment. *Endocr. J.* **2015**, *62*, 811–816. [CrossRef]
6. Goodman, J.R.; Gelbier, M.J.; Bennett, J.H.; Winter, G.B. Dental problems associated with hypophosphataemic vitamin D resistant rickets. *Int. J. Paediatr. Dent.* **1998**, *8*, 19–28. [CrossRef]
7. Sabandal, M.M.; Robotta, P.; Bürklein, S.; Schäfer, E. Review of the dental implications of X-linked hypophosphataemic rickets (XLHR). *Clin. Oral Investig.* **2015**, *19*, 759–768. [CrossRef]
8. Duplan, M.B.; Norcy, E.L.; Courson, F.; Chaussain, C. Dental and periodontal features and management in XLH children and adults. *Int. J. Bone Frag.* **2021**, *1*, 74–79. [CrossRef]
9. Baroncelli, G.I.; Mora, S. X-Linked Hypophosphatemic Rickets: Multisystemic Disorder in Children Requiring Multidisciplinary Management. *Front. Endocrinol.* **2021**, *12*, 688309. [CrossRef]
10. Nguyen, C.; Celestin, E.; Chambolle, D.; Linglart, A.; Biosse Duplan, M.; Chaussain, C.; Friedlander, L. Oral health-related quality of life in patients with X-linked hypophosphatemia: A qualitative exploration. *Endocr. Connect.* **2022**, *11*, e210564. [CrossRef]
11. Trombetti, A.; Al-Daghri, N.; Brandi, M.L.; Cannata-Andía, J.B.; Cavalier, E.; Chandran, M.; Chaussain, C.; Cipullo, L.; Cooper, C.; Haffner, D.; et al. Interdisciplinary management of FGF23-related phosphate wasting syndromes: A Consensus Statement on the evaluation, diagnosis and care of patients with X-linked hypophosphataemia. *Nat. Rev. Endocrinol.* **2022**, *18*, 366–384. [CrossRef] [PubMed]
12. Archard, H.O.; Witkop, C.J. Hereditary hypophosphatemia (vitamin D-resistant rickets) presenting primary dental manifestations. *Oral Surg.* **1966**, *22*, 184–193. [CrossRef]
13. Batra, P.; Tejani, Z.; Mars, M. X-linked hypophosphatemia: Dental and histologic findings. *J. Can. Dent. Assoc.* **2006**, *72*, 69–72. [PubMed]
14. Wato, K.; Okawa, R.; Matayoshi, S.; Ogaya, Y.; Nomura, R.; Nakano, K. X-linked hypophosphatemia diagnosed after identification of dental symptoms. *Ped. Dent. J.* **2020**, *30*, 115–119. [CrossRef]
15. Kinoshita, Y.; Fukumoto, S. X-Linked Hypophosphatemia and FGF23-Related Hypophosphatemic Diseases: Prospect for New Treatment. *Endocr. Rev.* **2018**, *39*, 274–291. [CrossRef]
16. Tajima, T.; Hasegawa, Y. Treatment of X-Linked Hypophosphatemia in Children. *Endocrines* **2022**, *3*, 522–529. [CrossRef]
17. Fukumoto, S. FGF23-related hypophosphatemic rickets/osteomalacia: Diagnosis and new treatment. *J. Mol. Endocrinol.* **2021**, *66*, R57–R65. [CrossRef]
18. Harris, R.; Sullivan, H.R. Dental Sequelae in Deciduous Dentition in Vitamin D Resistant Rickets. *Aust. Dent. J.* **1960**, *5*, 200–203. [CrossRef]

19. Baroncelli, G.I.; Angiolini, M.; Ninni, E.; Galli, V.; Saggese, R.; Giuca, M.R. Prevalence and pathogenesis of dental and periodontal lesions in children with X-linked hypophosphatemic rickets. *Eur. J. Paediatr. Dent.* **2006**, *7*, 61–66.
20. Robinson, M.E.; AlQuorain, H.; Murshed, M.; Rauch, F. Mineralized tissues in hypophosphatemic rickets. *Pediatr. Nephrol.* **2020**, *35*, 1843–1854. [CrossRef]
21. Chavez, M.B.; Kramer, K.; Chu, E.Y.; Thumbigere-Math, V.; Foster, B.L. Insights into dental mineralization from three heritable mineralization disorders. *J. Struct. Biol.* **2020**, *212*, 107597. [CrossRef]
22. Vital, S.O.; Gaucher, C.; Bardet, C.; Rowe, P.S.; George, A.; Linglart, A.; Chaussain, C. Tooth dentin defects reflect genetic disorders affecting bone mineralization. *Bone* **2012**, *50*, 989–997. [CrossRef] [PubMed]
23. Abe, K.; Ooshima, T.; Lily, T.S.; Yasufuku, Y.; Sobue, S. Structural deformities of deciduous teeth in patients with hypophosphatemic vitamin D-resistant rickets. *Oral Surg. Oral Med. Oral Pathol.* **1988**, *65*, 191–198. [CrossRef]
24. Abe, K.; Ooshima, T.; Sobue, S.; Moriwaki, Y. The crystallinity of human deciduous teeth in hypophosphataemic vitamin D-resistant rickets. *Arch. Oral Biol.* **1989**, *34*, 365–372. [CrossRef]
25. Abe, K.; Ooshima, T.; Masatomi, Y.; Sobue, S.; Moriwaki, Y. Microscopic and crystallographic examinations of the teeth of the X-linked hypophosphatemic mouse. *J. Dent. Res.* **1989**, *68*, 1519–1524. [CrossRef] [PubMed]
26. Ribeiro, T.R.; Costa, F.W.; Soares, E.C.; Williams, J.R., Jr.; Fonteles, C.S. Enamel and dentin mineralization in familial hypophosphatemic rickets: A micro-CT study. *Dentomaxillofac. Radiol.* **2015**, *44*, 20140347. [CrossRef]
27. Coyac, B.R.; Falgayrac, G.; Penel, G.; Schmitt, A.; Schinke, T.; Linglart, A.; McKee, M.D.; Chaussain, C.; Bardet, C. Impaired mineral quality in dentin in X-linked hypophosphatemia. *Connect. Tissue Res.* **2018**, *59*, 91–96. [CrossRef]
28. Clayton, D.; Chavez, M.B.; Tan, M.H.; Kolli, T.N.; Giovani, P.A.; Hammersmith, K.J.; Bowden, S.A.; Foster, B.L. Mineralization Defects in the Primary Dentition Associated With X-Linked Hypophosphatemic Rickets. *JBMR Plus* **2021**, *5*, e10463. [CrossRef]
29. De Menezes Oliveira, M.A.; Torres, C.P.; Gomes-Silva, J.M.; Chinelatti, M.A.; De Menezes, F.C.; Palma-Dibb, R.G.; Borsatto, M.C. Microstructure and mineral composition of dental enamel of permanent and deciduous teeth. *Microsc. Res. Tech.* **2010**, *73*, 572–577. [CrossRef]
30. Johansson, A.K.; Sorvari, R.; Birkhed, D.; Meurman, J.H. Dental erosion in deciduous teeth—An in vivo and in vitro study. *J. Dent.* **2001**, *29*, 333–340. [CrossRef]
31. McWhorter, A.G.; Seale, N.S. Prevalence of dental abscess in a population of children with vitamin D-resistant rickets. *Pediatr. Dent.* **1991**, *13*, 91–96.
32. Baroncelli, G.I.; Zampollo, E.; Manca, M.; Toschi, B.; Bertelloni, S.; Michelucci, A.; Isola, A.; Bulleri, A.; Peroni, D.; Giuca, M.R. Pulp chamber features, prevalence of abscesses, disease severity, and PHEX mutation in X-linked hypophosphatemic rickets. *J. Bone Miner. Metab.* **2021**, *39*, 212–223. [CrossRef] [PubMed]
33. Marin, A.; Morales, P.; Jiménez, M.; Borja, E.; Ivanovic-Zuvic, D.; Collins, M.T.; Florenzano, P. Characterization of Oral Health Status in Chilean Patients with X-Linked Hypophosphatemia. *Calcif. Tissue Int.* **2021**, *109*, 132–138. [CrossRef] [PubMed]
34. Ruppe, M.D. X-Linked Hypophosphatemia. *GeneReviews®*, 9 Feberuary 2012. University of Washington, Seattle, 1993–2022. Available online: https://www.ncbi.nlm.nih.gov/books/NBK83985/ (accessed on 13 April 2017).
35. Seow, W.K.; Romaniuk, K.; Sclavos, S. Micromorphologic features of dentin in vitamin D-resistant rickets: Correlation with clinical grading of severity. *Pediatr. Dent.* **1989**, *11*, 203–208. [PubMed]
36. Rakocz, M.; Keating, J.; Johnson, R. Management of the primary dentition in vitamin D-resistant rickets. *Oral Surg. Oral Med. Oral Pathol.* **1982**, *54*, 166–171. [CrossRef]
37. Seow, W.K.; Needleman, H.L.; Holm, I.A. Effect of familial hypophosphatemic rickets on dental development: A controlled, longitudinal study. *Pediatr. Dent.* **1995**, *17*, 346–350.
38. Al-Jundi, S.H.; Dabous, I.M.; Al-Jamal, G.A. Craniofacial morphology in patients with hypophosphataemic vitamin-D-resistant rickets: A cephalometric study. *J. Oral Rehabil.* **2009**, *36*, 483–490. [CrossRef]
39. Souza, M.A.; Junior, L.A.S.; Santos, M.A.; Vaisbich, M.H. Dental abnormalities and oral health in patients with Hypophosphatemic rickets. *Clinics* **2010**, *65*, 1023–1026. [CrossRef]
40. Murayama, T.; Iwatsubo, R.; Akiyama, S.; Amano, A.; Morisaki, I. Familial hypophosphatemic vitamin D-resistant rickets: Dental findings and histologic study of teeth. *Oral Surg. Oral Med. Oral Pathol. Oral Radiol. Endod.* **2000**, *90*, 310–316.
41. Andersen, M.G.; Beck-Nielsen, S.S.; Haubek, D.; Hintze, H.; Gjørup, H.; Poulsen, S. Periapical and endodontic status of permanent teeth in patients with hypophosphatemic rickets. *J. Oral Rehabil.* **2012**, *39*, 144–150. [CrossRef]
42. Connor, J.; Olear, E.A.; Insogna, K.L.; Katz, L.; Baker, S.; Kaur, R.; Simpson, C.A.; Sterpka, J.; Dubrow, R.; Zhang, J.H.; et al. Conventional Therapy in Adults With X-Linked Hypophosphatemia: Effects on Enthesopathy and Dental Disease. *J. Clin. Endocrinol. Metab.* **2015**, *100*, 3625–3632. [CrossRef] [PubMed]
43. Ye, L.; Liu, R.; White, N.; Alon, U.S.; Cobb, C.M. Periodontal status of patients with hypophosphatemic rickets: A case series. *J. Periodontol.* **2011**, *82*, 1530–1535. [CrossRef] [PubMed]
44. Duplan, M.B.; Coyac, B.R.; Bardet, C.; Zadikian, C.; Rothenbuhler, A.; Kamenicky, P.; Briot, K.; Linglart, A.; Chaussain, C. Phosphate and Vitamin D Prevent Periodontitis in X-Linked Hypophosphatemia. *J. Dent. Res.* **2017**, *96*, 388–395. [CrossRef]
45. Douyere, D.; Joseph, C.; Gaucher, C.; Chaussain, C.; Courson, F. Familial hypophosphatemic vitamin D-resistant rickets—Prevention of spontaneous dental abscesses on primary teeth: A case report. *Oral Surg. Oral Med. Oral Pathol. Oral Radiol. Endod.* **2009**, *107*, 525–530. [CrossRef] [PubMed]

46. Lee, B.N.; Jung, H.Y.; Chang, H.S.; Hwang, Y.C.; Hwang, I.N.; Oh, W.M. Dental management of patients with X-linked hypophosphatemia. *Restor. Dent. Endod.* **2017**, *42*, 146–151. [CrossRef] [PubMed]
47. Akif, D.; Tuba, A.A.; Esra, E.; Tulga, Ö.F. Dental Management of Hypophosphatemic Vitamin D Resistant Rickets. *J. Pediatr. Res.* **2018**, *5*, 221–224.
48. Breen, G.H. Prophylactic dental treatment for a patient with vitamin D-resistant rickets: Report of case. *ASDC J. Dent. Child.* **1986**, *53*, 38–43.
49. Seow, W.K.; Latham, S.C. The spectrum of dental manifestations in vitamin D-resistant rickets: Implications for management. *Pediatr. Dent.* **1986**, *8*, 245–250.
50. Laing, E.; Ashley, P.; Farhad, B.N.; Dalgit, S.G. Space maintenance. *Int. J. Pediatr. Dent.* **2009**, *19*, 155–162. [CrossRef]
51. Mortazavi, M.; Mesbahi, M. Comparison of zinc oxide and eugenol, and Vitapex for root canal treatment of necrotic primary teeth. *Int. J. Pediatr. Dent.* **2004**, *14*, 417–424. [CrossRef]
52. Lee, J.S. Ca(OH)$_2$ apexification of pulp necroses of the permanent incisors in a case of X-linked hypophosphataemic rickets—The 60-month check-up: A case report. *Ped. Dent. J.* **2021**, *31*, 112–116. [CrossRef]
53. Bradley, H.; Dutta, A.; Philpott, R. Presentation and non-surgical endodontic treatment of two patients with X-linked hypophosphatemia: A case report. *Int. Endod. J.* **2021**, *54*, 1403–1414. [CrossRef] [PubMed]
54. Rosen, E.; Beitlitum, I.; Tsesis, I. The preservation of teeth with root-originated fractures. *Evid. Based Endod.* **2018**, *3*, 2. [CrossRef]
55. Yoshino, K.; Ito, K.; Kuroda, M.; Sugihara, N. Prevalence of vertical root fracture as the reason for tooth extraction in dental clinics. *Clin. Oral Investig.* **2015**, *19*, 1405–1409. [CrossRef] [PubMed]
56. Makrygiannakis, M.A.; Dastoori, M.; Athanasiou, A.E. Orthodontic treatment of a nine-year-old patient with hypophosphatemic rickets diagnosed since the age of two: A case report. *Int. Orthod.* **2020**, *18*, 648–656. [CrossRef] [PubMed]
57. Gibson, C.; Mubeen, S.; Evans, R. X-linked hypophosphatemic rickets: Orthodontic considerations and management. A case report. *J. Orthod.* **2022**, *49*, 205–212. [CrossRef]
58. Kawakami, M.; Takano-Yamamoto, T. Orthodontic treatment of a patient with hypophosphatemic vitamin D-resistant rickets. *ASDC J. Dent. Child.* **1997**, *64*, 395–399.
59. Resnick, D. Implant placement and guided tissue regeneration in a patient with congenital vitamin D-resistant rickets. *J. Oral Implantol.* **1998**, *24*, 214–218. [CrossRef]
60. Larmas, M.; Hietala, E.L.; Similä, S.; Pajari, U. Oral manifestations of familial hypophosphatemic rickets after phosphate supplement therapy: A review of the literature and report of case. *ASDC J. Dent. Child.* **1991**, *58*, 328–334.
61. Seow, W.K. The effect of medical therapy on dentin formation in vitamin D-resistant rickets. *Pediatr. Dent.* **1991**, *13*, 97–102.
62. Chaussain-Miller, C.; Sinding, C.; Wolikow, M.; Lasfargues, J.J.; Godeau, G.; Garabédian, M. Dental abnormalities in patients with familial hypophosphatemic vitamin D-resistant rickets: Prevention by early treatment with 1-hydroxyvitamin D. *J. Pediatr.* **2003**, *142*, 324–331. [CrossRef] [PubMed]
63. Chaussain-Miller, C.; Sinding, C.; Septier, D.; Wolikow, M.; Goldberg, M.; Garabedian, M. Dentin structure in familial hypophosphatemic rickets: Benefits of vitamin D and phosphate treatment. *Oral Dis.* **2007**, *13*, 482–489. [CrossRef] [PubMed]
64. Beltes, C.; Zachou, E. Endodontic management in a patient with vitamin D-resistant Rickets. *J. Endod.* **2012**, *38*, 255–258. [CrossRef] [PubMed]
65. Linglart, A.; Biosse-Duplan, M.; Briot, K.; Chaussain, C.; Esterle, L.; Guillaume-Czitrom, S.; Kamenicky, P.; Nevoux, J.; Prié, D.; Rothenbuhler, A.; et al. Therapeutic management of hypophosphatemic rickets from infancy to adulthood. *Endocr. Connect.* **2014**, *3*, R13–R30. [CrossRef]
66. Econs, M.J. Conventional Therapy in Adults With XLH Improves Dental Manifestations, But Not Enthesopathy. *J. Clin. Endocrinol. Metab.* **2015**, *100*, 3622–3624. [CrossRef]
67. Okawa, R.; Hamada, M.; Takagi, M.; Matayoshi, S.; Nakano, K. A Case of X-Linked Hypophosphatemic Rickets with Dentin Dysplasia in Mandibular Third Molars. *Children* **2022**, *9*, 1304. [CrossRef]
68. Ward, L.M.; Glorieux, F.H.; Whyte, M.P.; Munns, C.F.; Portale, A.A.; Högler, W.; Simmons, J.H.; Gottesman, G.S.; Padidela, R.; Namba, N.; et al. Effect of Burosumab Compared With Conventional Therapy on Younger vs Older Children With X-linked Hypophosphatemia. *J. Clin. Endocrinol. Metab.* **2022**, *107*, e3241–e3253. [CrossRef]
69. Schour, I.; Massler, M. The development of the human dentition. *J. Am. Dent. Assoc.* **1941**, *28*, 1153–1160.
70. Petje, G.; Meizer, R.; Radler, C.; Aigner, N.; Grill, F. Deformity correction in children with hereditary hypophosphatemic rickets. *Clin. Orthop. Relat. Res.* **2008**, *466*, 3078–3085. [CrossRef]

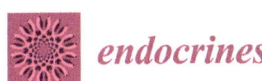

Review

X-Linked Hypophosphatemia Transition and Team Management

Takuo Kubota

Department of Pediatrics, Graduate School of Medicine, Osaka University, 2-2 Yamadaoka, Suita, Osaka 565-0871, Japan; tkubota@ped.med.osaka-u.ac.jp

Abstract: X-linked hypophosphatemia (XLH) is the most common form of inherited disorders that are characterized by renal phosphate wasting, but it is a rare chronic disease. XLH presents in multisystemic organs, not only in childhood, but also in adulthood. Multidisciplinary team management is necessary for the care of patients with XLH. Although XLH has often been perceived as a childhood disease, recent studies have demonstrated that it is a long-term and progressive disease throughout adulthood. In the past 20 years, the importance of the transition from pediatric care to adult care for patient outcomes in adulthood in many pediatric onset diseases has been increasingly recognized. This review describes transitional care and team management for patients with XLH.

Keywords: X-linked hypophosphatemia; transition; team management; transfer

1. Introduction

X-linked hypophosphatemia (XLH) is the most common form of inherited disorders that are characterized by renal phosphate wasting. XLH presents with a number of symptoms, not only in childhood, but also in adulthood. Despite the long-term and progressive disease burden continuing to adulthood, XLH is often perceived as a rare childhood disease [1–3]. A lack of recognition of the symptoms and signs of XLH in adulthood delays adequate intervention. Although the clinical manifestations of XLH may persist or recur in later life, standard clinical practice involves the discontinuation of conventional treatment when skeletal growth is completed. This is due to limited evidence for the benefits of continuing conventional treatment into adulthood [3,4]. The resumption of treatment based on symptoms results in gaps in care. Seamless follow-ups are needed. Moreover, since XLH presents in a number of organs, the multidisciplinary management of patients with XLH is essential to improve health outcomes. Therefore, appropriate transition is critical for patients with XLH. This review describes transitional care and team management for patients with XLH.

2. Team Management

XLH is a multisystem disorder with musculoskeletal and non-musculoskeletal complications (Table 1). The musculoskeletal complications of XLH include rickets, impaired growth, bone deformities, osteomalacia, bone pain, pseudofractures, enthesopathies, osteoarthritis, dental abscesses, muscle weakness, and gait abnormalities [5–7]. Non-musculoskeletal symptoms include delayed motor development, Chiari malformation, a diminished quality of life, and hearing loss. Several manifestations are more specific to either children or adults. Growth retardation, craniosynostosis, rickets, and delayed motor development are observed in children with XLH, whereas pseudofractures, osteoarthritis, extraosseous calcification—including enthesopathy and spinal stenosis, hearing loss, and disability appear in adulthood. Clinical practice recommendations for the diagnosis and management of XLH advocate regular check-ups for patients by multidisciplinary teams which are organized by an expert in metabolic bone disorders [1,5]. Several excellent studies on the management of XLH have recently been published [8–15]. Since clinical, biochemical, and radiographic features vary between individuals, monitoring and treatment need to

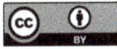

be personalized based on a patient's clinical manifestations, medical history, and stage of development [5,16]. Recommendations for follow-ups, the treatment and management of orthopedic conditions, dental health, hearing, and neurosurgical complications in patients with XLH have been described in detail and summarized [5]. XLH management goals have been summarized as follows: initiate and continue medical therapy; prevent and resolve rickets with early treatment; minimize the risk of developing skeletal deformities; monitor and improve growth and growth velocity; use guided growth procedures; ensure an understanding of therapies and self-administration; psychological, psychosocial, and mental well-being support; ongoing dental care; ongoing physical activity; healthy lifestyle and mobility; the ability to navigate healthcare and insurance systems; corrective surgeries as indicated; therapy self-administration; reproductive health; knowledge of XLH risks and symptoms; self-advocacy; education about therapies, including new developments; monitoring for spinal stenosis and enthesopathy; resolving pseudofractures; and preventing fractures [1]. A survey using online public open consultations with patients with XLH indicated that the disease burden becomes complicated and multifactorial with an increase in psychological issues [17].

Table 1. Clinical features and disease burden [6,16].

Bone, growth plate	Rickets * or osteomalacia, short stature
Cartilage	Early osteoarthritis
Kidney	Nephrocalcinosis, nephrolithiasis, chronic kidney disease, hypertension
Cardiovascular system	Hypertension, possible left ventricular hypertrophy
Ligament and tendons	Enthesopathy
Muscle	Muscle weakness, pain, stiffness
Skull	Craniosynostosis *, Arnold-Chiari type 1 malformations
Spine	Spinal stenosis
Teeth	Dental necrosis with severe abscesses, periodontitis, tooth loss
Ear	Hearing loss
QoL-related burden	Pain, physical deformities, dental complications, muscle weakness, stiffness, fatigue, mood alterations/depression, surgical procedures

*, specific to children.

Experts in metabolic bone diseases are commonly endocrinologists, nephrologists, and geneticists (pediatric and/or adult) who liaise with a patient's local health care providers (HCPs) (internist, general practitioner, pediatrician, and advanced practice providers), radiologists, orthopedic surgeons, physical therapists, rheumatologists, and dentists. As needed, the following professionals may be involved in patient care: neurosurgeons, otolaryngologists, ophthalmologists, audiologists, orthodontists, dieticians, rehabilitation specialists, pain management specialists, genetic counselors, occupational therapists, and social workers or psychologists [1]. Since XLH presents with a number of symptoms and signs in addition to the musculoskeletal system, the expert in metabolic bone diseases needs to be at the center of patient care and coordinate and collaborate with other professionals. Evidence for the disease burden of XLH during adulthood, as early as 20 years of age, is accumulating [2,18–24]. In addition, a new therapy targeting FGF23 has been developed and applied to clinical practice for children and adults [25–27]. The appropriate transition and effective transfer from pediatric HCPs to adult HCPs is essential for patients with XLH.

3. Transition

Increased survival from a wide range of chronic illnesses has resulted in greater numbers of children with disabilities reaching 20 years of age [28]. In 2002, a consensus statement by the American Academy of Pediatrics (AAP), the American Academy of Family Physicians (AAFP), and the American College of Physicians (ACP)—American Society of Internal Medicine was published, and the statement mentioned the importance of facilitating the transition of adolescents with special health care needs into adulthood [29]. In 2011, the AAP, AAFP, and ACP with the authoring group published a clinical report entitled "Supporting the Health Care Transition (HCT) from Adolescence to Adulthood in the Medical Home" [30]. This report describes the process for transition preparation, planning, tracking, and completion for all youths and young adults (AYAs) beginning in early adolescence and provides a structure for training and continuing education to understand the essence of adolescent transition. In 2018, the clinical report was updated to provide more practice-based guidance on key elements of the transition; however, the policy and algorithm was not changed [31]. HCT is defined as "the process of moving from a child model to an adult model of health care with or without a transfer to a new clinician". The purpose of HCT is to decrease the numbers of patients that are lost to follow-ups and improve the quality of care through organized navigation that is provided to AYA patients and their caregivers. Patients that are lost to the follow-up do not receive appropriate practice management. Experts in XLH are commonly endocrinologists, nephrologists, and geneticists, although this depends on the countries and institutes that see patients with XLH. In general, geneticists are thought to see patients in both childhood and adulthood, rather than endocrinologists and nephrologists, who are usually either pediatric- or adult-specific. In some situations, a clinician that is familiar with pediatric and adult patients with XLH may continue to follow the patients through their life and provide them with proper medical care.

Transition barriers, including a fear of a new health care system and/or hospital, inadequate planning, and system difficulties, are experienced by AYAs and their families [31]. The greatest barrier mentioned is the difficulties that are associated with leaving their pediatric clinicians with whom they have had a long-standing relationship. Clinicians also find many transition barriers, such as communication and/or consultation gaps, training limitations, care delivery, care coordination, staff support gaps, a lack of patient knowledge and engagement, and a lack of comfort with adult care. The most common impediments are the lack of communication and coordination and the different practice behaviors between clinicians. Core elements in HCT consist of transition policy, transition tracking and monitoring, transition readiness, transition planning, transfer and/or integration into adult-centered care, and transition completion and ongoing care with adult clinicians. The process of HCT may be divided into three stages: (1) setting the stage: the initiation of HCT planning and a transition readiness assessment; (2) moving forward: the ongoing provision of HCT services; (3) reaching the goal: the transfer to adult healthcare services [32]. Based on expert opinions and limited research evidence, HCT planning needs to start at approximately 10 to 12 years of age for children with chronic conditions. Fruitful HCT requires collaborations between pediatric and adult-focused providers and settings that encourage AYA to continue to increase skills, even into their mid-20s. Effective HCT needs to be delivered in a similar culture and linguistic background based on the unique necessities of each AYA. An assessment of HCT readiness will direct interventions that lead to better outcomes and quality of life for AYAs.

4. Transition in Rare Diseases

Since HCT requires the efforts and contributions of pediatric and adult care providers, as well as the patient and parent, the benefits of HCT programs have been evaluated. Four randomized controlled trials, including cystic fibrosis, inflammatory bowel disease, type 1 diabetes, heart disease, and spina bifida, which aimed to improve the transition of care for adolescents from pediatric to adult health services, suggested positive effects on patients' knowledge of their condition, self-efficacy, and confidence [33]. A systematic review evaluating 43 studies on multiple chronic conditions demonstrated that HCT interventions often achieved positive outcomes, with the most common being adherence to care and the use of ambulatory care in adult settings [34]. In contrast, despite the well-depicted transition position statement, patients with type 1 diabetes have experienced gaps in care during the transition period between pediatric and adult care. Five recommendations for the effective receivership of AYAs with type 1 diabetes have been established: communication between pediatric and adult HCPs; an objective assessment of patient knowledge; the patient and adult provider relationship; support for psychosocial needs for AYAs; and a team-based approach [35].

Difficulties are associated with the application of traditional health care models for common diseases to rare diseases, which have specific challenges. A survey revealed educational and knowledge gaps in HCPs that were related to rare endocrine conditions [36]. Medical self-management skills, including medical knowledge, practical skills, and communication in adolescents with rare endocrine conditions were recently reported to be insufficient [37]. The authors recommended three elements to improve transition readiness: the repeated provision of individualized medical information; the use of a transition checklist; and training communication ability with the help of parents, caregivers, and/or e-technology. HCT models have been reported for rare diseases, such as hemophilia [38], sickle cell disease [39], and phenylketonuria [40]. Key barriers to rare diseases include a lack of access to disease experts, limited knowledge on the disease course, and few patient–clinician research collaborations for the diseases [41]. A care continuum model for patients with rare diseases has been proposed that emphasizes the implementation of telehealth using modern e-technologies to reduce these barriers. A technology program using web and texting interventions in adolescents with chronic diseases was shown to improve the performance of disease management tasks, health-related self-efficacy, and patient-initiated communications [42]. The integration of telemedicine (an audiovisual interaction between a patient and HCP using computers, mobile devices, or telephones) may promote the care of AYAs with rare diseases, such as XLH, by improving access to disease experts, which may be limited due to physical distance and/or COVID-19-related restrictions, and supporting HCT [1]. Telemedicine appointments have been substituted for face-to-face visits with permission from the national health insurance system. Although telemedicine has allowed HCPs to deliver care to their patients during the COVID-19 pandemic, management challenges for endocrine conditions, including no physical examination and laboratory and radiographic evaluations, have been described [43].

Among rare bone disorders, HCT to adult-focused care for osteogenesis imperfecta (OI) has been reported. OI is a rare inherited disorder that is characterized by decreased bone mass and bone fragility and needs a multidisciplinary care team for patient management. Therefore, HCT for patients with OI is similar to that for XLH. The OI Foundation, the only voluntary US national health organization for OI, lists goals for the physician caring for a young adult with OI: "Maintain the current health status, preserve or improve the level of function, assure the continuity of medical and surgical care, and provide psychosocial support with referral to counseling and other services if needed" based on the relevant documents [44,45] (https://oif.org/wp-content/uploads/2019/08/Fact_Sheet_Transition_from_Pediatric_to_Adult_Care.pdf, accessed on 4 July 2022). They also show important transition topics for AYAs with OI, as follows: "Taking responsibility for one's own health care, being knowledgeable about OI in general and how it changes after puberty, knowing their personal health history, being able to communicate confidently with physicians, understanding how their health insurance works, and having identified adult care resources who are informed about OI. An interprofessional expert task force at Shriners Hospitals for Children in Canada reviewed the literature, developed guidelines for HCT for children with OI to adult healthcare services, and created a transfer summary tool [46]. The transfer tool includes "contact information, general information, psychosocial information, general medical information, family history, medical diagnosis and history, currently prescribed medications, recent laboratory results and x-rays, rehabilitation services, medical equipment, orthotics and assistive devices, functional capabilities and independence level, follow-up requirements, other professionals involved and community services, and general concerns". The goals for the physician, the issues for the young person, and the transfer tool in OI provide important insights for establishing HCT for patients with XLH, because OI is a rare inherited musculoskeletal disorder with occasional non-musculoskeletal manifestations, such as XLH.

5. Transition in XLH

Regarding HCT for XLH, patient advocacy organizations for XLH, such as the XLH Network in the US and XLHuk in the UK, and for various rare diseases, such as the Genetic and Rare Diseases Information Center and National Organization for Rare Disorders in the US, provide patients with information on their disease. The international XLH alliance, consisting of more than 23 organizations worldwide, has been established to amplify the voices of patients with XLH and set a global multi-disciplinary standard of care and research. The XLH Network developed a toolkit on the transition from pediatric to adult care for patients and their caregivers (http://www.xlhnetwork.org/application/files/1916/0311/3210/XLH_TRANSITIONS_TOOLKIT.pdf, accessed on 4 July 2022), as well as the "Voice of the Patient Report", about the symptoms and treatment of XLH (http://www.xlhnetwork.org/application/files/5515/9317/2550/VOP_Report.pdf, accessed on 4 July 2022). Gianni et al. emphasized that the transition to adult care is a responsibility that is shared by the pediatric and adult teams involved in XLH, because XLH involves lifetime multi-organ morbidities that are associated with age [3]. Dahir et al. provided expert recommendations on HCT for patients with XLH [1]. Three areas of competency have been described: patient foundational knowledge, information transfer, and timelines and supportive behaviors to drive engagement. The timelines of transfer include transition readiness tracking, the initiation of assessments on transition readiness, transition planning, transfer of care, and post transfer (Table 2). Even though ages are mentioned in the timelines, HCT plans need to be individualized. Of note, age- and sex-specific patterns in growth velocity and bone mineral acquisition are distinct between girls and boys, especially in adolescence [47]. Girls reach both peak height velocity and peak bone-mass gain at a younger age than boys. The difference of the patterns in growth and bone accretion between females and males needs to be considered in HCT. It is important to begin the transition process in early adolescence and regularly assess transition readiness. The transition documents for patients with XLH include patient information, healthcare information, disease history, XLH complications, treatment history, the support of advocacy groups, and education, such as XLH symptoms emerging in adulthood [1].

Table 2. Simple timelines of transfer [1].

12 years: transition readiness tracking	- Pediatric practice approach to transitioning to adult care - Educate patients about self-advocacy, self-care, shared decision-making, and self-sufficiency - Educate parents about guidance on encouraging children to succeed in disease ownership
14 years: initiate assessments of transition readiness	- Assess understanding of symptoms, treatment goals, lab results, making appointments, available resources, and legal and insurance age-related changes - Educate patients about disease and management - Assess transition readiness yearly from the ages of 13 to 17 years
17 years: transition planning	- Discuss the optimal time of transition - Checklist of medical, laboratory, and imaging histories for adult providers - Discuss potential dosing changes (pediatric to adult) - Identify adult providers - Connect with advocacy groups

Table 2. *Cont.*

18–26 years: transfer of care	- Confirm the first adult provider appointment - Establish a process to orient adolescents/young adults into practice
3–6 months post-transfer	- Confirm the transfer of care - Continue collaborations between pediatric and adult providers

6. Conclusions

XLH is the most common form of inherited disorders that are characterized by renal phosphate wasting, but it is a rare multisystem disease that is often perceived as a childhood disease. However, recent studies demonstrated that XLH is a long-term and progressive disease throughout adulthood with a worsening disease burden. The lifelong multidisciplinary care of patients with XLH is necessary. Therefore, HCT plays a vital role in patient care and management for continuous adult care. Pediatric and adult HCPs both need to act in HCT to improve the outcomes of AYAs with XLH. HCT will prevent the loss of AYAs to follow-ups during the transition to adult care and will also improve healthcare conditions throughout life.

Funding: This article was funded by the Ministry of Health, Labour and Welfare, Japan (Grant No. 21FC1010) for English editing.

Institutional Review Board Statement: Not applicable.

Informed Consent Statement: Not applicable.

Data Availability Statement: Not applicable.

Conflicts of Interest: TK has received research grants from Teijin Pharma and received honorarium from Kyowa Kirin.

References

1. Dahir, K.; Dhaliwal, R.; Simmons, J.; Imel, E.A.; Gottesman, G.S.; Mahan, J.D.; Prakasam, G.; Hoch, A.I.; Ramesan, P.; de Ferris, M.D.-G. Health Care Transition From Pediatric- to Adult-Focused Care in X-linked Hypophosphatemia: Expert Consensus. *J. Clin. Endocrinol. Metab.* **2021**, *107*, 599–613. [CrossRef] [PubMed]
2. Seefried, L.; Smyth, M.; Keen, R.; Harvengt, P. Burden of disease associated with X-linked hypophosphataemia in adults: A systematic literature review. *Osteoporos. Int.* **2020**, *32*, 7–22. [CrossRef]
3. Giannini, S.; Bianchi, M.; Rendina, D.; Massoletti, P.; Lazzerini, D.; Brandi, M. Burden of disease and clinical targets in adult patients with X-linked hypophosphatemia. A comprehensive review. *Osteoporos. Int.* **2021**, *32*, 1937–1949. [CrossRef]
4. Connor, J.; Olear, E.A.; Insogna, K.; Katz, L.; Baker, S.; Kaur, R.; Simpson, C.A.; Sterpka, J.; Dubrow, R.; Zhang, J.H.; et al. Conventional Therapy in Adults With X-Linked Hypophosphatemia: Effects on Enthesopathy and Dental Disease. *J. Clin. Endocrinol. Metab.* **2015**, *100*, 3625–3632. [CrossRef] [PubMed]
5. Haffner, D.; Emma, F.; Eastwood, D.M.; Duplan, M.B.; Bacchetta, J.; Schnabel, D.; Wicart, P.; Bockenhauer, D.; Santos, F.; Levtchenko, E.; et al. Clinical practice recommendations for the diagnosis and management of X-linked hypophosphataemia. *Nat. Rev. Nephrol.* **2019**, *15*, 435–455. [CrossRef] [PubMed]
6. Beck-Nielsen, S.S.; Mughal, Z.; Haffner, D.; Nilsson, O.; Levtchenko, E.; Ariceta, G.; Collantes, C.D.L.; Schnabel, D.; Jandhyala, R.; Mäkitie, O. FGF23 and its role in X-linked hypophosphatemia-related morbidity. *Orphanet J. Rare Dis.* **2019**, *14*, 58. [CrossRef]
7. Linglart, A.; Duplan, M.B.; Briot, K.; Chaussain, C.; Esterle, L.; Guillaume-Czitrom, S.; Kamenicky, P.; Nevoux, J.; Prié, D.; Rothenbuhler, A.; et al. Therapeutic management of hypophosphatemic rickets from infancy to adulthood. *Endocr. Connect.* **2014**, *3*, R13–R30. [CrossRef]
8. Dahir, K.; Roberts, M.S.; Krolczyk, S.; Simmons, J.H. X-Linked Hypophosphatemia: A New Era in Management. *J. Endocr. Soc.* **2020**, *4*, bvaa151. [CrossRef]
9. Lambert, A.-S.; Zhukouskaya, V.; Rothenbuhler, A.; Linglart, A. X-linked hypophosphatemia: Management and treatment prospects. *Jt. Bone Spine* **2019**, *86*, 731–738. [CrossRef]
10. Laurent, M.R.; De Schepper, J.; Trouet, D.; Godefroid, N.; Boros, E.; Heinrichs, C.; Bravenboer, B.; Velkeniers, B.; Lammens, J.; Harvengt, P.; et al. Consensus Recommendations for the Diagnosis and Management of X-Linked Hypophosphatemia in Belgium. *Front. Endocrinol.* **2021**, *12*, 641543. [CrossRef]

11. Padidela, R.; Cheung, M.S.; Saraff, V.; Dharmaraj, P. Clinical guidelines for burosumab in the treatment of XLH in children and adolescents: British paediatric and adolescent bone group recommendations. *Endocr. Connect.* **2020**, *9*, 1051–1056. [CrossRef] [PubMed]
12. Baroncelli, G.I.; Mora, S. X-Linked Hypophosphatemic Rickets: Multisystemic Disorder in Children Requiring Multidisciplinary Management. *Front. Endocrinol.* **2021**, *12*, 688309. [CrossRef] [PubMed]
13. Rothenbuhler, A.; Schnabel, D.; Högler, W.; Linglart, A. Diagnosis, treatment-monitoring and follow-up of children and adolescents with X-linked hypophosphatemia (XLH). *Metabolism* **2020**, *103*, 153892. [CrossRef] [PubMed]
14. Lecoq, A.-L.; Brandi, M.L.; Linglart, A.; Kamenický, P. Management of X-linked hypophosphatemia in adults. *Metabolism* **2020**, *103*, 154049. [CrossRef]
15. Saraff, V.; Nadar, R.; Högler, W. New Developments in the Treatment of X-Linked Hypophosphataemia: Implications for Clinical Management. *Pediatr. Drugs* **2020**, *22*, 113–121. [CrossRef]
16. Trombetti, A.; Al-Daghri, N.; Brandi, M.L.; Cannata-Andía, J.B.; Cavalier, E.; Chandran, M.; Chaussain, C.; Cipullo, L.; Cooper, C.; Haffner, D.; et al. Interdisciplinary management of FGF23-related phosphate wasting syndromes: A Consensus Statement on the evaluation, diagnosis and care of patients with X-linked hypophosphataemia. *Nat. Rev. Endocrinol.* **2022**, *18*, 366–384. [CrossRef]
17. Ferizović, N.; Marshall, J.; Williams, A.E.; Mughal, M.Z.; Shaw, N.; Mak, C.; Gardiner, O.; Hossain, P.; Upadhyaya, S. Exploring the Burden of X-Linked Hypophosphataemia: An Opportunistic Qualitative Study of Patient Statements Generated During a Technology Appraisal. *Adv. Ther.* **2020**, *37*, 770–784. [CrossRef]
18. Hawley, S.; Shaw, N.J.; Delmestri, A.; Prieto-Alhambra, D.; Cooper, C.; Pinedo-Villanueva, R.; Javaid, M.K. Prevalence and Mortality of Individuals With X-Linked Hypophosphatemia: A United Kingdom Real-World Data Analysis. *J. Clin. Endocrinol. Metab.* **2020**, *105*, e871–e878. [CrossRef]
19. Steele, A.; Gonzalez, R.; Garbalosa, J.C.; Steigbigel, K.; Grgurich, T.; Parisi, E.J.; Feinn, R.S.; Tommasini, S.M.; Macica, C.M. Osteoarthritis, Osteophytes, and Enthesophytes Affect Biomechanical Function in Adults With X-linked Hypophosphatemia. *J. Clin. Endocrinol. Metab.* **2020**, *105*, e1798–e1814. [CrossRef]
20. Herrou, J.; Picaud, A.S.; Lassalle, L.; Pacot, L.; Chaussain, C.; Merzoug, V.; Hervé, A.; Gadion, M.; Rothenbuhler, A.; Kamenický, P.; et al. Prevalence of Enthesopathies in Adults With X-linked Hypophosphatemia: Analysis of Risk Factors. *J. Clin. Endocrinol. Metab.* **2021**, *107*, e224–e235. [CrossRef]
21. Orlando, G.; Bubbear, J.; Clarke, S.; Keen, R.; Roy, M.; Anilkumar, A.; Schini, M.; Walsh, J.S.; Javaid, M.K.; Ireland, A. Physical function and physical activity in adults with X-linked hypophosphatemia. *Osteoporos. Int.* **2022**, *33*, 1485–1491. [CrossRef] [PubMed]
22. Cheung, M.; Rylands, A.J.; Williams, A.; Bailey, K.; Bubbear, J. Patient-Reported Complications, Symptoms, and Experiences of Living With X-Linked Hypophosphatemia Across the Life-Course. *J. Endocr. Soc.* **2021**, *5*, bvab070. [CrossRef] [PubMed]
23. Skrinar, A.; Dvorak-Ewell, M.; Evins, A.; Macica, C.; Linglart, A.; Imel, E.A.; Theodore-Oklota, C.; Martin, J.S. The Lifelong Impact of X-Linked Hypophosphatemia: Results From a Burden of Disease Survey. *J. Endocr. Soc.* **2019**, *3*, 1321–1334. [CrossRef] [PubMed]
24. Javaid, M.K.; Ward, L.; Pinedo-Villanueva, R.; Rylands, A.J.; Williams, A.; Insogna, K.; Imel, E.A. Musculoskeletal Features in Adults With X-linked Hypophosphatemia: An Analysis of Clinical Trial and Survey Data. *J. Clin. Endocrinol. Metab.* **2021**, *107*, e1249–e1262. [CrossRef] [PubMed]
25. Carpenter, T.O.; Whyte, M.P.; Imel, E.A.; Boot, A.M.; Högler, W.; Linglart, A.; Padidela, R.; Hoff, W.V.; Mao, M.; Chen, C.-Y.; et al. Burosumab Therapy in Children with X-Linked Hypophosphatemia. *N. Engl. J. Med.* **2018**, *378*, 1987–1998. [CrossRef]
26. Insogna, K.L.; Briot, K.; Imel, E.A.; Kamenický, P.; Ruppe, M.D.; Portale, A.A.; Weber, T.; Pitukcheewanont, P.; Cheong, H.I.; de Beur, S.J.; et al. A Randomized, Double-Blind, Placebo-Controlled, Phase 3 Trial Evaluating the Efficacy of Burosumab, an Anti-FGF23 Antibody, in Adults With X-Linked Hypophosphatemia: Week 24 Primary Analysis. *J. Bone Miner. Res.* **2018**, *33*, 1383–1393. [CrossRef]
27. Imel, E.A.; Glorieux, F.H.; Whyte, M.P.; Munns, C.F.; Ward, L.M.; Nilsson, O.; Simmons, J.; Padidela, R.; Namba, N.; Cheong, H.I.; et al. Burosumab versus conventional therapy in children with X-linked hypophosphataemia: A randomised, active-controlled, open-label, phase 3 trial. *Lancet* **2019**, *393*, 2416–2427. [CrossRef]
28. Blum, R.W. Transition to adult health care: Setting the stage. *J. Adolesc. Health* **1995**, *17*, 3–5. [CrossRef]
29. Blum, R.W.; Hirsch, D.; Kastner, T.A.; Quint, R.D.; Sandler, A.D.; Anderson, S.M.; Britto, M.; Brunstrom, J.; Buchanan, G.A.; Burke, R.; et al. A consensus statement on health care transitions for young adults with special health care needs. *Pediatrics* **2002**, *110*, 1304–1306.
30. Cooley, W.C.; Sagerman, P.J. Supporting the Health Care Transition From Adolescence to Adulthood in the Medical Home. *Pediatrics* **2011**, *128*, 182–200. [CrossRef]
31. White, P.H.; Cooley, W.C.; Boudreau, A.D.A.; Cyr, M.; Davis, B.E.; Dreyfus, D.E.; Forlenza, E.; Friedland, A.; Greenlee, C.; Mann, M.; et al. Supporting the Health Care Transition From Adolescence to Adulthood in the Medical Home. *Pediatrics* **2018**, *142*, e20182587. [CrossRef] [PubMed]
32. Mahan, J.D.; Betz, C.L.; Okumura, M.J.; Ferris, M.E. Self-management and Transition to Adult Health Care in Adolescents and Young Adults: A Team Process. *Pediatr. Rev.* **2017**, *38*, 305–319. [CrossRef] [PubMed]
33. Campbell, F.; Biggs, K.; Aldiss, S.K.; O'Neill, P.M.; Clowes, M.; McDonagh, J.; While, A.; Gibson, F. Transition of care for adolescents from paediatric services to adult health services. *Cochrane Database Syst. Rev.* **2016**, *4*, CD009794. [CrossRef] [PubMed]

34. Gabriel, P.; McManus, M.; Rogers, K.; White, P. Outcome Evidence for Structured Pediatric to Adult Health Care Transition Interventions: A Systematic Review. *J. Pediatr.* **2017**, *188*, 263–269.e15. [CrossRef] [PubMed]
35. Iyengar, J.; Thomas, I.H.; Soleimanpour, S.A. Transition from pediatric to adult care in emerging adults with type 1 diabetes: A blueprint for effective receivership. *Clin. Diabetes Endocrinol.* **2019**, *5*, 3. [CrossRef]
36. Iotova, V.; Schalin-Jäntti, C.; Bruegmann, P.; Broesamle, M.; Bratina, N.; Tillmann, V.; Hiort, O.; Pereira, A.M. Educational and knowledge gaps within the European reference network on rare endocrine conditions. *Endocr. Connect.* **2021**, *10*, 37–44. [CrossRef]
37. van Alewijk, L.; Davidse, K.; Pellikaan, K.; van Eck, J.; Hokken-Koelega, A.C.S.; Sas, T.C.; Hannema, S.; van der Lely, A.J.; de Graaff, L.C. Transition readiness among adolescents with rare endocrine conditions. *Endocr. Connect.* **2021**, *10*, 432–446. [CrossRef]
38. Bidlingmaier, C.; Olivieri, M.; Schilling, F.H.; Kurnik, K.; Pekrul, I. Health Care Transition of Adolescents and Young Adults with Haemophilia: The Situation in Germany and the Munich experience. *Hamostaseologie* **2020**, *40*, 097–104. [CrossRef]
39. Inusa, B.P.D.; Stewart, C.E.; Mathurin-Charles, S.; Porter, J.; Hsu, L.L.-Y.; Atoyebi, W.; De Montalembert, M.; Diaku-Akinwumi, I.; Akinola, N.O.; Andemariam, B.; et al. Paediatric to adult transition care for patients with sickle cell disease: A global perspective. *Lancet Haematol.* **2020**, *7*, e329–e341. [CrossRef]
40. Beazer, J.; Breck, J.; Eggerding, C.; Gordon, P.; Hacker, S.; Thompson, A. Strategies to engage lost to follow-up patients with phenylketonuria in the United States: Best practice recommendations. *Mol. Genet. Metab. Rep.* **2020**, *23*, 100571. [CrossRef]
41. Augustine, E.F.; Dorsey, E.R.; Saltonstall, P.L. The Care Continuum: An Evolving Model for Care and Research in Rare Diseases. *Pediatrics* **2017**, *140*, e20170108. [CrossRef] [PubMed]
42. Huang, J.S.; Terrones, L.; Tompane, T.; Dillon, L.; Pian, M.; Gottschalk, M.; Norman, G.J.; Bartholomew, L.K. Preparing Adolescents With Chronic Disease for Transition to Adult Care: A Technology Program. *Pediatrics* **2014**, *133*, e1639–e1646. [CrossRef] [PubMed]
43. Regelmann, M.O.; Conroy, R.; Gourgari, E.; Gupta, A.; Guttmann-Bauman, I.; Heksch, R.; Kamboj, M.K.; Krishnan, S.; Lahoti, A.; Matlock, K.; et al. Pediatric Endocrinology in the Time of COVID-19: Considerations for the Rapid Implementation of Telemedicine and Management of Pediatric Endocrine Conditions. *Horm. Res. Paediatr.* **2020**, *93*, 343–350. [CrossRef] [PubMed]
44. Dogba, M.J.; Rauch, F.; Wong, T.; Ruck, J.; Glorieux, F.H.; Bedos, C. From pediatric to adult care: Strategic evaluation of a transition program for patients with osteogenesis imperfecta. *BMC Health Serv. Res.* **2014**, *14*, 489. [CrossRef]
45. Shapiro, J.R.; Germain-Lee, E.L. Osteogenesis imperfecta: Effecting the transition from adolescent to adult medical care. *J. Musculoskelet. Neuronal Interact.* **2012**, *12*, 24–27.
46. Carrier, J.I.; Siedlikowski, M.; Chougui, K.; Plourde, S.-A.; Mercier, C.; Thevasagayam, G.; Lafrance, M.; Wong, T.; Bilodeau, C.; Michalovic, A.; et al. A Best Practice Initiative to Optimize Transfer of Young Adults With Osteogenesis Imperfecta From Child to Adult Healthcare Services. *Clin. Nurse Spéc.* **2018**, *32*, 323–335. [CrossRef] [PubMed]
47. Weaver, C.M.; Gordon, C.M.; Janz, K.F.; Kalkwarf, H.J.; Lappe, J.M.; Lewis, R.; O'Karma, M.; Wallace, T.C.; Zemel, B.S. The National Osteoporosis Foundation's position statement on peak bone mass development and lifestyle factors: A systematic review and implementation recommendations. *Osteoporos. Int.* **2016**, *27*, 1281–1386. [CrossRef]

Review

Treatment of X-Linked Hypophosphatemia in Children

Toshihiro Tajima [1,*] and Yukihiro Hasegawa [2]

1. Jichi Children's Medical Center Tochigi, Jichi Medical University, Shimotsuke, Tochigi 329-0498, Japan
2. Division of Endocrinology and Metabolism, Tokyo Metropolitan Children's Medical Center, Tokyo 183-8561, Japan
* Correspondence: t-tajima@jichi.ac.jp

Abstract: The conventional treatment for X-linked hypophosphatemia (XLH), consisting of phosphorus supplementation and a biologically active form of vitamin D (alfacalcidol or calcitriol), is used to treat rickets and leg deformities and promote growth. However, patients' adult height often remains less than −2 SD. Moreover, adverse events, such as renal calcification and hyperparathyroidism, may occur. The main pathology in XLH is caused by excessive production of fibroblast growth factor 23 (FGF23). Several studies have demonstrated that treatment with burosumab, a blocking neutralizing antibody against FGF23, is better than conventional therapy for severe XLH and has no serious, short-term side effects. Thus, treatment with burosumab may be an option for severe XLH. The present article reviews the conventional and burosumab therapies. In addition to the fact that the long-term efficacy of antibody-based treatment has not been demonstrated, there are other, unresolved issues concerning the burosumab treatment of XLH.

Keywords: phosphorus; active form of Vitamin D; renal calcification; fibroblast growth factor 23 (FGF23); burosumab

1. Introduction

Hereditary hypo-phosphatemic disorders caused by elevated fibroblast growth factor-23 (FGF23) includes X-linked hypo-phosphatemic rickets (XLH) and autosomal-dominant hypo-phosphatemic rickets (ADHR) [1–4]. Osteoblasts and osteocytes produce and secrete FGF23, which binds to KLOTHO-FGF receptor 1 (FGFR1) in the target organs [3,4]. FGF23 suppresses the expression of type 2a and 2c sodium-phosphate cotransporters in renal proximal tubules, inhibiting phosphate reabsorption [3,4]. Moreover, FGF23 downregulates the expression of 1α-hydroxylase (CYP27B1), which converts 25-hydroxyvitamin D to 1, 25 $(OH)_2$ hydroxyvitamin D [3,4]. Thus, the symptoms of XLH and ADHR consist of rickets, short stature, osteo-malacia, bone pain, and dental diseases caused by renal phosphate wasting and low or inappropriately normal 1, 25 $(OH)_2$-hydroxyvitamin D levels [1,2].

The frequency of XLH is 1.7 per 100,000 children [1–3]. XLH arises from mutations of the phosphate-regulating endopeptidase homolog X-linked (PHEX) gene (Xp22.11), and its inheritance is X-linked dominant [3,4]. Males and females are equally affected, but the clinical severity is often variable even in familial cases [3,4]. The PHEX protein, a protease expressed in osteocytes and odontoblasts, does not degrade FGF23 [3,4]. Although the exact mechanism underlying elevated FGF23 in XLH is not completely understood, it is speculated that the sensing of phosphate in osteocytes may be disturbed [3,4].

The treatment target in X-linked hypophosphatemia (XLH) in childhood is to improve rickets, restore growth, alleviate bone pain, improve physical activity, and maintain dental health [1,2,5–9]. Infants in whom the condition is diagnosed at birth via family screening should be treated as soon as possible, as the outcomes are better the earlier therapy is begun [1,2,10].

The conventional therapy for XLH consists of oral phosphorus supplementation and alfacalcidol or calcitriol [1,2,5–9]. Recently burosumab, an IgG1 monoclonal antibody targeting FGF23, was developed and authorized for use by the European Medicines Agency and Food and Drug Administration [1–3,10–12], and several studies of its use in the treatment of severe XLH have already been published [13–17].

The present review provides a descriptive summary of oral phosphorus supplementation and alfacalcidol or calcitriol therapy, issues related to this treatment, and the prospects of burosumab as an alternative therapy for XLH.

2. Conventional Therapy

As mentioned above, the conventional therapy for XLH consists of oral phosphorus supplementation and alfacalcidol or calcitriol. Oral phosphorus supplementation compensates for renal phosphate wasting, and alfacalcidol or calcitriol compensates for impaired 1, 25 $(OH)_2$-hydroxyvitamin D production caused by excess fibroblast growth factor 23 (FGF23) [1,2,18].

The phosphorus is administered in the form of a sodium-based and/or potassium-based salt preparation. Table 1 summarizes the dosage of phosphorus and alfacalcidol or calcitriol [7].

Table 1. Dosage of phosphorus and alfacalcidol or calcitriol.

	Dose (Ref. [2])	Number of Doses per Day
Phosphorus	20–60 mg/kg/day (initial dose)	4–6 times/day
Alfacalcidol	0.03–0.05 mg/kg/day	Once a day
Calcitriol	0.02–0.03 mg/kg/day	One or two doses

Oral phosphorus 20–60 mg/kg/day is recommended as the initial dosage, depending on the age of the patient and the severity of the clinical symptoms [1,2]. It may be advisable to begin with a low dosage. However, to avoid gastrointestinal side effects, such as abdominal pain and diarrhea, and hyperparathyroidism, the dosage should not exceed 80 mg/kg/day [1,2]. When phosphorus is administered orally, it is poorly absorbed by the intestinal tract and returns to the original value after a few hours [2]. Therefore, multiple, daily doses of phosphorus are needed. In children, four to six divided doses daily are preferable [2]. The serum phosphate level should not be used to adjust the dosage of phosphorus supplementation [2].

Alfacalcidol or calcitriol is administered with oral phosphorus supplementation to compensate for impaired 1, 25 $(OH)_2$ hydroxyvitamin D production caused by excess FGF23 [1,2,5–8]. Alfacalcidol and calcitriol increase the absorption of phosphorus from the intestines. Initially, alfacalcidol 0.03–0.05 mg/kg/day should be administered once daily, and calcitriol 0.02–0.03 mg/kg/day could be administered in one or two doses daily [2]. The alfacalcidol and calcitriol dosage are often higher in toddlers and adolescents than in children [1,2,5,6] and should be adjusted so that it does not exceed (0.35 mg/mg) in urinary calcium/creatine [2]. If necessary, water intake is recommended to reduce the urinary calcium concentration [1]. Calculating the dosage should also take into consideration the degree of ALP decrease as well [1,2]. While administering a large amount of alfacalcidol or calcitriol is effective for improving rickets and growth velocity, it can lead to hypercalcemia, increased urinary calcium excretion, and renal calcification [1,2,5–8]. However, if the dosage is too low, it will be ineffective in improving rickets or the growth velocity. Thus, fine-tuning the alfacalcidol and calcitriol dosage is often difficult.

Regarding adult height, Miyamoto et al. [19] reported that the adult height of patients with XLH who received conventional therapy was -1.69 SD. Linglart et al. [8,20] reported that the mean adult height in female and male patients with XLH was -1.3 SD and -1.9 SD, respectively. However, 25–40% of patients with well-controlled XLH show an adult height below -2 SD despite receiving optimized conventional therapy [21–26].

Cheung et al. [27] reported that pediatric patients with conventional therapy showed lower cortical volumetric bone mineral density (vBMD) of the radius as determined by peripheral quantitative computed tomography (pQCT) than control subjects. Neto et al. [28] also reported a lower vBMD of the radius and tibia in pediatric patients with conventional therapy. In Hyp mice, early supplementation with calcitriol and phosphate improved bone microarchitecture on micro-CT to a greater extent than in non-treated Hyp mice [29]. In Hyp mice, the abnormal PHEX function may directly cause the cartilage abnormalities [30,31]. Taken together, conventional therapy may be only partially effective for bone mineralization.

3. Possible Complications under Conventional Therapy

Three to five phosphorus doses are normally administered. Phosphorus supplementation stimulates the gastrointestinal system and can cause diarrhea [1,2], possibly leading to decreased compliance. Furthermore, alfacalcidol and calcitriol have a relatively narrow therapeutic window, as mentioned previously, and may thus increase urinary calcium excretion. Increased urinary calcium excretion and hyper-phosphaturia lead to nephrocalcinosis and nephrolithiasis [3–6]. Renal calcification reportedly occurs in 30–70% of patients with XLH [1,32–34] as a manifestation of secondary hyperparathyroidism [1,2,8,35–37], which is caused by the high dose of oral phosphorus and/or an active form of vitamin D. In addition, FGF23 contributes to the progression of secondary hyperparathyroidism by reducing 1, 25 $(OH)_2$ hydroxyvitamin D synthesis and subsequently decreasing active intestinal calcium transport [1,2,8]. Furthermore, hyperparathyroidism in XLH patients has been reported to cause hypertension [36,37]. According to Alon et al. [36]. eight of 41 patients with XLH aged 20–29 years experienced hypertension during treatment. Secondary and tertiary hyperparathyroidism were observed in all eight of these patients, and nephrocalcinosis was observed in seven patients. Nakamura et al. [37] also reported that six of 22 adult patients with XLH experienced hypertension, and that the average age at hypertension onset was 29 years. All six patients had secondary or tertiary hyperparathyroidism, and two patients had renal dysfunction. Monitoring of blood pressure is necessary for XLH patients with hyperparathyroidism.

4. Clinical Trials of Burosumab

As mentioned above, the conventional therapy is effective, but leg deformities and diminished adult height persist in some patients with XLH despite long-term therapy.

Recently, burosumab, an anti-FGF23 antibody, was developed as a drug for decreasing excess FGF23 [3,11,12], which is central to the pathology of XLH [1–3]. Burosumab is a recombinant immunoglobulin G1 monoclonal antibody that binds intact and fragmented FGF23 at the N-terminal domain [12]. N-terminal antibodies to FGF23 can prevent the interaction of FGF23 and FGF receptor 1c [12]. Blood levels of burosumab peak in seven to 11 days on average, and its half-life in blood is 16 to 19 days [38,39]. The pharmacokinetics are the same for adults and children [39].

Aono et al. [12] reported the effects of antiFGF23 antibody in Hyp mice. The antibodies were administered to 4-week-old mice once a week for one month. As a result, the serum phosphate and 1, 25 $(OH)_2$ hydroxyvitamin D levels increased. Improvement of bone deformities and mineralization were observed. Blocking FGF23 with antibodies can cause a rapid increase in 1, 25 $(OH)_2$ hydroxyvitamin D, leading to hypercalcemia and possible renal calcification. However, in the previously cited study of Hyp mice, no nephrocalcinosis was observed.

Table 2 summarizes the results of several clinical trials of burosumab [13–17]. In all the trials, changes in rickets were assessed using the Rickets Severity Score (RSS) and Radiographic Global Impression of Change (RGI-C). The RSS consists of ten sores, with 0 indicating no rickets, and 10 indicating the greatest severity [40]. The RGI-C is an ordinal scale in which −3 indicates severe exacerbation and +3 indicates a complete cure [41].

Table 2. The effect on radiographic changes and height change of burosumab.

	Ref [13]	Ref [14]	Ref [15]	Ref [16] [1]	Ref [17]
Number of patients (age)	52 (5–12 years)	13 (1–4 year)	61 (1–12 years)	52 (5–12 years)	15 (1–12 years)
Burosumab dose	N = 26 Q2W [2] (initial 0.1 mg/kg, titrated to mean 0.98 mg/kg) N = 26 Q4W [3] (initial 0.2 mg/kg, titrated mean 1.5 mg/kg)	0.8–1.2 mg/kg Q2W	N = 29 Burosumab 0.8–1.2 mg/kg Q2W N = 32 Conventional therapy	0.8–1.2 mg/kg Q2W	0.8–1.2 mg/kg Q2W
Change of RSS Mean ± SD	At base line Q2W 1.9 ± 1.2 Q4W 1.7 ± 1.0 At 64 weeks Q2W 0.8 ± 0.6 Q4W 0.9 ± 0.5	At base line 2.9 ± 1.2 At 64 weeks 0.9 ± 0.5 [4]	At base line Burosumab 3.2 ± 1.1 Conventional therapy 3.2 ± 1.0 At 64 weeks Burosumab 1.0 ± 0.7 [4] Conventional therapy 2.2 ± 0.8 [4]	At 160 weeks RSS decreased in 41/52 patients	At base line 1.3 ± 1.2
Change of RGC-I LSM [5] ± SE	Q2W 0.8 ± 0.6 at 64 weeks Q4W 0.9 ± 0.5 at 64 weeks	0.9 ± 0.5 (RGI-C score ≥+2 13/13) patients) [6]	Burosumab at 64 weeks 1.0 ± 0.7 [4] (RGI-C score ≥+2 25/29 patients) [6] Conventional at 64 weeks 2.2 ± 0.8 [4] (RGI-C score ≥+2 6/32 patients)	LSM (SE) from base line to week 160 +1.89 ± 0.1 (RGI-C score ≥+2 23/41 patients at 160 weeks) [6]	Global RGC-I At 40 weeks 1.5 ± 0.8 At the end of treatment (average 121.7 weeks) 2.1 ± 0.7
Effect on length of height change after burosumab	Mean change of height Z score Q2W +0.19 at 64 weeks Q4W +0.12 at 64 weeks	Mean (SD) recumbent length or standing height Z score −1.38 ± 1.1 at base line −1.64 ± 1.09 at 63 weeks	LSM (SE) at 64 weeks Burosumab 0.17 ± 0.07 Conventional therapy 0.02 ± 0.04	Mean (SD) height Z score Q4W→Q2W −2.05 ± 0.96 at base line −1.85 ± 0.85 at 160 weeks Q2W→Q2W −1.72 ± 1.03 at base line −1.38 ± 1.06 at 160 weeks	No change of height Z score from baseline

[1]. Shown here is a study examining the continued treatment of the 52 patients previously enrolled in a study by Carpenter et al. [13] with burosumab for up to 160 weeks. [2]. Q2W, every two weeks. [3]. Q4W, every four weeks. [4]. These data were provided by ref. [42]. [5]. LSM, lean squared mean. [6]. The number of patients with ≥ 2 points at the end of the study.

The first, open-label, uncontrolled study included 52 patients with XLH (aged 5–12 years) who were followed to week 64 [13]. All the patients switched from the conventional therapy to burosumab. At base line, 94% of the patients had active rickets (RSS > 0). The subjects were divided into biweekly and four-weekly administration groups. The initial dosage was 0.1 mg/kg in the biweekly group and 0.2 mg/kg in the four-weekly group. The dosage was gradually increased to reach the lower limit of the reference value for fasting serum phosphorus level by age at week 2 after administration.

Increased serum phosphorus, renal phosphate reabsorption, 1, 25 (OH) 2D, and decreased serum ALP were observed in both groups. The mean fasting serum phosphorus level initially increased from the baseline value at all time-points in both groups and was able to be maintained in the biweekly group during the treatment period whereas in the four-weekly group it decreased steadily even at week 64 until the next dose.

While the biweekly group showed a decrease in the mean RSS, the four-weekly group showed a smaller decrease, indicating greater improvement in the former group. A small increase in the mean standing height Z score was also observed in the biweekly group and the four-weekly group. Furthermore, the score for physical functioning and pain improved in both groups. Based on these findings, burosumab was considered effective for children with XLH, and biweekly administration of burosumab was considered most appropriate.

Secondly, an open-label study of 13 patients (aged 1 to 4 years) [14] switching conventional therapy to burosumab treatment at baseline found that 12 of the patients had a RSS of at least 1.5, indicating severe rickets. As a result, the RSS improved by week 64. However, the length and height Z scores worsened. The authors stated that a precise assessment of length and height can be difficult at this age; however, most patients' height Z score continued to follow the growth curves.

Third, a randomized control study enrolled 61 children with XLH (aged 1 to 12 years) with an RSS score > 2 (relatively severe) who switched from the conventional therapy to burosumab or continued the conventional therapy [15]. The patients in both groups had already received the conventional therapy for an average of 4.3 years and 3.3 years, respectively. Burosumab administration was begun at 0.8 mg/kg every two weeks, then increased to 1.2 mg/kg.

At week 64, improvement in RGC-I and RSS was better in the burosumab group than in the conventional therapy group. The increase in the length and height Z scores at week 64 was also significantly greater in the burosumab group than in the conventional therapy group. Therefore, in patients with relatively severe XLH, burosumab is more effective than conventional therapy.

A study which examined continuation of burosumab therapy in the 52 patients previously enrolled in a study by Carpenter et al. [13] for up to 160 weeks [16] was reported. Most patients showed improvement in radiographic findings of rickets. Although the height Z score improved, the change from the baseline was moderate.

Namba et al. [17] recently reported the results of a Phase 3 and 4 open-label trial. Fifteen children (aged 1 to 12 years) received an average of six years of the conventional therapy. As in previous reports, RSS, RGI-S and growth rate tended to improve at week 124.

5. Safety of Burosumab

No previous studies based on clinical trials reported any short-term serious adverse events leading to the discontinuation of burosumab [13–16]. A recent, longitudinal study reported that adverse events related to burosumab occurred in 73% of the patients enrolled [16]. The most common adverse event was a reaction at the injection site [13–17], which occurred in about half the patients receiving burosumab but resolved one to two days after the injection. The second most common burosumab-related adverse event was pain in the extremities (10%). One patient experienced two serious adverse events requiring hospitalization (fever and muscle pain at week 48 and headache at week 182) but the therapy was nonetheless continued [16].

Six patients were positive for antidrug antibodies at the baseline while 40 patients remained negative for the 160-week course [16]. Three of the six patients with antidrug antibodies were also positive for neutralizing antibody. These patients experienced a reaction at the injection site but achieved improved RSS and maintained their serum phosphorus level. None of the patients had increased serum calcium, excessive urinary calcium excretion or increased serum PTH even after 160 weeks of therapy [16].

A study comparing burosumab with the conventional therapy found no renal calcification or hyperparathyroidism in a burosumab-therapy group [15] but reported a higher number of dental abscesses in this group than in a conventional therapy group [15], corroborating previous findings of the efficacy of the conventional therapy against dental diseases [1,2,8]. Further study is needed to clarify these issues.

6. Indications for Burosumab Treatment in Children

A recent consensus statement has suggested that burosumab therapy should be considered as the first-line therapy in children with XLH aged 1 year or older (6 months in some countries, such as the USA) and adolescents with radiographic findings of bone disease [2]. The consensus also recommended that the treatment be continued until epiphyseal closure [2]. While clinical trials have so far shown burosumab to be more effective than conventional therapy in severe XLH, the effect of burosumab on mild XLH is still unknown. Further, the annual cost of burosumab therapy is enormous (about US $200,000). Therefore, conventional therapy should be attempted first in mild cases [2].

The initial burosumab dosage is 0.8 mg/kg administered subcutaneously every two weeks [2]. The dosage should be adjusted so that the fasting serum phosphorus concentration is at the lower end of the normal reference range by age [2]. The fasting phosphate level should be measured 12–14 days after the injection to avoid hyperphosphatemia [2].

7. Future Prospects for Burosumab Treatment

Table 3 summarizes the unsolved questions in burosumab therapy.

Table 3. Open questions to be considered in burosumab treatment.

- Treatment of infants
- Biochemical markers for dose setting (fasting serum phosphorus level, tubular reabsorption of phosphorus, urine calcium/creatinine, PTH, etc.)
- Long-term effect on healing of rickets, adult height, dental health, bone pain, and physical function
- Long-term safety

Further, long-term follow up is needed to assess the long-term impact of the therapy on rickets, adult height, and safety.

8. Summary

The present review summarized the current methods of treating XLH. The conventional therapy consisting of phosphorus supplementation and alfacalcidol or calcitriol is effective for improving rickets and growth rate, but some patients fail to respond adequately, resulting in leg deformities and reduced adult height. Moreover, adverse events sometimes occur with the conventional therapy. Burosumab is more effective than the conventional therapy in severe XLH, but some unresolved issues, including the fact that final height data have not yet been collected, remain. More evidence from future studies should clarify these issues.

Author Contributions: Writing—review and editing, T.T. and Y.H. All authors have read and agreed to the published version of the manuscript.

Funding: This research received no external funding.

Institutional Review Board Statement: Not applicable.

Informed Consent Statement: Not applicable.

Acknowledgments: We are indebted to James R. Valera for his assistance with editing this manuscript.

Conflicts of Interest: The authors declare no conflict of interest.

References

1. Haffner, D.; Emma, F.; Eastwood, D.M.; Duplan, M.B.; Bacchetta, J.; Schnabel, D.; Wicart, P.; Bockenhauer, D.; Santos, F.; Levtchenko, E.; et al. Clinical practice recommendations for the diagnosis and management of X-linked hypophosphataemia. *Nat. Rev. Nephrol.* **2019**, *15*, 435–455. [CrossRef] [PubMed]
2. Trombetti, A.; Al-Daghri, N.; Brandi, M.L.; Cannata-Andía, J.B.; Cavalier, E.; Chandran, M.; Chaussain, C.; Cipullo, L.; Cooper, C.; Haffner, D.; et al. Interdisciplinary management of FGF23-related phosphate wasting syndromes: A Consensus Statement on the evaluation, diagnosis and care of patients with X-linked hypophosphataemia. *Nat. Rev. Endocrinol.* **2022**, *18*, 366–384. [CrossRef] [PubMed]
3. Takashi, Y.; Kawanami, D.; Fukumoto, S. FGF23 and Hypophosphatemic Rickets/Osteomalacia. *Curr. Osteoporos. Rep.* **2021**, *19*, 669–675. [CrossRef] [PubMed]
4. Michigami, T. Advances in understanding of phosphate homeostasis and related disorders. *Endocr. J.* **2022**, EJ22-0239. [CrossRef] [PubMed]
5. Glorieux, F.H.; Marie, P.J.; Pettifor, J.M.; Delvin, E.E. Bone response to phosphate salts, ergocalciferol, and calcitriol in hypophosphatemic vitamin D-resistant rickets. *N. Engl. J. Med.* **1980**, *303*, 1023–1031. [CrossRef]
6. Petersen, D.J.; Boniface, A.M.; Schranck, F.W.; Rupich, R.C.; Whyte, M.P. X-linked hypophosphatemic rickets: A study (with literature review) of linear growth response to calcitriol and phosphate therapy. *J. Bone Miner. Res.* **1992**, *7*, 583–597. [CrossRef]
7. Carpenter, T.O.; Imel, E.A.; Holm, I.A.; De Beur, S.M.J.; Insogna, K.L. A clinician's guide to X-linked hypophosphatemia. *J. Bone Miner. Res.* **2011**, *26*, 1381–1388. [CrossRef]

8. Linglart, A.; Duplan, M.B.; Briot, K.; Chaussain, C.; Esterle, L.; Guillaume-Czitrom, S.; Kamenicky, P.; Nevoux, J.; Prié, D.; Rothenbuhler, A.; et al. Therapeutic management of hypophosphatemic rickets from infancy to adulthood. *Endocr. Connect.* **2014**, *3*, R13–R30. [CrossRef] [PubMed]
9. Rafaelsen, S.; Johansson, S.; Ræder, H.; Bjerknes, R. Hereditary hypophosphatemia in Norway: A retrospective population-based study of genotypes, phenotypes, and treatment complications. *Eur. J. Endocrinol.* **2016**, *174*, 125–136. [CrossRef] [PubMed]
10. Mäkitie, O.; Doria, A.; Kooh, S.W.; Cole, W.G.; Daneman, A.; Sochett, E. Early Treatment Improves Growth and Biochemical and Radiographic Outcome in X-Linked Hypophosphatemic Rickets. *J. Clin. Endocrinol. Metab.* **2003**, *88*, 3591–3597.
11. Yamazaki, Y.; Tamada, T.; Kasai, N.; Urakawa, I.; Aono, Y.; Hasegawa, H.; Fujita, T.; Kuroki, R.; Yamashita, T.; Fukumoto, S.; et al. Anti-FGF23 Neutralizing Antibodies Show the Physiological Role and Structural Features of FGF23. *J. Bone Miner. Res.* **2008**, *23*, 1509–1518. [CrossRef] [PubMed]
12. Aono, Y.; Yamazaki, Y.; Yasutake, J.; Kawata, T.; Hasegawa, H.; Urakawa, I.; Fujita, T.; Wada, M.; Yamashita, T.; Fukumoto, S.; et al. Therapeutic Effects of Anti-FGF23 Antibodies in Hypophosphatemic Rickets/Osteomalacia. *J. Bone Miner. Res.* **2009**, *24*, 1879–1888. [CrossRef] [PubMed]
13. Carpenter, T.O.; Whyte, M.P.; Imel, E.A.; Boot, A.M.; Högler, W.; Linglart, A.; Padidela, R.; Van't Hoff, W.; Mao, M.; Chen, C.Y.; et al. Burosumab therapy in children with X-linked hypophosphatemia. *N. Engl. J. Med.* **2018**, *378*, 1987–1998. [CrossRef] [PubMed]
14. Whyte, M.P.; Carpenter, T.O.; Gottesman, G.S.; Mao, M.; Skrinar, A.; Martin, J.S.; Imel, E.A. Efficacy and safety of burosumab in children aged 1–4 years with X-linked hypophosphataemia: A multicentre, open-label, phase 2 trial. *Lancet Diabetes Endocrinol.* **2019**, *7*, 189–199. [CrossRef]
15. Imel, E.A.; Glorieux, F.H.; Whyte, M.P.; Munns, C.F.; Ward, L.M.; Nilsson, O.; Simmons, J.H.; Padidela, R.; Namba, N.; Cheong, H.I.; et al. Burosumab versus conventional therapy in children with X-linked hypophosphataemia: A randomised, active-controlled, open-label, phase 3 trial. *Lancet* **2019**, *393*, 2416–2427. [CrossRef]
16. Linglart, A.; Imel, E.A.; Whyte, M.P.; Portale, A.A.; Högler, W.; Boot, A.M.; Padidela, R.; Van't Hoff, W.; Gottesman, G.S.; Chen, A.; et al. Sustained efficacy and safety of burosumab, a monoclonal antibody to FGF23, in children with X-linked hypophosphatemia. *J. Clin. Endocrinol. Metab.* **2022**, *107*, 813–824. [CrossRef] [PubMed]
17. Namba, N.; Kubota, T.; Muroya, K.; Tanaka, H.; Kanematsu, M.; Kojima, M.; Orihara, S.; Kanda, H.; Seino, Y.; Ozono, K. Safety and Efficacy of Burosumab in Pediatric Patients With X-linked Hypophosphatemia: A Phase 3/4 Open-Label Trial. *J. Endocr. Soc.* **2022**, *6*, bvac021. [CrossRef]
18. Harrell, R.M.; Lyles, K.W.; Harrelson, J.M.; Friedman, N.E.; Drezner, M.K. Healing of bone disease in X-linked hypophosphatemic rickets/osteomalacia. Induction and maintenance with phosphorus and calcitriol. *J. Clin. Investig.* **1985**, *75*, 1858–1868. [CrossRef] [PubMed]
19. Miyamoto, J.; Koto, S.; Hasegawa, Y. Final Height of Japanese Patients with X-Linked Hypophosphatemic Rickets Effect of Vitamin D and Phosphate Therapy. *Endocr. J.* **2000**, *47*, 163–167. [CrossRef]
20. Heude, B.; Scherdel, P.; Werner, A.; Le Guern, M.; Gelbert, N.; Walther, D.; Arnould, M.; Bellaïche, M.; Chevallier, B.; Cheymol, J.; et al. A big-data approach to producing descriptive anthropometric references: A feasibility and validation study of paediatric growth charts. *Lancet Digit. Health* **2019**, *1*, e413–e423. [CrossRef]
21. Sochett, E.; Doria, A.S.; Henriques, F.; Kooh, S.W.; Daneman, A.; Mäkitie, O. Growth and Metabolic Control during Puberty in Girls with X-Linked Hypophosphataemic Rickets. *Horm. Res. Paediatr.* **2004**, *61*, 252–256. [CrossRef] [PubMed]
22. Ariceta, G.; Langman, C.B. Growth in X-linked hypophosphatemic rickets. *Eur. J. Pediatr.* **2006**, *166*, 303–309. [CrossRef] [PubMed]
23. Zivicnjak, M.; Schnabel, D.; Billing, H.; Staude, H.; Filler, G.; Querfeld, U.; Schumacher, M.; Pyper, A.; Schroder, C.; Bramswig, J.; et al. Age-related stature and linear body segments in children with X-linked hypophosphatemic rickets. *Pediatr. Nephrol.* **2011**, *26*, 2231–2232. [CrossRef] [PubMed]
24. Quinlan, C.; Guegan, K.; Offiah, A.; Neill, R.O.; Hiorns, M.P.; Ellard, S.; Bockenhauer, D.; Hoff, W.V.; Waters, A.M. Growth in PHEX-associated X-linked hypophosphatemic rickets: The importance of early treatment. *Pediatr. Nephrol.* **2012**, *27*, 581–588. [CrossRef]
25. Santos, F.; Fuente, R.; Mejia, N.; Mantecon, L.; Gil-Peña, H.; Ordoñez, F.A. Hypophosphatemia and growth. *Pediatr. Nephrol.* **2013**, *28*, 595–603. [CrossRef]
26. Mao, M.; Carpenter, T.O.; Whyte, M.P.; Skrinar, A.; Chen, C.-Y.; Martin, J.S.; Rogol, A.D. Growth Curves for Children with X-linked Hypophosphatemia. *J. Clin. Endocrinol. Metab.* **2020**, *105*, 3243–3249. [CrossRef]
27. Cheung, M.; Roschger, P.; Klaushofer, K.; Veilleux, L.-N.; Roughley, P.; Glorieux, F.H.; Rauch, F. Cortical and Trabecular Bone Density in X-Linked Hypophosphatemic Rickets. *J. Clin. Endocrinol. Metab.* **2013**, *98*, E954–E961. [CrossRef]
28. Colares Neto, G.P.; Pereira, R.M.R.; Alvarenga, J.C.; Takayama, L.; Funari, M.F.A.; Martin, R.M. Evaluation of bone mineral density and microarchitectural parameters by DXA and HR-pQCT in 37 children and adults with X-linked hypophosphatemic rickets. *Osteoporos. Int.* **2017**, *28*, 1685–1692. [CrossRef]
29. Cauliez, A.; Zhukouskaya, V.V.; Hilliquin, S.; Sadoine, J.; Slimani, L.; Miceli-Richard, C.; Briot, K.; Linglart, A.; Chaussain, C.; Bardet, C. Impact of Early Conventional Treatment on Adult Bone and Joints in a Murine Model of X-Linked Hypophosphatemia. *Front. Cell Dev. Biol.* **2021**, *8*, 591417. [CrossRef]
30. Miao, D.; Bai, X.; Panda, D.K.; Karaplis, A.C.; Goltzman, D.; McKee, M.D. Cartilage abnormalities are associated with abnormal Phex expression and with altered matrix protein and MMP-9 localization in Hyp mice. *Bone* **2004**, *34*, 638–647. [CrossRef]

31. Fuente, R.; García-Bengoa, M.; Fernández-Iglesias, Á.; Gil-Peña, H.; Santos, F.; López, J.M. Cellular and Molecular Alterations Underlying Abnormal Bone Growth in X-Linked Hypophosphatemia. *Int. J. Mol. Sci.* **2022**, *23*, 934. [CrossRef] [PubMed]
32. Alon, U.S.; Lovell, H.B.; Donaldson, D.L. Nephrocalcinosis, hyperparathyroidism, and renal failure in familial hypophosphatemic rickets. *Clin. Pediatr.* **1992**, *31*, 180–183. [CrossRef] [PubMed]
33. Latta, K.; Hisano, S.; Chan, J.C.M. Therapeutics of X-linked hypophosphatemic rickets. *Pediatr. Nephrol.* **1993**, *7*, 744–748. [CrossRef] [PubMed]
34. DeLacey, S.; Liu, Z.; Broyles, A.; El-Azab, S.A.; Guandique, C.F.; James, B.C.; Imel, E.A. Hyperparathyroidism and parathyroidectomy in X-linked hypophosphatemia patients. *Bone* **2019**, *127*, 386–392. [CrossRef]
35. Lecoq, A.-L.; Chaumet-Riffaud, P.; Blanchard, A.; Dupeux, M.; Rothenbuhler, A.; Lambert, B.; Durand, E.; Boros, E.; Briot, K.; Silve, C.; et al. Hyperparathyroidism in Patients With X-Linked Hypophosphatemia. *J. Bone Miner. Res.* **2020**, *35*, 1263–1273. [CrossRef]
36. Alon, U.S.; Monzavi, R.; Lilien, M.; Rasoulpour, M.; Geffner, M.E.; Yadin, O. Hypertension in hypophosphatemic rickets—Role of secondary hyperparathyroidism. *Pediatr. Nephrol.* **2003**, *18*, 155–158. [CrossRef]
37. Nakamura, Y.; Takagi, M.; Takeda, R.; Miyai, K.; Hasegawa, Y. Hypertension is a characteristic complication of X-linked hypophosphatemia. *Endocr. J.* **2017**, *64*, 283–289. [CrossRef]
38. Zhang, X.; Imel, E.; Ruppe, M.D.; Weber, T.J.; Klausner, M.A.; Ito, T.; Vergeire, M.; Humphrey, J.; Glorieux, F.H.; Portale, A.A.; et al. Pharmacokinetics and pharmacodynamics of a human monoclonal anti-FGF23 antibody (KRN23) in the first multiple ascending-dose trial treating adults with X-linked hypophosphatemia. *J. Clin. Pharmacol.* **2016**, *56*, 176–185. [CrossRef]
39. Zhang, X.; Peyret, T.; Gosselin, N.H.; Marier, J.F.; Imel, E.A.; Carpenter, T.O. Population pharmacokinetic and pharmacodynamic analyses from a 4-month intradose escalation and its subsequent 12-month dose titration studies for a human monoclonal anti-FGF23 antibody (KRN23) in adults with X-linked hypophosphatemia. *J. Clin. Pharmacol.* **2016**, *56*, 429–438. [CrossRef]
40. Thacher, T.; Pettifor, J.; Tebben, P.J.; Creo, A.L.; Skrinar, A.; Mao, M.; Chen, C.-Y.; Chang, T.; Martin, J.S.; Carpenter, T.O. Rickets severity predicts clinical outcomes in children with X-linked hypophosphatemia: Utility of the radiographic Rickets Severity Score. *Bone* **2019**, *122*, 76–81. [CrossRef]
41. Whyte, M.P.; Fujita, K.P.; Moseley, S.; Thompson, D.D.; McAlister, W.H. Validation of a Novel Scoring System for Changes in Skeletal Manifestations of Hypophosphatasia in Newborns, Infants, and Children: The Radiographic Global Impression of Change Scale. *J. Bone Miner. Res.* **2018**, *33*, 868–874. [CrossRef] [PubMed]
42. Imel, E.A. Burosumab for Pediatric X-Linked Hypophosphatemia. *Curr. Osteoporos. Rep.* **2021**, *19*, 271–277. [CrossRef] [PubMed]

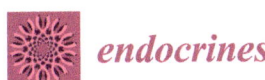

Review

Complications and Treatments in Adult X-Linked Hypophosphatemia

Yasuo Imanishi [1,*], Tetsuo Shoji [2] and Masanori Emoto [1]

1. Department of Metabolism, Endocrinology and Molecular Medicine, Osaka Metropolitan University Graduate School of Medicine, Osaka 545-8585, Japan
2. Department of Vascular Medicine, Osaka Metropolitan University Graduate School of Medicine, Osaka 545-8585, Japan
* Correspondence: imanishig@gmail.com

Abstract: X-linked hypophosphatemia (XLH) is a rare inherited disorder involving elevated levels of fibroblast growth factor (FGF) 23, and is caused by loss-of-function mutations in the *PHEX* gene. FGF23 induces renal phosphate wasting and suppresses the activation of vitamin D, resulting in defective bone mineralization and rachitic changes in the growth plate and osteomalacia. Conventional treatment with combinations of oral inorganic phosphate and active vitamin D analogs enhances bone calcification, but the efficacy of conventional treatment is insufficient for adult XLH patients to achieve an acceptable quality of life. Burosumab, a fully human monoclonal anti-FGF23 antibody, binds and inhibits FGF23, correcting hypophosphatemia and hypovitaminosis D. This review describes a typical adult with XLH and summarizes the results of clinical trials of burosumab in adults with XLH.

Keywords: burosumab; FGF23; hypophosphatemic rickets; XLH

1. Introduction

X-linked hypophosphatemia (XLH) is caused by loss-of-function mutations in the phosphate-regulating gene with homologies to endopeptidases on the X chromosome (PHEX) [1]. XLH was first described in 1937 as a type of rickets resistant to physiologic doses of natural vitamin D [2]. XLH is the most frequent cause of inherited hypophosphatemic rickets, with an incidence of 3.9 per 100,000 live births and a prevalence of 4.8 per 100,000 persons [3–5].

Fibroblast growth factor 23 (FGF23) is an osteocyte-derived hormone that regulates phosphate and vitamin D homeostasis. Elevated circulating FGF23 causes renal phosphate wasting and suppresses the production of activated vitamin D, resulting in hypophosphatemia and impaired bone mineralization [6–10]. Physiologically, FGF23 is important in calcium-phosphate homeostasis, as well as in regulating parathyroid hormone (PTH) and dihydroxy vitamin D levels [11]. Mutations in *PHEX* enhance circulating FGF23 levels, resulting in hypophosphatemic rickets [12,13]. Hypophosphatemic rickets/osteomalacia caused by excessive FGF23 activity has also been observed in individuals with autosomal dominant hypophosphatemic rickets [14], tumor-induced osteomalacia [12,13], fibrous dysplasia with McCune-Albright syndrome [15], sporadic fibrous dysplasia [16], and repeated intravenous iron infusion [17,18].

Conventional treatment for hypophosphatemic ricket/osteomalacia consists of combinations of active vitamin D analogs and multiple daily doses of oral inorganic phosphate [19]. However, both active vitamin D and phosphate enhance FGF23 secretion [11]. Clinical trials have shown that burosumab, a humanized monoclonal anti-FGF23 antibody, is safe and effective in pediatric patients with XLH [20–22].

This review will first describe an adult XLH patient, enabling an understanding of the complications that frequent occur in these patients. This review will also focus on the effects of treatment, comparing conventional treatments with burosumab.

2. Case Presentation

A 48-year-old woman was referred to our hospital for incidental hypophosphatemia at a medical checkup. She was short in stature (119.5 cm), with a body weight of 32.5 kg and bowed legs. She could not walk alone until age 5 years. She had been diagnosed with malnutrition of unknown causes and did not receive any treatment for her rickets. Her mother was also short in stature with bowed legs, but her father and five brothers did not exhibit short stature or bone abnormalities. Her serum phosphate concentration was 0.8 mg/dL, and she was diagnosed with XLH. She was started on treatment with alfacalcidol and inorganic phosphate, resulting in a gradual reduction of alkaline phosphatase levels. Her renal function was normal (serum creatinine 0.5 mg/dL). Analyses at age 58 years showed that her intact FGF23 level was 38.7 pg/mL and her tubular maximal reabsorption of phosphate to glomerular filtration rate (TmP/GFR) was 1.28 mg/dL, indicating a diagnosis of FGF23-related hypophosphatemia [23].

She began to experience numbness in her legs at age 54 years. She was diagnosed with ossification of the posterior longitudinal ligament (OPLL) of the cervical spine. She was advised by an orthopedic surgeon to undergo recommended surgical treatment but refused it for a long time. Finally, her gait became spastic at age 64 years, and she underwent vertebral resection (Figure 1). Her symptoms, such as cervicodynia, stiff neck, and pain/paresthesia of the upper limbs, improved but not completely. She also developed hearing loss at this age.

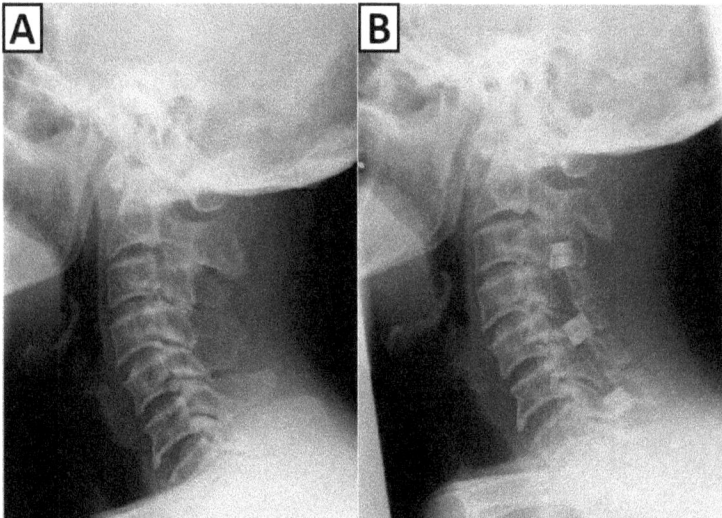

Figure 1. Cervical X-rays of the patient before (**A**) and after (**B**) vertebral resection for OPLL. After the operation, her symptoms partially improved.

At age 66 years, this patient experienced a left tibial pseudofracture and at age 67 years, she experienced pseudofractures on right tibia and left fibula. Conservative treatment of the pseudofracture of the left tibia was ineffective and intramedullary nail surgery was performed (Figure 2). After these lower limb fractures, she could not walk independently outside her house. Although her bone mineral density at age 66 years was not osteoporotic but osteopenic, both at the lumbar spine (L2–4 0.906 g/cm^2, T-score −0.9) and the femoral neck (0.602 g/cm^2, T-score −1.7), her vertebral fracture gradually progressed from this age, with multiple vertebral fractures resulting in a circle back at age 71 years.

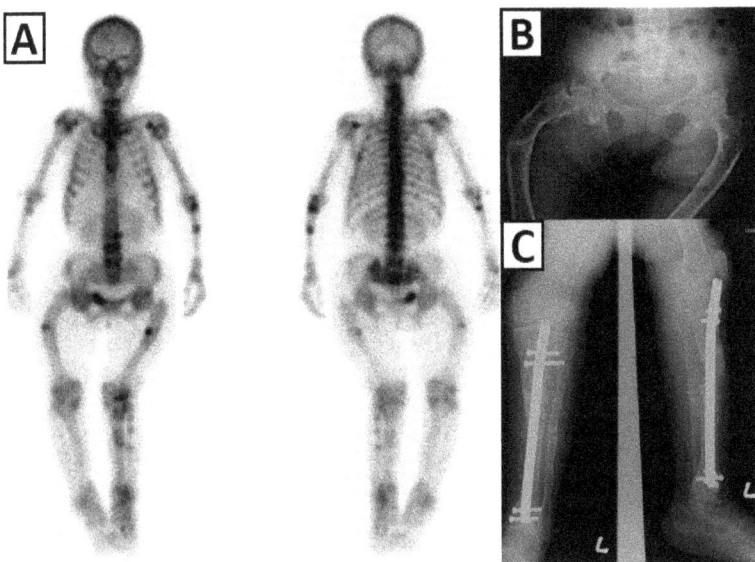

Figure 2. Bone scintigraphy of the patient at age 67 years (**A**). X-rays of both femurs (**B**) and left lower legs (**C**) after intramedullary nail surgery. The accumulations of radioisotope indicated fracture/pseudofracture of the left forearm, lumbar spines, and both legs. Along with bowing, beaking was observed at both femurs, findings consistent with the results of bone scintigraphy. After the surgery, she experienced partial easing of pain in her lower extremities, but calcifications of the pseudofracture regions were delayed.

Her blood pressure gradually increased during this time, and she was started on a calcium channel blocker at age 64 years. Her renal function also gradually decreased, with her serum creatinine concentration at age 75 years being above 1.0 mg/dL. Her doses of alfacalcidol and inorganic phosphate were reduced, with both stopped at age 75 years, resulting in a decrease in renal function. Because her renal function at age 79 years became very low (Cre 6.86 mg/dL, eGFR 4.98 mL/min), she was started on hemodialysis. Before starting hemodialysis, she exhibited secondary hyperparathyroidism (SHPT) with hyperphosphatemia (serum Ca 9.1 mg/dL, Pi 4.9 mg/dL, ALP (IFCC) 212 U/L, and whole PTH 821.3 pg/mL).

3. Complications in Adult XLH Patients

The patient described above had been diagnosed with adult XLH with severe complications, such as short stature, lower limb deformity and gait difficulty, OPLL, bone fragility, and hearing loss, complications often encountered in adult XLH patients. Renal insufficiency and SHPT were also observed, with these complications resulting from conventional treatment with inorganic phosphate and active vitamin D.

3.1. Short Stature

Short stature and growth retardation are typical phenotypes of XLH. At birth, patients with XLH are not abnormally small [24], but adult XLH patients are smaller than healthy subjects [25]. Despite treatment with oral inorganic phosphate and active vitamin D, including agents such as calcitriol and alfacalcidol, many patients show suboptimal growth [26]. Pubertal growth spurt is almost normal in patients with XLH [27], suggesting that some of the height deficit in treated patients results from late diagnosis and treatment onset.

Although initiating treatment in early infancy increases adult heights in patients with XLH, these heights are not completely normalized compared with healthy subjects [28]. Recombinant human growth hormone (rhGH) has also been used to improve growth velocity in pediatric XLH patients [29], with the combination of rhGH and conventional treatments in pediatric patients improving final height and bone mineral density (BMD) [30]. However, rhGH therapy is ineffective in adult XLH patients with epiphyseal line closure.

3.2. Lower Limb Deformity and Gait Difficulty

Long bone deformities, including bowing and maltorsion of the lower limbs, are common in patients with XLH, with many of these patients requiring multiple surgical procedures to correct these deformities [31,32]. A cross-sectional study in East Asian patients with XLH showed that 59.4% of adult XLH patients complained walking difficulties and that 25.0% required a walking device [33]. Because of these deformities, most patients with XLH experience gait and joint problems, reducing their quality of life (QoL) [34,35]. Gait analyses with a motion capture system showed that gait quality was lower in 29 XLH patients than in healthy individuals [36]. Factors associated with poor gait quality include the severity of lower limb deformity, high body mass index (BMI > 30 kg/m^2), and the presence of enthesopathies.

Poor muscle strength is also associated with gait difficulties. An analysis of calf muscle quantity and quality by peripheral quantitative computed tomography and jumping mechanography in 34 patients with hypophosphatemic rickets showed that muscle size was normal, but muscle density and peak muscle force and power were lower than in age-matched healthy volunteers [37]. Lower muscle quality and limb deformities contribute to gait difficulty. Most renal transplant recipients develop hypophosphatemia after transplantation due to the inappropriate secretion of FGF-23 and PTH in spite of improved renal function [38]. Administration of inorganic phosphate to hypophosphatemic patients after renal transplantation restored their serum phosphate levels and the composition of muscular phosphate components, such as adenosine 5'-triphosphate, and systemic acid/base homeostasis [39]. Hypophosphatemia itself may cause poor muscle quality in patients with XLH.

3.3. Spinal Complications

Spinal complications, such as ossified ligamentum flavum (OLF), posterior longitudinal ligament (OPLL), and Chiari malformation, have been observed frequently in adult XLH patients. For example, seven (11.8%) of 59 adult XLH patients were reported to have symptoms attributable to the spine clinically and/or radiologically [40]. Spinal complications observed in these patients included OLF, OPLL, Chiari malformation, cervical discectomy, cervical disc prolapse, and spinal cord syrinx. Surgical intervention (osteotomy) was frequently required. High rates of spinal ligament ossification, hip and knee osteophytes, and enthesopathy in the Achilles tendon have also been reported in Japanese adults with XLH [41].

3.4. Bone Fragility

High rates of fractures and/or pseudofractures have been reported in adult XLH patients [25,33,42]. For example, a cross-sectional survey of Japanese adults with XLH found that 34.4% had experienced a fracture, with the most commonly fractured bone being the femur (25.0%) [33]. In addition, some patients experienced more than one fracture.

BMD of the lumbar spine and hip assessed by dual-energy X-ray absorptiometry (DXA) was found to be higher in adult XLH patients than in an age-matched reference group [25,43,44]. A histologic analysis of adult patients with hypophosphatemic rickets showed that trabecular calcified and osteoid volumes were elevated, as was osteoid seam thickness [45]. Significant discrepancies between BMDs of the lumbar spine and hip have been observed in some patients, suggesting that extra-skeletal calcifications may interfere with BMD, especially of the lumbar spine. Bone microstructure is a component of bone quality that affects bone fragility [46] and can be evaluated noninvasively in patients with osteoporosis using high-resolution peripheral quantitative computed tomography (HR-pQCT) [47]. Although DXA showed that areal BMD was higher in 37 female XLH patients than in matched healthy controls, HR-pQCT found that volumetric BMD and microarchitectural parameters were lower in the XLH patients than in controls [48]. These findings suggested that bone quality is poor in patients with XLH.

Histopathologic assessments of transiliac bone biopsy specimens from 16 adult XLH patients showed osteomalacia in almost all of these patients, including the absence of tetracycline double-labeling and increased osteoid surfaces [43]. Only 4 of 16 patients had been administered calcitriol when bone biopsies were performed, whereas 14 had previously been treated with vitamin D_2 and/or inorganic phosphate. Fifteen patients were found to have osteoid halos around their osteocytes, a finding typically observed in patients with vitamin D-resistant rickets [49]. Evaluation of the relationship between the severity of bone pain and the degree of osteomalacia, as determined by osteoid volumes, showed a clear threshold, with relative osteoid volumes > 25% being associated with bone pain. Histomorphometric evaluation of bone biopsies from patients with vitamin D-resistant rickets showed the presence of osteomalacia, even in asymptomatic patients [45]. Taken together, this evidence indicates that BMD does not reflect bone fragility.

3.5. Hearing Loss

Approximately 30% of adult patients with XLH experience hearing impairment [41,50], although otologic phenotype and age at presentation vary [50]. Hearing loss was not significantly associated with the severity of biochemical and skeletal abnormalities. These patients should therefore undergo routine otologic examinations.

4. Conventional Treatment of Patients with XLH

The goals of treatment of adult XLH patients include reducing bone pain and improving fracture and/or pseudofracture healing [19]. These symptoms, as well as osteomalacia, may be ameliorated by conventional treatments, such as active vitamin D and inorganic phosphate [51–54].

A 2-year randomized prospective study evaluated the efficacy and safety of 20 versus 40 ng/kg body weight (BW)/day of calcitriol in 68 children with XLH [55]. Higher doses had greater effects on Thacher rickets severity scores, reductions in serum alkaline phosphatase concentrations, and increases in height and serum phosphate concentrations. However, conventional treatment did not improve dental disease, arthritic complications, enthesopathy, and ligament calcification in adult XLH patients [19].

The risks of long-term conventional therapy with, for example, active vitamin D and inorganic phosphate, include hypercalcemia, hypercalciuria, nephrolithiasis, and nephrocalcinosis, all conditions that can cause chronic kidney disease (Table 1). The severity of nephrocalcinosis was shown to be significantly associated with the dose of inorganic phosphate [56]. Active vitamin D can contribute to the development of nephrolithiasis and nephrocalcinosis. Routine monitoring of serum and urinary parameters is necessary to avoid the side effects of conventional therapy.

Table 1. Problems of conventional treatments in adult XLH patients.

Poor adherence to medication
Gastrointestinal side effects
Secondary hyperparathyroidism
Ectopic calcification
Renal insufficiency
Insufficient effect

Although hyperparathyroidism has been linked to long-term oral administration of inorganic phosphate, it has also been reported in untreated patients. Hyperparathyroidism may be caused not only by inorganic phosphate administration but by FGF23 inactivation of calcitriol. PTH levels are high in more than 80% of patients with XLH [57], with an observational study in adult XLH patients showing that hyperparathyroidism was associated with disruption of the physiological regulation of PTH secretion [58]. Ten percent of these patients developed hypercalcemic hyperparathyroidism and underwent parathyroidectomy.

5. Burosumab Treatment of Adult XLH Patients

5.1. Preclinical Findings

Two types of anti-FGF23 antibodies were developed, FN1 and FC1, which recognize the amino- and carboxy-terminal regions, respectively, of FGF23 [59]. Both FN1 and FC1 inhibited FGF23 activity. Specifically, FN1 masked putative FGF receptor-binding sites in the amino-terminal domain of FGF23, whereas FC1 interfered with the association between FGF23 and Klotho by binding to the carboxy-terminal domain of FGF23. In Hyp mice, a model of human XLH, anti-FGF23 antibody, consisting of a 1:1 mixture of FN1 and FC1, improved hypophosphatemia by attenuating hyper-phosphaturia and low $1,25(OH)_2D$ levels, thereby improving growth and muscle strength [60,61].

5.2. Clinical Findings in Adults with XLH

Burosumab (KRN23), a recombinant human monoclonal IgG1 antibody that binds to the amino-terminal domain of FGF23, was developed for the treatment of FGF23-related hypophosphatemic rickets/osteomalacia, such as XLH [20–22,62] and tumor-induced osteomalacia (TIO) [63,64]. A phase 1 double-blind, placebo-controlled study tested the effects of a single intravenous or subcutaneous dose of burosumab in adults with XLH, finding that single doses of burosumab temporarily increased the ratio of TmP/GFR, as well as increasing serum phosphate and $1,25(OH)_2D$ levels [65]. Serum phosphate levels peaked 0.5–4 days after intravenous administration and 8–15 days after subcutaneous administration of burosumab. The pharmacokinetics and pharmacodynamics of burosumab in adult XLH patients [66,67] were analyzed using preclinical [60] and clinical [65] data. Because the effects of subcutaneous injection lasted longer than those of intravenous injection, subcutaneous administration was regarded as more suitable for clinical use [65].

A phase 1/2 open-label dose-escalation study evaluated the efficacy of subcutaneous burosumab in adults with XLH [68]. Twenty-eight adults with XLH participated in a 4-month dose-escalation study (0.05–0.6 mg/kg every 28 days), and 22 of 28 joined a 12-month extension study (0.1–1 mg/kg every 28 days). Burosumab administration resulted in prolonged improvements in TmP/GFR, serum phosphate, and serum $1,25(OH)_2D$ levels, with a favorable safety profile [68]. Moreover, burosumab was reported to improve patient perception of their physical functioning and stiffness due to their disease, as determined by the SF-36v2 Health Survey and the Western Ontario and McMaster Osteoarthritis Index (WOMAC), respectively, as well as to improve health-related QOL [69].

A large, double-blind, placebo-controlled, phase 3 trial found that burosumab improved patient-reported outcomes in 134 symptomatic adults with XLH [70]. Patients were administered burosumab 1 mg/kg or placebo subcutaneously every 4 weeks for 24 weeks, followed by open-label treatment with burosumab for an additional 24 weeks. Burosumab significantly improved WOMAC physical function and stiffness compared with placebo, and, also, accelerated active fracture healing [70]. None of the patients in this trial experienced treatment-related serious adverse events, nephrocalcinosis, or meaningful changes from baseline in serum and urinary calcium concentrations and intact PTH concentrations. During the open-label extension phase of this trial, the ability of burosumab to improve phosphate homeostasis was sustained for up to 48 weeks [71]. In addition, patient-reported outcomes, such as WOMAC, Brief Pain Inventory-Short Form (BPI-SF), and Brief Fatigue

Inventory (BFI) scores, were improved, as was ambulatory function, as measured by the 6 min walk test (6MWT), for up to 96 weeks [72].

An open-label, single-arm, international phase 3 trial evaluated the histomorphometric effects of burosumab in 14 adults with XLH [73]. Eleven of fourteen patients completed treatment with 1.0 mg/kg burosumab every 4 weeks for 48 weeks and underwent paired transiliac bone biopsies before and after burosumab treatment. Burosumab improved all osteomalacia-related histomorphometric parameters. such as osteoid volume/bone volume, osteoid thickness, osteoid surface/bone surface, and mineralization lag time [73]. Analyses of BMD distribution in these biopsied samples showed that mineralization in bones of patients with XLH is very heterogeneous and that burosumab treatment increased mineral matrix volume rather than overall mineralization [74].

6. Conclusions

XLH is a hereditary disorder with many complications. Conventional treatment consists of combined oral administration of inorganic phosphate and active vitamin D analogs. These treatments, however, do not restore normal phosphate levels, and their outcomes, including QOL, are not optimal [75].

Several clinical studies showed that burosumab was superior to conventional treatment in adults with XLH. Clinical trials showed that burosumab consistently improved phosphate homeostasis, fracture and pseudofracture healing, and patient-reported outcomes. Burosumab is a promising treatment that can improve QOL in adult XLH patients.

Author Contributions: Original draft preparation, Y.I.; review and editing, T.S., M.E. All authors have read and agreed to the published version of the manuscript.

Funding: This research received no external funding.

Institutional Review Board Statement: Not applicable.

Informed Consent Statement: Not applicable.

Data Availability Statement: Not applicable.

Conflicts of Interest: Y.I. have received honoraria for serving as an advisory board member or for speaker fees from Kyowa Kirin International plc. T.S. and M.E. have no COI.

References

1. HYP-Consortium. A gene (PEX) with homologies to endopeptidases is mutated in patients with X-linked hypophosphatemic rickets. *Nat. Genet.* **1995**, *11*, 130–136. [CrossRef] [PubMed]
2. Albright, F.; Butler, A.; Bloomberg, E. Rickets resistant to vitamin D therapy. *Am. J. Dis. Child.* **1937**, *54*, 529–547. [CrossRef]
3. Beck-Nielsen, S.S.; Brock-Jacobsen, B.; Gram, J.; Brixen, K.; Jensen, T.K. Incidence and prevalence of nutritional and hereditary rickets in southern Denmark. *Eur. J. Endocrinol.* **2009**, *160*, 491–497. [CrossRef] [PubMed]
4. Endo, I.; Fukumoto, S.; Ozono, K.; Namba, N.; Inoue, D.; Okazaki, R.; Yamauchi, M.; Sugimoto, T.; Minagawa, M.; Michigami, T.; et al. Nationwide survey of fibroblast growth factor 23 (FGF23)-related hypophosphatemic diseases in Japan: Prevalence, biochemical data and treatment. *Endocr. J.* **2015**, *62*, 811–816. [CrossRef]
5. Rafaelsen, S.; Johansson, S.; Raeder, H.; Bjerknes, R. Hereditary hypophosphatemia in Norway: A retrospective population-based study of genotypes, phenotypes, and treatment complications. *Eur. J. Endocrinol.* **2016**, *174*, 125–136. [CrossRef] [PubMed]
6. Shimada, T.; Mizutani, S.; Muto, T.; Yoneya, T.; Hino, R.; Takeda, S.; Takeuchi, Y.; Fujita, T.; Fukumoto, S.; Yamashita, T. Cloning and characterization of FGF23 as a causative factor of tumor-induced osteomalacia. *Proc. Natl. Acad. Sci. USA* **2001**, *98*, 6500–6505. [CrossRef]
7. Shimada, T.; Hasegawa, H.; Yamazaki, Y.; Muto, T.; Hino, R.; Takeuchi, Y.; Fujita, T.; Nakahara, K.; Fukumoto, S.; Yamashita, T. FGF-23 is a potent regulator of vitamin D metabolism and phosphate homeostasis. *J. Bone Miner. Res.* **2004**, *19*, 429–435. [CrossRef]
8. Shimada, T.; Muto, T.; Urakawa, I.; Yoneya, T.; Yamazaki, Y.; Okawa, K.; Takeuchi, Y.; Fujita, T.; Fukumoto, S.; Yamashita, T. Mutant FGF-23 responsible for autosomal dominant hypophosphatemic rickets is resistant to proteolytic cleavage and causes hypophosphatemia in vivo. *Endocrinology* **2002**, *143*, 3179–3182. [CrossRef]
9. Shimada, T.; Kakitani, M.; Yamazaki, Y.; Hasegawa, H.; Takeuchi, Y.; Fujita, T.; Fukumoto, S.; Tomizuka, K.; Yamashita, T. Targeted ablation of Fgf23 demonstrates an essential physiological role of FGF23 in phosphate and vitamin D metabolism. *J. Clin. Investig.* **2004**, *113*, 561–568. [CrossRef]

10. Shimada, T.; Urakawa, I.; Yamazaki, Y.; Hasegawa, H.; Hino, R.; Yoneya, T.; Takeuchi, Y.; Fujita, T.; Fukumoto, S.; Yamashita, T. FGF-23 transgenic mice demonstrate hypophosphatemic rickets with reduced expression of sodium phosphate cotransporter type IIa. *Biochem. Biophys. Res. Commun.* **2004**, *314*, 409–414. [CrossRef]
11. Imanishi, Y.; Inaba, M.; Kawata, T.; Nishizawa, Y. Cinacalcet in hyperfunctioning parathyroid diseases. *Ther. Apher. Dial.* **2009**, *13* (Suppl S1), S7–S11. [CrossRef] [PubMed]
12. Jonsson, K.B.; Zahradnik, R.; Larsson, T.; White, K.E.; Sugimoto, T.; Imanishi, Y.; Yamamoto, T.; Hampson, G.; Koshiyama, H.; Ljunggren, O.; et al. Fibroblast growth factor 23 in oncogenic osteomalacia and X-linked hypophosphatemia. *N. Engl. J. Med.* **2003**, *348*, 1656–1663. [CrossRef] [PubMed]
13. Yamazaki, Y.; Okazaki, R.; Shibata, M.; Hasegawa, Y.; Satoh, K.; Tajima, T.; Takeuchi, Y.; Fujita, T.; Nakahara, K.; Yamashita, T.; et al. Increased circulatory level of biologically active full-length FGF-23 in patients with hypophosphatemic rickets/osteomalacia. *J. Clin. Endocrinol. Metab.* **2002**, *87*, 4957–4960. [CrossRef] [PubMed]
14. ADHR-Consortium. Autosomal dominant hypophosphataemic rickets is associated with mutations in FGF23. *Nat. Genet.* **2000**, *26*, 345–348. [CrossRef] [PubMed]
15. Riminucci, M.; Collins, M.T.; Fedarko, N.S.; Cherman, N.; Corsi, A.; White, K.E.; Waguespack, S.; Gupta, A.; Hannon, T.; Econs, M.J.; et al. FGF-23 in fibrous dysplasia of bone and its relationship to renal phosphate wasting. *J. Clin. Investig.* **2003**, *112*, 683–692. [CrossRef]
16. Kobayashi, K.; Imanishi, Y.; Koshiyama, H.; Miyauchi, A.; Wakasa, K.; Kawata, T.; Goto, H.; Ohashi, H.; Koyano, H.M.; Mochizuki, R.; et al. Expression of FGF23 is correlated with serum phosphate level in isolated fibrous dysplasia. *Life Sci.* **2006**, *78*, 2295–2301. [CrossRef]
17. Wolf, M.; Koch, T.A.; Bregman, D.B. Effects of iron deficiency anemia and its treatment on fibroblast growth factor 23 and phosphate homeostasis in women. *J. Bone Miner. Res.* **2013**, *28*, 1793–1803. [CrossRef]
18. Vilaca, T.; Velmurugan, N.; Smith, C.; Abrahamsen, B.; Eastell, R. Osteomalacia as a Complication of Intravenous Iron Infusion: A Systematic Review of Case Reports. *J. Bone Miner Res.* **2022**, *37*, 1188–1199. [CrossRef]
19. Carpenter, T.O.; Imel, E.A.; Holm, I.A.; Jan de Beur, S.M.; Insogna, K.L. A clinician's guide to X-linked hypophosphatemia. *J. Bone Miner. Res.* **2011**, *26*, 1381–1388. [CrossRef]
20. Carpenter, T.O.; Whyte, M.P.; Imel, E.A.; Boot, A.M.; Hogler, W.; Linglart, A.; Padidela, R.; Van't Hoff, W.; Mao, M.; Chen, C.Y.; et al. Burosumab Therapy in Children with X-Linked Hypophosphatemia. *N. Engl. J. Med.* **2018**, *378*, 1987–1998. [CrossRef]
21. Imel, E.A.; Glorieux, F.H.; Whyte, M.P.; Munns, C.F.; Ward, L.M.; Nilsson, O.; Simmons, J.H.; Padidela, R.; Namba, N.; Cheong, H.I.; et al. Burosumab versus conventional therapy in children with X-linked hypophosphataemia: A randomised, active-controlled, open-label, phase 3 trial. *Lancet* **2019**, *393*, 2416–2427. [CrossRef]
22. Lim, R.; Shailam, R.; Hulett, R.; Skrinar, A.; Nixon, A.; Williams, A.; Nixon, M.; Thacher, T.D. Validation of the Radiographic Global Impression of Change (RGI-C) score to assess healing of rickets in pediatric X-linked hypophosphatemia (XLH). *Bone* **2021**, *148*, 115964. [CrossRef] [PubMed]
23. Fukumoto, S.; Ozono, K.; Michigami, T.; Minagawa, M.; Okazaki, R.; Sugimoto, T.; Takeuchi, Y.; Matsumoto, T. Pathogenesis and diagnostic criteria for rickets and osteomalacia–proposal by an expert panel supported by the Ministry of Health, Labour and Welfare, Japan, the Japanese Society for Bone and Mineral Research, and the Japan Endocrine Society. *J. Bone Miner. Metab.* **2015**, *33*, 467–473. [CrossRef] [PubMed]
24. Schutt, S.M.; Schumacher, M.; Holterhus, P.M.; Felgenhauer, S.; Hiort, O. Effect of GH replacement therapy in two male siblings with combined X-linked hypophosphatemia and partial GH deficiency. *Eur. J. Endocrinol.* **2003**, *149*, 317–321. [CrossRef]
25. Beck-Nielsen, S.S.; Brusgaard, K.; Rasmussen, L.M.; Brixen, K.; Brock-Jacobsen, B.; Poulsen, M.R.; Vestergaard, P.; Ralston, S.H.; Albagha, O.M.; Poulsen, S.; et al. Phenotype presentation of hypophosphatemic rickets in adults. *Calcif. Tissue Int.* **2010**, *87*, 108–119. [CrossRef]
26. Zivicnjak, M.; Schnabel, D.; Billing, H.; Staude, H.; Filler, G.; Querfeld, U.; Schumacher, M.; Pyper, A.; Schroder, C.; Bramswig, J.; et al. Age-related stature and linear body segments in children with X-linked hypophosphatemic rickets. *Pediatr. Nephrol.* **2011**, *26*, 223–231. [CrossRef]
27. Weglage, J.; Funders, B.; Wilken, B.; Schubert, D.; Schmidt, E.; Burgard, P.; Ullrich, K. Psychological and social findings in adolescents with phenylketonuria. *Eur. J. Pediatr.* **1992**, *151*, 522–525. [CrossRef]
28. Makitie, O.; Doria, A.; Kooh, S.W.; Cole, W.G.; Daneman, A.; Sochett, E. Early treatment improves growth and biochemical and radiographic outcome in X-linked hypophosphatemic rickets. *J. Clin. Endocrinol. Metab.* **2003**, *88*, 3591–3597. [CrossRef]
29. Wilson, D.M.; Lee, P.D.; Morris, A.H.; Reiter, E.O.; Gertner, J.M.; Marcus, R.; Quarmby, V.E.; Rosenfeld, R.G. Growth hormone therapy in hypophosphatemic rickets. *Am. J. Dis. Child.* **1991**, *145*, 1165–1170. [CrossRef]
30. Baroncelli, G.I.; Bertelloni, S.; Ceccarelli, C.; Saggese, G. Effect of growth hormone treatment on final height, phosphate metabolism, and bone mineral density in children with X-linked hypophosphatemic rickets. *J. Pediatr.* **2001**, *138*, 236–243. [CrossRef]
31. Petje, G.; Meizer, R.; Radler, C.; Aigner, N.; Grill, F. Deformity correction in children with hereditary hypophosphatemic rickets. *Clin. Orthop. Relat. Res.* **2008**, *466*, 3078–3085. [CrossRef] [PubMed]
32. Horn, A.; Wright, J.; Bockenhauer, D.; Van't Hoff, W.; Eastwood, D.M. The orthopaedic management of lower limb deformity in hypophosphataemic rickets. *J. Child. Orthop.* **2017**, *11*, 298–305. [CrossRef] [PubMed]
33. Ito, N.; Kang, H.G.; Nishida, Y.; Evins, A.; Skrinar, A.; Cheong, H.I. Burden of disease of X-linked hypophosphatemia in Japanese and Korean patients: A cross-sectional survey. *Endocr. J.* **2022**, *69*, 373–383. [CrossRef] [PubMed]

34. Skrinar, A.; Dvorak-Ewell, M.; Evins, A.; Macica, C.; Linglart, A.; Imel, E.A.; Theodore-Oklota, C.; San Martin, J. The Lifelong Impact of X-Linked Hypophosphatemia: Results From a Burden of Disease Survey. *J. Endocr. Soc.* **2019**, *3*, 1321–1334. [CrossRef] [PubMed]
35. Seefried, L.; Smyth, M.; Keen, R.; Harvengt, P. Burden of disease associated with X-linked hypophosphataemia in adults: A systematic literature review. *Osteoporos. Int.* **2021**, *32*, 7–22. [CrossRef]
36. Mindler, G.T.; Kranzl, A.; Stauffer, A.; Kocijan, R.; Ganger, R.; Radler, C.; Haeusler, G.; Raimann, A. Lower Limb Deformity and Gait Deviations Among Adolescents and Adults With X-Linked Hypophosphatemia. *Front. Endocrinol.* **2021**, *12*, 754084. [CrossRef]
37. Veilleux, L.N.; Cheung, M.; Ben Amor, M.; Rauch, F. Abnormalities in muscle density and muscle function in hypophosphatemic rickets. *J. Clin. Endocrinol. Metab.* **2012**, *97*, E1492–E1498. [CrossRef]
38. Baia, L.C.; Heilberg, I.P.; Navis, G.; de Borst, M.H.; NIGRAM investigators. Phosphate and FGF-23 homeostasis after kidney transplantation. *Nat. Rev. Nephrol.* **2015**, *11*, 656–666. [CrossRef]
39. Ambuhl, P.M.; Meier, D.; Wolf, B.; Dydak, U.; Boesiger, P.; Binswanger, U. Metabolic aspects of phosphate replacement therapy for hypophosphatemia after renal transplantation: Impact on muscular phosphate content, mineral metabolism, and acid/base homeostasis. *Am. J. Kidney Dis.* **1999**, *34*, 875–883. [CrossRef]
40. Chesher, D.; Oddy, M.; Darbar, U.; Sayal, P.; Casey, A.; Ryan, A.; Sechi, A.; Simister, C.; Waters, A.; Wedatilake, Y.; et al. Outcome of adult patients with X-linked hypophosphatemia caused by PHEX gene mutations. *J. Inherit. Metab. Dis.* **2018**, *41*, 865–876. [CrossRef]
41. Kato, H.; Koga, M.; Kinoshita, Y.; Taniguchi, Y.; Kobayashi, H.; Fukumoto, S.; Nangaku, M.; Makita, N.; Ito, N. Incidence of Complications in 25 Adult Patients With X-linked Hypophosphatemia. *J. Clin. Endocrinol. Metab.* **2021**, *106*, e3682–e3692. [CrossRef] [PubMed]
42. Berndt, M.; Ehrich, J.H.; Lazovic, D.; Zimmermann, J.; Hillmann, G.; Kayser, C.; Prokop, M.; Schirg, E.; Siegert, B.; Wolff, G.; et al. Clinical course of hypophosphatemic rickets in 23 adults. *Clin. Nephrol.* **1996**, *45*, 33–41.
43. Reid, I.R.; Hardy, D.C.; Murphy, W.A.; Teitelbaum, S.L.; Bergfeld, M.A.; Whyte, M.P. X-linked hypophosphatemia: A clinical, biochemical, and histopathologic assessment of morbidity in adults. *Medicine* **1989**, *68*, 336–352. [CrossRef]
44. Rosenthall, L. DEXA bone densitometry measurements in adults with X-linked hypophosphatemia. *Clin. Nucl. Med.* **1993**, *18*, 564–566. [CrossRef]
45. Marie, P.J.; Glorieux, F.H. Bone histomorphometry in asymptomatic adults with hereditary hypophosphatemic vitamin D-resistant osteomalacia. *Metab. Bone Dis. Relat. Res.* **1982**, *4*, 249–253. [CrossRef]
46. NIH Consensus Development Panel on Osteoporosis Prevention, Diagnosis, and Therapy. Osteoporosis prevention, diagnosis, and therapy. *JAMA* **2001**, *285*, 785–795. [CrossRef]
47. Liu, X.S.; Stein, E.M.; Zhou, B.; Zhang, C.A.; Nickolas, T.L.; Cohen, A.; Thomas, V.; McMahon, D.J.; Cosman, F.; Nieves, J.; et al. Individual trabecula segmentation (ITS)-based morphological analyses and microfinite element analysis of HR-pQCT images discriminate postmenopausal fragility fractures independent of DXA measurements. *J. Bone Miner. Res.* **2012**, *27*, 263–272. [CrossRef]
48. Colares Neto, G.P.; Pereira, R.M.; Alvarenga, J.C.; Takayama, L.; Funari, M.F.; Martin, R.M. Evaluation of bone mineral density and microarchitectural parameters by DXA and HR-pQCT in 37 children and adults with X-linked hypophosphatemic rickets. *Osteoporos. Int.* **2017**, *28*, 1685–1692. [CrossRef]
49. Fanconi, A.; Fischer, J.A.; Prader, A. Serum parathyroid hormone concentrations in hypophosphataemic vitamin D resistant rickets. *Helv Paediatr. Acta* **1974**, *29*, 187–194.
50. Ivanovic-Zuvic, D.; Santander, M.J.; Jimenez, M.; Novoa, I.; Winter, M.; Florenzano, P. Characterization of otologic involvement in patients with X-Linked Hypophosphatemia. *Clin. Otolaryngol.* **2021**, *46*, 1251–1256. [CrossRef]
51. Glorieux, F.H.; Marie, P.J.; Pettifor, J.M.; Delvin, E.E. Bone response to phosphate salts, ergocalciferol, and calcitriol in hypophosphatemic vitamin D-resistant rickets. *N. Engl. J. Med.* **1980**, *303*, 1023–1031. [CrossRef]
52. Costa, T.; Marie, P.J.; Scriver, C.R.; Cole, D.E.; Reade, T.M.; Nogrady, B.; Glorieux, F.H.; Delvin, E.E. X-linked hypophosphatemia: Effect of calcitriol on renal handling of phosphate, serum phosphate, and bone mineralization. *J. Clin. Endocrinol. Metab.* **1981**, *52*, 463–472. [CrossRef]
53. Harrell, R.M.; Lyles, K.W.; Harrelson, J.M.; Friedman, N.E.; Drezner, M.K. Healing of bone disease in X-linked hypophosphatemic rickets/osteomalacia. Induction and maintenance with phosphorus and calcitriol. *J. Clin. Investig.* **1985**, *75*, 1858–1868. [CrossRef]
54. Sullivan, W.; Carpenter, T.; Glorieux, F.; Travers, R.; Insogna, K. A prospective trial of phosphate and 1,25-dihydroxyvitamin D3 therapy in symptomatic adults with X-linked hypophosphatemic rickets. *J. Clin. Endocrinol. Metab.* **1992**, *75*, 879–885.
55. Jin, C.; Zhang, C.; Ni, X.; Zhao, Z.; Xu, L.; Wu, B.; Chi, Y.; Jiajue, R.; Jiang, Y.; Wang, O.; et al. The efficacy and safety of different doses of calcitriol combined with neutral phosphate in X-linked hypophosphatemia: A prospective study. *Osteoporos. Int.* **2022**, *33*, 1385–1395. [CrossRef]
56. Verge, C.F.; Lam, A.; Simpson, J.M.; Cowell, C.T.; Howard, N.J.; Silink, M. Effects of therapy in X-linked hypophosphatemic rickets. *N. Engl. J. Med.* **1991**, *325*, 1843–1848. [CrossRef]
57. DeLacey, S.; Liu, Z.; Broyles, A.; El-Azab, S.A.; Guandique, C.F.; James, B.C.; Imel, E.A. Hyperparathyroidism and parathyroidectomy in X-linked hypophosphatemia patients. *Bone* **2019**, *127*, 386–392. [CrossRef]

58. Lecoq, A.L.; Chaumet-Riffaud, P.; Blanchard, A.; Dupeux, M.; Rothenbuhler, A.; Lambert, B.; Durand, E.; Boros, E.; Briot, K.; Silve, C.; et al. Hyperparathyroidism in Patients With X-Linked Hypophosphatemia. *J. Bone Miner. Res.* **2020**, *35*, 1263–1273. [CrossRef]
59. Yamazaki, Y.; Tamada, T.; Kasai, N.; Urakawa, I.; Aono, Y.; Hasegawa, H.; Fujita, T.; Kuroki, R.; Yamashita, T.; Fukumoto, S.; et al. Anti-FGF23 neutralizing antibodies show the physiological role and structural features of FGF23. *J. Bone Miner. Res.* **2008**, *23*, 1509–1518. [CrossRef]
60. Aono, Y.; Yamazaki, Y.; Yasutake, J.; Kawata, T.; Hasegawa, H.; Urakawa, I.; Fujita, T.; Wada, M.; Yamashita, T.; Fukumoto, S.; et al. Therapeutic effects of anti-FGF23 antibodies in hypophosphatemic rickets/osteomalacia. *J. Bone Miner. Res.* **2009**, *24*, 1879–1888. [CrossRef]
61. Aono, Y.; Hasegawa, H.; Yamazaki, Y.; Shimada, T.; Fujita, T.; Yamashita, T.; Fukumoto, S. Anti-FGF-23 neutralizing antibodies ameliorate muscle weakness and decreased spontaneous movement of Hyp mice. *J. Bone Miner. Res.* **2011**, *26*, 803–810. [CrossRef] [PubMed]
62. Padidela, R.; Whyte, M.P.; Glorieux, F.H.; Munns, C.F.; Ward, L.M.; Nilsson, O.; Portale, A.A.; Simmons, J.H.; Namba, N.; Cheong, H.I.; et al. Patient-Reported Outcomes from a Randomized, Active-Controlled, Open-Label, Phase 3 Trial of Burosumab Versus Conventional Therapy in Children with X-Linked Hypophosphatemia. *Calcif. Tissue Int.* **2021**, *108*, 622–633. [CrossRef]
63. Imanishi, Y.; Ito, N.; Rhee, Y.; Takeuchi, Y.; Shin, C.S.; Takahashi, Y.; Onuma, H.; Kojima, M.; Kanematsu, M.; Kanda, H.; et al. Interim Analysis of a Phase 2 Open-Label Trial Assessing Burosumab Efficacy and Safety in Patients With Tumor-Induced Osteomalacia. *J. Bone Miner. Res.* **2021**, *36*, 262–270. [CrossRef] [PubMed]
64. Jan de Beur, S.M.; Miller, P.D.; Weber, T.J.; Peacock, M.; Insogna, K.; Kumar, R.; Rauch, F.; Luca, D.; Cimms, T.; Roberts, M.S.; et al. Burosumab for the Treatment of Tumor-Induced Osteomalacia. *J. Bone Miner. Res.* **2021**, *36*, 627–635. [CrossRef] [PubMed]
65. Carpenter, T.O.; Imel, E.A.; Ruppe, M.D.; Weber, T.J.; Klausner, M.A.; Wooddell, M.M.; Kawakami, T.; Ito, T.; Zhang, X.; Humphrey, J.; et al. Randomized trial of the anti-FGF23 antibody KRN23 in X-linked hypophosphatemia. *J. Clin. Investig.* **2014**, *124*, 1587–1597. [CrossRef] [PubMed]
66. Zhang, X.; Imel, E.A.; Ruppe, M.D.; Weber, T.J.; Klausner, M.A.; Ito, T.; Vergeire, M.; Humphrey, J.; Glorieux, F.H.; Portale, A.A.; et al. Pharmacokinetics and pharmacodynamics of a human monoclonal anti-FGF23 antibody (KRN23) in the first multiple ascending-dose trial treating adults with X-linked hypophosphatemia. *J. Clin. Pharmacol.* **2016**, *56*, 176–185. [CrossRef]
67. Zhang, X.; Peyret, T.; Gosselin, N.H.; Marier, J.F.; Imel, E.A.; Carpenter, T.O. Population pharmacokinetic and pharmacodynamic analyses from a 4-month intradose escalation and its subsequent 12-month dose titration studies for a human monoclonal anti-FGF23 antibody (KRN23) in adults with X-linked hypophosphatemia. *J. Clin. Pharmacol.* **2016**, *56*, 429–438. [CrossRef]
68. Imel, E.A.; Zhang, X.; Ruppe, M.D.; Weber, T.J.; Klausner, M.A.; Ito, T.; Vergeire, M.; Humphrey, J.S.; Glorieux, F.H.; Portale, A.A.; et al. Prolonged Correction of Serum Phosphorus in Adults With X-Linked Hypophosphatemia Using Monthly Doses of KRN23. *J. Clin. Endocrinol. Metab.* **2015**, *100*, 2565–2573. [CrossRef]
69. Ruppe, M.D.; Zhang, X.; Imel, E.A.; Weber, T.J.; Klausner, M.A.; Ito, T.; Vergeire, M.; Humphrey, J.S.; Glorieux, F.H.; Portale, A.A.; et al. Effect of four monthly doses of a human monoclonal anti-FGF23 antibody (KRN23) on quality of life in X-linked hypophosphatemia. *Bone Rep.* **2016**, *5*, 158–162. [CrossRef]
70. Insogna, K.L.; Briot, K.; Imel, E.A.; Kamenicky, P.; Ruppe, M.D.; Portale, A.A.; Weber, T.; Pitukcheewanont, P.; Cheong, H.I.; Jan de Beur, S.; et al. A Randomized, Double-Blind, Placebo-Controlled, Phase 3 Trial Evaluating the Efficacy of Burosumab, an Anti-FGF23 Antibody, in Adults With X-Linked Hypophosphatemia: Week 24 Primary Analysis. *J. Bone Miner. Res.* **2018**, *33*, 1383–1393. [CrossRef]
71. Portale, A.A.; Carpenter, T.O.; Brandi, M.L.; Briot, K.; Cheong, H.I.; Cohen-Solal, M.; Crowley, R.; Jan De Beur, S.; Eastell, R.; Imanishi, Y.; et al. Continued Beneficial Effects of Burosumab in Adults with X-Linked Hypophosphatemia: Results from a 24-Week Treatment Continuation Period After a 24-Week Double-Blind Placebo-Controlled Period. *Calcif. Tissue Int.* **2019**, *105*, 271–284. [CrossRef] [PubMed]
72. Briot, K.; Portale, A.A.; Brandi, M.L.; Carpenter, T.O.; Cheong, H.I.; Cohen-Solal, M.; Crowley, R.K.; Eastell, R.; Imanishi, Y.; Ing, S.; et al. Burosumab treatment in adults with X-linked hypophosphataemia: 96-week patient-reported outcomes and ambulatory function from a randomised phase 3 trial and open-label extension. *RMD Open* **2021**, *7*, e001714. [CrossRef]
73. Insogna, K.L.; Rauch, F.; Kamenicky, P.; Ito, N.; Kubota, T.; Nakamura, A.; Zhang, L.; Mealiffe, M.; San Martin, J.; Portale, A.A. Burosumab Improved Histomorphometric Measures of Osteomalacia in Adults With X-Linked Hypophosphatemia: A Phase 3, Single-Arm, International Trial. *J. Bone Miner. Res.* **2019**, *34*, 2183–2191. [CrossRef] [PubMed]
74. Fratzl-Zelman, N.; Hartmann, M.A.; Gamsjaeger, S.; Rokidi, S.; Paschalis, E.P.; Blouin, S.; Zwerina, J. Bone matrix mineralization and response to burosumab in adult patients with X -linked hypophosphatemia: Results from the phase 3, single-arm international trial. *J. Bone Miner. Res.*. 2022 in press. [CrossRef] [PubMed]
75. Linglart, A.; Biosse-Duplan, M.; Briot, K.; Chaussain, C.; Esterle, L.; Guillaume-Czitrom, S.; Kamenicky, P.; Nevoux, J.; Prie, D.; Rothenbuhler, A.; et al. Therapeutic management of hypophosphatemic rickets from infancy to adulthood. *Endocr. Connect.* **2014**, *3*, R13–R30. [CrossRef] [PubMed]

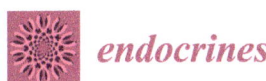

Case Report

The Possible Outcomes of Poor Adherence to Conventional Treatment in Patients with X-Linked Hypophosphatemic Rickets/Osteomalacia

Hiroaki Zukeran [1,*], Kento Ikegawa [1], Chikahiko Numakura [2] and Yukihiro Hasegawa [1]

[1] Division of Endocrinology and Metabolism, Tokyo Metropolitan Children Medical Center, 2-8-29 Musashidai, Fuchu-shi 183-8561, Tokyo, Japan
[2] Department of Pediatrics, Yamagata University School of Medicine, 2-2-2 Iidanishi, Yamagata-shi 990-9585, Yamagata, Japan
* Correspondence: hzukeran0325.63@gmail.com; Tel.: +81-42-300-5111

Highlights:

What are the main findings?

- Adherence to conventional treatment is essential but challenging for patients with XLH.
- Conventional treatment should continue even after XLH-children have stopped their growth.

What is the implication of the main findings?

- Burosumab is a novel treatment strategy for pediatric patients with poor adherence to conventional treatment.

Abstract: X-linked hypophosphatemic rickets/osteomalacia is an inherited disease caused by the loss of function in *PHEX*. Elevated plasma FGF23 in patients with XLH leads to hypophosphatemia. The conventional treatment for XLH, consisting of oral phosphate and active vitamin D, is often poorly adhered to for various reasons, such as the requirement to take multiple daily doses of phosphate. Burosumab, an anti-FGF23 antibody, is a new drug that directly targets the mechanism underlying XLH. We report herein three adult patients with poor adherence to the conventional treatment. In Patient 1, adherence was poor throughout childhood and adolescence. The treatment of Patients 2 and 3 became insufficient after adolescence. All of the patients suffered from gait disturbance caused by pain, fractures, and lower extremity deformities early in life. We prescribed burosumab for the latter two patients, and their symptoms, which were unaffected by resuming conventional treatment, dramatically improved with burosumab. Maintaining adherence to the conventional treatment is crucial but challenging for patients with XLH. Starting burosumab therapy from childhood or adolescence in pediatric patients with poor adherence may help prevent the early onset of complications.

Keywords: X-linked hypophosphatemic rickets/osteomalacia; conventional treatment; adherence; burosumab

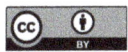

1. Introduction

X-linked hypophosphatemic rickets/osteomalacia (XLH) is an X-linked dominant disorder caused by loss of function in the phosphate-regulating gene with homologies to endopeptidase on the X chromosome (PHEX). Inactivating mutations in PHEX raise plasma concentrations of fibroblast growth factor 23 (FGF23), although the mechanism is not fully understood. Excess FGF23 leads to hypophosphatemia by impairing renal phosphate reabsorption, and decreasing 1,25-dihydroxyvitamin D synthesis [1–3].

The conventional treatment, consisting of oral phosphate and active vitamin D, has some efficacy, but most pediatric patients still have lower limb deformities, diminished growth, and bone or joint pain. Moreover, because the serum phosphate level returns to a low baseline value within a few hours of phosphate intake, patients must take phosphate several times a day, which contributes to poor adherence [4,5].

The effect of the conventional treatment in adults is also insufficient. Adult patients suffer from bone or joint pain and stiffness, fractures, osteoarthritis, and enthesopathy. Moreover, various complications related to the conventional treatment, such as nephrocalcinosis and hyperparathyroidism, may also occur. Owing to the burden of these symptoms, the quality of life (QOL) of patients with XLH is low [6,7].

Burosumab, a human monoclonal anti-FGF23 antibody approved for use in Japan in December 2019, is the first drug that directly targets the underlying mechanism of XLH. Burosumab is administered via subcutaneous injection every four weeks in adult patients, and every two weeks in pediatric patients [2,3]. Randomized controlled trials with pediatric patients with XLH demonstrated that burosumab therapy was more effective than the conventional treatment in improving rickets, lower limb deformity, growth, and mobility [8,9]. Studies with adult patients demonstrated that burosumab therapy also contributed to healing fractures and improving QOL [10–12].

Herein, we reported three male patients with XLH whose conventional treatment during childhood and adolescence was insufficient. Patient 1 showed a serious outcome that may have contributed to poor adherence to conventional treatment. The other patients demonstrated favorable outcomes after receiving burosumab therapy.

2. Case Presentation

2.1. Patient 1

The patient presented with hypotonia at the age of 1 year and 7 months, and a bone X-ray revealed rachitic changes in his wrists and knees. Laboratory results confirmed the hypophosphatemia (2.7 mg/dL [normal range: 3.9–6.2 mg/dL]), elevated ALP (642 IU/L, IFCC [normal range: 139–471 IU/L]), and a decreased ratio of the maximum tubular reabsorption to glomerular filtration rate (TmP/GFR) (2.0 mg/dL [normal range: 4.5–6.1 mg/dL]). Based on these findings, he was suspected of having XLH. There was no family history of rickets. A gene analysis at the age of 16 confirmed a frameshift mutation in *PHEX* (c.2473insACTC).

The conventional treatment, consisting of oral phosphate (30 mg/kg) and active vitamin D (0.1 µg/kg), was delayed until the age of 3 years. Even after our diagnosis, his parents refused to acknowledge for some time that he had XLH. After he began walking, genu valgum and waddling gait became apparent. At that time, he stopped attending school because of the embarrassment of having short stature and began acting out violently towards his family. Adherence to conventional treatment was extremely poor throughout childhood and adolescence, hence the lower extremity deformities and short stature failed to improve, and scoliosis developed. He had three genu valgum orthopedic surgery between the ages of 12 and 15. During the third surgery at the age of 15, intramedullary nails were inserted into his left femur. However, there was not much improvement, and the waddling gait persisted. His adult height was 140 cm (-5.3 SD [13]). He continued the oral phosphate and active vitamin D therapy without effect until he decided to discontinue the treatment at the age of 25. Figure 1 shows the severe scoliosis and deformities in his extremities at the age of 33.

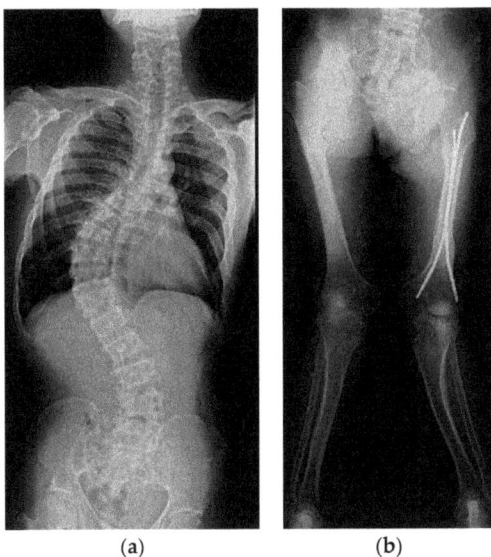

Figure 1. Bone X-rays at the age of 33. (**a**): Severe scoliosis. (**b**): Malalignment of the lower extremities, including differences in the length of the femurs and bowing of the tibias. (Intramedullary nails were inserted into the left femur).

2.2. Patient 2

The patient was referred to our hospital at the age of 11 months because he was unable to crawl. His family history was unremarkable. A physical examination revealed a rachitic rosary and mild thoracic deformity. A laboratory examination demonstrated hypophosphatemia (2.4 mg/dL [normal range: 3.9–6.2 mg/dL]), and a decreased TmP/GFR ratio (2.1 mg/dL [normal range: 4.5–6.1 mg/dL]). No abnormal findings were observed on the other routine tests. Radiographs demonstrated cupping and flaring of the radii and ulnae, indicating XLH. Conventional treatment was started (phosphate 40 mg/kg, active vitamin D 0.1 μg/kg), and his motor development delay and bone deformities improved as a result. At the age of 12, a gene analysis detected a mutation in *PHEX* (IVS9+1 G > A).

His adherence to therapy began worsening from around the age of 17 until he finally stopped visiting the hospital at the age of 21. Although he resumed the phosphate and active vitamin D therapy one year later, he experienced tibial fractures without trauma where technetium-99m bone scan demonstrated abnormal uptake (Figure 2). The lower leg pain was too severe to allow him to walk normally and prevented him from taking a six-minute walk test (6MWT).

Burosumab 0.8 mg per actual weight (1.0 mg per ideal weight) for four weeks was started at the age of 25. The patient reported that, shortly after starting burosumab administration, his pain diminished and was almost completely remitted within six months. One year and two months later, although he was still unable to walk at the average speed for his age, the patient achieved 240 m on a 6MWT and (reference range: 584–686 m [14]). Laboratory data at five months after the start of burosumab therapy found elevated serum inorganic phosphate and TmP/GFR ratio and decreased intact PTH (Table 1). Unfortunately, no blood samples were taken in the first month after burosumab therapy, as recommended in most guidelines [2,3]. A technetium-99m bone scan twelve months after the start of burosumab therapy demonstrated marked improvement (Figure 2).

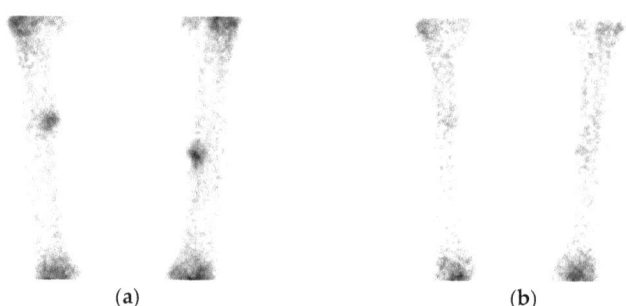

(a) (b)

Figure 2. Technetium-99m bone scans of the bilateral tibiae. (a) Before burosumab therapy: abnormal uptake indicating fractures. (b) Twelve months after the start of burosumab therapy: minimal abnormal uptake.

Table 1. Laboratory data on Patient 2 before and after the start of burosumab therapy (Tx).

		At Start of Tx	Five Months after Tx	Reference Range
TmP/GFR	(mg/dL)	0.87	1.76	2.3–4.3
Serum inorganic phosphorus	(mg/dL)	1.3	2.0	2.3–4.5
Serum calcium	(mg/dL)	9.2	9.5	8.2–10.4
Serum intact PTH	(pg/mL)	140.9	80.2	10.3–65.9
Serum alkaline phosphatase	(IU/L)	143	179	110–330
Urinary calcium/creatinine		0.04	0.05	-

2.3. Patient 3

The patient was brought to the hospital at the age of 1 year and 8 months for waddling gait. There was nothing remarkable in his family history. A physical examination revealed genu varum. Laboratory examination found hypophosphatemia (2.2 mg/dL [normal range: 3.9–6.2 mg/dL]), a decreased TmP/GFR ratio (0.6 mg/dL [normal range: 4.5–6.1 mg/dL]), and normal serum 25-hydroxyvitamin D (36 ng/mL). A bone X-ray found wrist and knee rickets. These findings implied XLH, and conventional treatment was begun (phosphate 40 mg/kg, active vitamin D 0.1 µg/kg). The treatment corrected the genu varum, and his gait normalized.

The patient reported difficulty adhering to the regimen of multiple daily phosphate doses during childhood. At the age of 11, with the end of his growth spurt, he discontinued the treatment. Although he continued receiving active vitamin D, the genu varum recurred one year after discontinuing phosphate therapy. At the age of 25, he began experiencing pain in his hip joints. He resumed phosphate therapy at the age of 35 without effect. The pain extended from the hip joints to the lower extremities and lower back.

At the age of 41, he was referred to our hospital. Gene analysis detected a mutation in *PHEX* (c.1735G > A). Six months after the referral, a bone X-ray demonstrated a vertebral compression fracture, and the patient was barely able to walk owing to the severe pain. Burosumab 0.7 mg per actual weight (1.0 mg per ideal weight) for four weeks was prescribed, almost completely eliminating the pain after eight months. One year later, he achieved 364 m on a 6MWT. His serum inorganic phosphorus was higher at one month before the start of burosumab therapy when he was receiving the conventional treatment than five months later. Table 2 shows the sequential changes in the laboratory data, including elevated TmP/GFR. The serum inorganic phosphorus value was highest before burosumab because the sample was obtained after phosphate administration.

Table 2. Sequential laboratory data on Patient 3: one month before Tx, at the start of Tx, and five months after Tx.

		One Month before Tx	At Start of Tx	Five Months after Tx	Reference Range
TmP/GFR	(mg/dL)	1.75	-	2.11	2.3–4.3
Serum inorganic phosphorus	(mg/dL)	2.9	1.7	2.7	2.3–4.5
Serum calcium	(mg/dL)	9.7	9.6	9.6	8.2–10.4
Serum intact PTH	(pg/mL)	-	80.7	91.2	10.3–65.9
Serum alkaline phosphatase	(IU/L)	187	169	152	110–330
Urinary calcium/creatinine		0.04	-	0.07	-

3. Discussion

The present report described three adult patients with gait disturbance caused by pain, fractures, and lower extremity deformities early in life. Although the disease expression and outcomes are highly variable, the poor outcomes in present cases may be related to inadequate conventional treatment in childhood and adolescence.

Adherence to the conventional treatment during childhood and adolescence is essential for patients with XLH. Patient 1 suffered from severe lower extremity deformities, and attained a markedly low adult height owing to his poor adherence to therapy throughout childhood and adolescence, and the delayed start of therapy. Before the conventional treatment became available, untreated adult patients were consigned to having severe bone deformities [15–17]. A recent report described a male patient with XLH, which had been misdiagnosed as achondroplasia until the mistake was discovered at the age of 51. Severe deformities developed in the patient's lower extremities and spine, and his final adult height was 127 cm [18].

One of the tremendous burdens of XLH in childhood and adolescence associated with the conventional treatment is the frequent dosing [2,5]. In Patient 2, the worsening of adherence to therapy during adolescence contributed to the formation of fractures and onset of pain in early adulthood. Although no studies have focused on treatment adherence in patients with XLH, the burden of frequent daily phosphate dosing is likely to contribute to discouraging adherence.

Conventional treatment should continue to be administered even after growth is complete. Patient 3 discontinued phosphate after his growth spurt, possibly contributing to his poor prognosis in adulthood. Continuing the conventional treatment into adulthood is controversial because the complications of enthesopathy and osteoarthritis are not alleviated by conventional treatment, and there are concerns about possible side effects, such as hyperparathyroidism and nephrocalcinosis [1,19,20]. Indeed, the 2022 consensus statement [3] does not recommend treating asymptomatic adult patients. However, in our previous report, ten patients with XLH who discontinued the conventional treatment at around the age of 20 became symptomatic (fractures and severe pain) within two to ten years, and resuming the therapy ameliorated their clinical symptoms [21]. These findings suggested that, even if patients are asymptomatic, the symptoms may re-emerge after treatment discontinuation. Continuing the conventional treatment into adulthood can prevent severe complications in patients with child-onset XHL.

Burosumab dramatically improved the pain and gait disorder caused by poor outcomes of the conventional treatment during adolescence and adulthood in Patients 2 and 3, whose symptoms failed to show any improvement after resuming the conventional treatment. Burosumab is recommended for adult patients with persistent bone and/or joint pain, fractures, pseudofractures, or an insufficient response to the conventional treatment [2,3].

On the other hand, the criteria for prescribing burosumab in pediatric patients are unclear. The criteria advocated by one guideline [22] are specific: burosumab is to be administered to pediatric patients with clinical symptoms, such as chronic pain, growth delay, and bone deformity. These criteria do not address poor adherence. Although the 2019 consensus statement [2] recommends burosumab for pediatric patients who are unable to adhere to conventional treatment, it also states that no conclusive recommendations can be given because the data on the long-term outcomes and cost-effectiveness of burosumab are pending. As mentioned above, conventional treatment is burdensome and difficult for the patient to adhere. To improve adherence in patients with chronic diseases such as XLH, the treatment burden needs continually to be assessed. Depending on the assessment, the treatment may need to be modified [23].

In conclusion, adequate adherence to conventional treatment is crucial but challenging for patients with XLH. Initiating burosumab therapy from childhood in pediatric patients with poor adherence may help prevent complications from appearing early in life. Since XLH is a rare disease and the present report describes only three patients, further long-term studies are required.

Author Contributions: Y.H. conceptualized the study. H.Z. wrote the original draft, and Y.H., K.I. and C.N. edited it. All authors have read and agreed to the published version of the manuscript.

Funding: This study received no external funding.

Institutional Review Board Statement: Ethical review and approval were waived for this study.

Informed Consent Statement: Informed consent was obtained from all the subjects mentioned in this report.

Data Availability Statement: Not applicable.

Acknowledgments: We thank our patients for consenting to participate in this report and James R. Valera for his assistance with editing this manuscript.

Conflicts of Interest: The authors declare no conflict of interest.

References

1. Carpenter, T.O.; Imel, E.A.; Holm, I.A.; Jan de Beur, S.M.; Insogna, K.L. A Clinician's Guide to X-Linked Hypophosphatemia. *J. Bone Miner Res.* **2011**, *26*, 1381–1388. [CrossRef] [PubMed]
2. Haffner, D.; Emma, F.; Eastwood, D.M.; Duplan, M.B.; Bacchetta, J.; Schnabel, D.; Wicart, P.; Bockenhauer, D.; Santos, F.; Levtchenko, E.; et al. Clinical Practice Recommendations for the Diagnosis and Management of X-Linked Hypophosphataemia. *Nat. Rev. Nephrol.* **2019**, *15*, 435–455. [CrossRef] [PubMed]
3. Trombetti, A.; Al-Daghri, N.; Brandi, M.L.; Cannata-Andía, J.B.; Cavalier, E.; Chandran, M.; Chaussain, C.; Cipullo, L.; Cooper, C.; Haffner, D.; et al. Interdisciplinary Management of FGF23-Related Phosphate Wasting Syndromes: A Consensus Statement on the Evaluation, Diagnosis and Care of Patients with X-Linked Hypophosphataemia. *Nat. Rev. Endocrinol.* **2022**, *18*, 366–384. [CrossRef] [PubMed]
4. Linglart, A.; Biosse-Duplan, M.; Briot, K.; Chaussain, C.; Esterle, L.; Guillaume-Czitrom, S.; Kamenicky, P.; Nevoux, J.; Prié, D.; Rothenbuhler, A.; et al. Therapeutic Management of Hypophosphatemic Rickets from Infancy to Adulthood. *Endocr. Connect.* **2014**, *3*, R13–R30. [CrossRef] [PubMed]
5. Ferizović, N.; Marshall, J.; Williams, A.E.; Mughal, M.Z.; Shaw, N.; Mak, C.; Gardiner, O.; Hossain, P.; Upadhyaya, S. Exploring the Burden of X-Linked Hypophosphataemia: An Opportunistic Qualitative Study of Patient Statements Generated During a Technology Appraisal. *Adv. Ther.* **2020**, *37*, 770–784. [CrossRef]
6. Skrinar, A.; Dvorak-Ewell, M.; Evins, A.; Macica, C.; Linglart, A.; Imel, E.A.; Theodore-Oklota, C.; San Martin, J. The Lifelong Impact of X-Linked Hypophosphatemia: Results From a Burden of Disease Survey. *J. Endocr. Soc.* **2019**, *3*, 1321–1334. [CrossRef]
7. Ito, N.; Kang, H.G.; Nishida, Y.; Evins, A.; Skrinar, A.; Cheong, H.I. Burden of Disease of X-Linked Hypophosphatemia in Japanese and Korean Patients: A Cross-Sectional Survey. *Endocr. J.* **2021**, *69*, 373–383. [CrossRef]
8. Imel, E.A.; Glorieux, F.H.; Whyte, M.P.; Munns, C.F.; Ward, L.; Nilsson, O.; Simmons, J.H.; Padidela, R.; Namba, N.; Cheong, H.I.; et al. Burosumab versus Continuation of Conventional Therapy in Children with X-Linked Hypophosphatemia: A Randomised, Active-Controlled, Open-Label, Phase 3 Trial. *Lancet* **2019**, *393*, 2416–2427. [CrossRef]
9. Padidela, R.; Whyte, M.P.; Glorieux, F.H.; Munns, C.F.; Ward, L.M.; Nilsson, O.; Portale, A.A.; Simmons, J.H.; Namba, N.; Cheong, H.I.; et al. Patient-Reported Outcomes from a Randomized, Active-Controlled, Open-Label, Phase 3 Trial of Burosumab Versus Conventional Therapy in Children with X-Linked Hypophosphatemia. *Calcif. Tissue Int.* **2021**, *108*, 622–633. [CrossRef] [PubMed]
10. Insogna, K.L.; Briot, K.; Imel, E.A.; Kamenický, P.; Ruppe, M.D.; Portale, A.A.; Weber, T.; Pitukcheewanont, P.; Cheong, H.I.; Jan de Beur, S.; et al. A Randomized, Double-Blind, Placebo-Controlled, Phase 3 Trial Evaluating the Efficacy of Burosumab, an Anti-FGF23 Antibody, in Adults With X-Linked Hypophosphatemia: Week 24 Primary Analysis. *J. Bone Miner Res.* **2018**, *33*, 1383–1393. [CrossRef]

11. Portale, A.A.; Carpenter, T.O.; Brandi, M.L.; Briot, K.; Cheong, H.I.; Cohen-Solal, M.; Crowley, R.; Jan De Beur, S.; Eastell, R.; Imanishi, Y.; et al. Continued Beneficial Effects of Burosumab in Adults with X-Linked Hypophosphatemia: Results from a 24-Week Treatment Continuation Period After a 24-Week Double-Blind Placebo-Controlled Period. *Calcif. Tissue Int.* **2019**, *105*, 271–284. [CrossRef]
12. Insogna, K.L.; Rauch, F.; Kamenický, P.; Ito, N.; Kubota, T.; Nakamura, A.; Zhang, L.; Mealiffe, M.; San Martin, J.; Portale, A.A. Burosumab Improved Histomorphometric Measures of Osteomalacia in Adults with X-Linked Hypophosphatemia: A Phase 3, Single-Arm, International Trial. *J. Bone Miner Res.* **2019**, *34*, 2183–2191. [CrossRef]
13. Suwa, S. Growth Charts for Height and Weight of Japanese from Birth to 17 Years Based on a Cross-Sectional of National Data. *Clin. Pediatr. Endocrinol.* **1993**, *2*, 11. [CrossRef]
14. Halliday, S.J.; Wang, L.; Yu, C.; Vickers, B.P.; Newman, J.H.; Fremont, R.D.; Huerta, L.E.; Brittain, E.L.; Hemnes, A.R. Six-Minute Walk Distance in Healthy Young Adults. *Respir. Med.* **2020**, *165*, 105933. [CrossRef] [PubMed]
15. Pedersen, H.E.; McCarroll, H.R. Vitamin-resistant rickets. *J. Bone Jt. Surg. Am.* **1951**, *33*, 203–220. [CrossRef] [PubMed]
16. Pierce, D.S.; Wallace, W.M.; Herndon, C.H. Long-term treatment of vitamin-D resistant rickets. *J. Bone Jt. Surg. Am.* **1964**, *46*, 978–997. [CrossRef]
17. Tapia, J.; Stearns, G.; Ponseti, I.V. Vitamin-D resistant rickets: A long-term clinical study of 11 patients. *J. Bone Jt. Surg. Am.* **1964**, *46*, 935–958. [CrossRef]
18. Chin, Y.A.; Zhao, Y.; Tay, G.; Sim, W.; Chow, C.Y.; Chandran, M. Delayed Diagnosis, Difficult Decisions: Novel Gene Deletion Causing X-Linked Hypophosphatemia in a Middle-Aged Man with Achondroplastic Features and Tertiary Hyperparathyroidism. *Case Rep. Endocrinol.* **2021**, *2021*, 9944552. [CrossRef]
19. Connor, J.; Olear, E.A.; Insogna, K.L.; Katz, L.; Baker, S.; Kaur, R.; Simpson, C.A.; Sterpka, J.; Dubrow, R.; Zhang, J.H.; et al. Conventional Therapy in Adults With X-Linked Hypophosphatemia: Effects on Enthesopathy and Dental Disease. *J. Clin. Endocrinol. Metab.* **2015**, *100*, 3625–3632. [CrossRef] [PubMed]
20. Mäkitie, O.; Kooh, S.W.; Sochett, E. Prolonged High-Dose Phosphate Treatment: A Risk Factor for Tertiary Hyperparathyroidism in X-Linked Hypophosphatemic Rickets. *Clin. Endocrinol.* **2003**, *58*, 163–168. [CrossRef]
21. Suzuki, E.; Yamada, M.; Ariyasu, D.; Izawa, M.; Miyamoto, J.; Koto, S.; Hasegawa, Y. Patients with Hypophosphatemic Osteomalacia Need Continuous Treatment during Adulthood. *Clin. Pediatr. Endocrinol.* **2009**, *18*, 29–33. [CrossRef] [PubMed]
22. Laurent, M.R.; De Schepper, J.; Trouet, D.; Godefroid, N.; Boros, E.; Heinrichs, C.; Bravenboer, B.; Velkeniers, B.; Lammens, J.; Harvengt, P.; et al. Consensus Recommendations for the Diagnosis and Management of X-Linked Hypophosphatemia in Belgium. *Front. Endocrinol.* **2021**, *12*, 641543. [CrossRef] [PubMed]
23. Heckman, B.W.; Mathew, A.R.; Carpenter, M.J. Treatment Burden and Treatment Fatigue as Barriers to Health. *Curr. Opin. Psychol.* **2015**, *5*, 31–36. [CrossRef] [PubMed]

Disclaimer/Publisher's Note: The statements, opinions and data contained in all publications are solely those of the individual author(s) and contributor(s) and not of MDPI and/or the editor(s). MDPI and/or the editor(s) disclaim responsibility for any injury to people or property resulting from any ideas, methods, instructions or products referred to in the content.

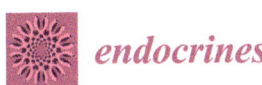

Review

Orthopedic Complications and Management in Children with X-Linked Hypophosphatemia

Chikahisa Higuchi

Department of Orthopaedic Surgery, Osaka Women's and Children's Hospital, Izumi 594-1101, Osaka, Japan; chiguchi@wch.opho.jp; Tel.: +81-725-56-1220

Abstract: X-linked hypophosphatemia is an inheritable disease of renal phosphate wasting that results in clinically manifestations associated with rickets or osteomalacia. The various symptoms in the skeletal system are well recognized, such as short stature; lower limb deformities; and bone, joint, or muscle pain, and it is often difficult to control these symptoms, despite the use of medication therapy in growing children. In addition, lower limb deformities can lead to degenerative osteoarthritis and dysfunction of lower limbs at the skeletal maturity. To prevent from future manifestation of those symptoms, orthopedic surgeries are applicable to growing patients with severe skeletal deformities or without response to conventional medication. Bone deformities are treated by acute or gradual corrective osteotomies and temporally hemiepiphysiodesis using guided growth method. The clinicians should choose the right procedure based on age, symptoms and state of deformities of the patient.

Keywords: X-linked hypophosphatemia; deformity correction; mechanical axis

1. Introduction

X-linked hypophosphatemia (XLH, OMIM #307800) is a rare genetic disorder caused by renal phosphate wasting and is the most common form of hypophosphatemic rickets and osteomalacia. This disease causes fibroblast growth factor 23 (FGF23)-related hypophosphatemia. FGF23 is a circulating hormone for phosphate regulation throughout the whole body, and the elevation of this growth factor leads to renal wasting of phosphate and low serum phosphate. The responsible gene for XLH is identified on PHEX (phosphate-regulating protein with homology to endopeptidases on the X chromosome) [1,2]. A decrease or absence of PHEX activity induces an increase in FGF23. On the other hand, bone is mainly composed of hydroxyapatite and collagens, and hydroxyapatite contains phosphate in its own structure. Therefore, skeletal complications are caused as phosphate regulation is out of order in the PHEX/FGF23 axis. This condition causes rickets, which is characterized by the impairment of the maturation of growth plates in patients during childhood, as well as osteomalacia, which is characterized by the disturbance of mineralization in osteoids in adulthood. Lower limb deformities and various sequelae such as gait alterations or pain in the lower limbs, which are the main complaints of patients with rickets [3], have been reported in affected children and adults [4–6] and are associated with impairment of quality of life [7].

The diagnosis of patients with XLH is generally made in childhood, and the treatment with medication is continued throughout the lifetime. Oral phosphate and active vitamin D are generally administered, with active vitamin D being included in the conventional treatment. This treatment promotes the growth and improvement of skeletal deformities such as bowlegs and alleviates bone, joint, and muscle pain. The good control of phosphate caused by the medication reduces the need for orthopedic surgeries [8–10]. However, the responses to this medical treatment are varied, and operative procedures for bone deformities can be chosen in unsuccessful cases of medication [11–13]. Burosumab, an

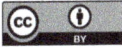

anti-fibroblast growth factor 23 antibody, is approved for this disease [14–16] and expected to be efficacious for various symptoms, including bone deformities. However, there are only two papers on the efficacy for bone deformities of this new medication at present.

This article reviews the orthopedic complications and recent orthopedic interventions in children with XLH.

2. Orthopedic Features and Treatments in Infancy and Early Childhood

XLH is a dominant disorder. If a parent or siblings of a newborn infant has been diagnosed with XLH, the baby can be expected to have XLH and a careful investigation of hypophosphatemia would be performed by a pediatrician. However, in the absence of the family history of XLH, this disorder should be suspected based on physical and radiographic findings as described below.

2.1. Bowlegs

The most characteristic orthopedic feature of XLH is a bowleg in childhood, especially after the start of standing and walking in early childhood. Weight-bearing leads lower limbs to more serious deformities than physiological varus or valgus knee deformities in XLH patients. Bowlegs in early childhood occur due to several causes, including vitamin D deficiency, Blount disease (epiphysitis in the proximally medial tibia), physiological factors, and so on. The clinicians should make a differential diagnosis between XLH and these conditions using various examinations.

Plain radiographic images of lower limbs should be examined for the differential diagnoses at the initial visit. The widening of epiphyseal plates and an unclear demarcation line between the epiphyseal plate and metaphysis are characteristically demonstrated in patients with rickets, and these factors should lead to a strong suspicion of rickets. However, these characteristic findings are detected in various forms of rickets. In particular, it is essential to differentiate between XLH and rickets caused by vitamin D insufficiency. In addition, these features are not always obvious upon first examination, and follow-up examinations are necessary for the diagnosis. In general, pediatricians commonly perform radiographic examinations of the wrist and knee joints in patients with rickets. From the point of view of orthopedists, radiographic images of the whole lower limbs should additionally be obtained not in a supine position but a standing position to evaluate the degree of a patient's varus deformity and functional disability in a standing posture. For the evaluation of limb deformities and functional disability, a mechanical axis deviation (MAD) is the most valuable parameter (Figure 1) [17]. The mechanical axis is defined as the line between the center of the femoral head and the center of the ankle joint on plain radiographic images of whole lower limbs in a standing individual. It represents a main weight-bearing point on the knee joint. An MAD shows the displacement of the mechanical axis from the center of the knee joint, and a large deviation to the medial or lateral side indicates severe deformity of the limb alignment.

The ideal mechanical axis line passes through the center of the knee joint and the ideal MAD is 0 mm. This parameter is useful for the objective assessment of the improvement or aggravation of limb deformities during follow-up examinations [18].

If the clinicians find radiographic evidence of rickets, they can add a radiographic survey of the growth plate around the wrist or knee joints for an assessment of pathological conditions using the Ricket Severity Score (RSS), which is a quantitative method based on the degree of metaphyseal fraying, concavity, and the rate of affected physis [19]. Recently, the Radiographic Global Impression of Change (RGI-C) score, which was developed in the evaluation of changes in hypophosphatasia [20], has been used to assess the healing of rickets in pediatric XLH patients [21]. If the patient has less obvious findings in the radiographic images, the clinicians should follow the changes of the genu varum with age. The various deformities around knee joints do not get better in most rachitic cases, while almost all physiological bowlegs improve. The development of a varus deformity is useful for the differential diagnosis between rickets and other conditions.

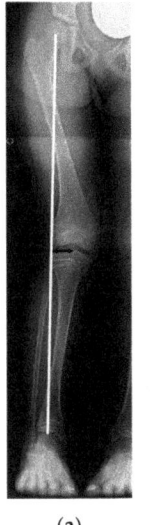 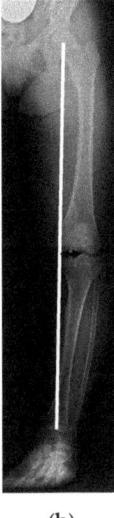

(a) (b)

Figure 1. Mechanical axis deviation (MAD) and varus or valgus deformity of a lower limb. The mechanical axis is defined as the line between the center of the femoral head and the center of the ankle joint (white line). Mechanical axis deviation is defined as the displacement of the mechanical axis from the center of the knee joint. (**a**) Valgus deformity of the lower limb exists because of the lateral displacement of the MAD. (**b**) Varus deformity of the lower limb exists because of the medial displacement of the MAD.

Laboratory abnormalities, which include hypophosphatemia and elevated alkaline phosphatase activity, must be checked in cases of rickets, including XLH. Recently, the FGF23 level and a mutation analysis of the PHEX gene can be examined and are very useful for reaching a definite diagnosis of XLH. Most orthopedists ask the expert pediatricians for investigations of bone metabolisms or genetics if they suspect rickets.

For patients with rickets in early childhood, medication treatment with phosphate and active vitamin D is first chosen. Therefore, orthopedic surgeons mainly check whether limb deformities, especially bowlegs, develop or not via plain radiography. If the deformity, mostly a varus deformity, is not improved or gets worse despite medication, the orthopedists should intervene in the management of the limb deformities. The orthopedic interventions include orthotic management and surgical treatment in this period. The effectiveness of orthoses such as a knee–ankle–foot orthosis (long leg brace) is not evident and is controversial. An orthopedic book describes no efficacy of orthotic management for vitamin-D-resistant rickets [22]. In particular, there has been no report of efficacious evidence in rickets of XLH. On the other hand, a few Japanese papers reported that orthotic treatment was efficacious in a small number of rachitic patients, including individuals with XLH [23]. Therefore, the application of orthoses is at each doctor's discretion in Japan for severe bowlegs caused by various pathologies, such as XLH or vitamin D deficiency. The author has no experience of the application of orthoses to rickets patients because of improvements in deformities caused by medication.

Osteotomies are performed in patients with XLH who have a severe deformity or less improvement of deformities via medication [24]. Most osteotomies are applied to the femur and tibia or fibula (Figure 2). Deformities of these long bones exist both around growth plates, i.e., the metaphysis, epiphysis, and diaphysis, and many deformity sites can exist in one lower limb. Therefore, it is difficult and unrealistic to correct a deformed bone to a normally morphological shape. The purpose of osteotomies is the acquisition of a better appearance and better function of the lower limbs. However, the clinicians should keep in mind that better function takes precedence over a better appearance. In early childhood, osteotomies around the inflection point of each bone are performed to improve the mechanical axis to as normal of a range as possible. However, the correction of deformities by osteotomies in early childhood is related with high recurrence rates and complications [12,25,26]. Petje et al. reported a recurrence rate of 90% after the first corrective osteotomy under adequate administration of phosphate [12]. Therefore, it is difficult to decide the time of the first surgical procedure, and two- or three-stage procedures should be planned during growth.

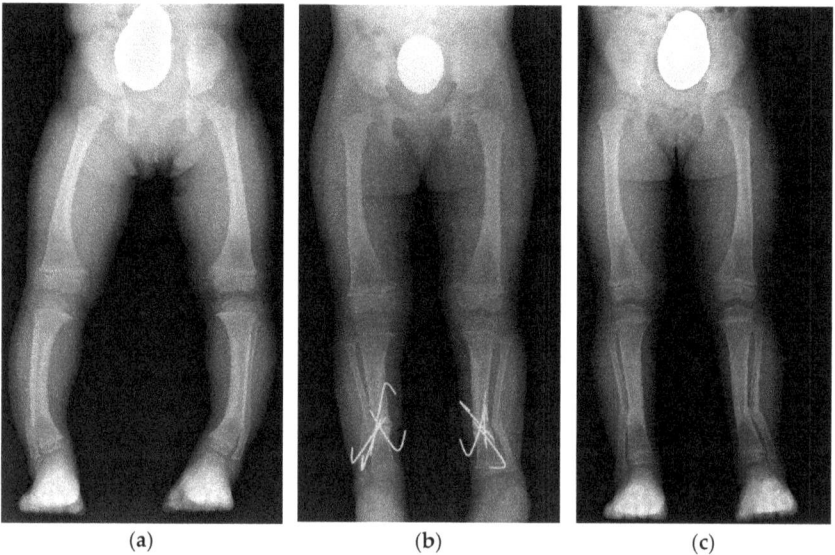

Figure 2. A case of correction osteotomy: (**a**) varus deformities of bilateral lower legs before correction osteotomy; (**b**) corrected lower legs after bilateral osteotomy with wire fixation; (**c**) correction of MAD after bone healing at osteotomy site.

2.2. Short Stature

One of the clinical symptoms in XLH is well known to be a growth impairment, especially short stature. Many pediatric orthopedists have encountered XLH patients with bowlegs and short stature. Several studies previously assessed the height in small populations of children with XLH [27,28], and Mao et al. recently reported growth curves for a relatively large population of children with XLH. They suggested that the height velocity decreased during the growth period compared to the normal population and that there was a notable decline in age- and sex-matched height Z-scores after walking age [29]. Short stature in XLH is proportional, although bowlegs are prominent. An orthopedic intervention is unnecessary and the treatment with phosphate and calcitriol should be selected for slow growth. Growth hormone therapy is also applied for short stature in XLH. Some papers have reported on the efficacious administration of recombinant human growth hormone, while others have suggested no significant benefits.

Burosumab, a recombinant human monoclonal antibody for FGF23, may be promising for the improvement of short stature in XLH patients [30].

3. Orthopedic Features and Treatments in Late Childhood and Adolescence

The physical and radiographic findings in late childhood and adolescence are similar to those in early childhood. However, the skeletal deformities are more various in these periods than in early childhood and patients are more likely to complain of their symptoms by themselves.

3.1. Lower Limb Deformity

Deformities around the knee joints are prominent in late childhood and adolescence, as are bowlegs in early childhood. However, those deformities are complicated in those generations, while varus deformities are more typical in early childhood. For example, some patients have varus or valgus deformities in bilateral knee joints and the others have a varus deformity in one lower limb and a valgus deformity in the other. The latter deformity is known as a windswept lower leg deformity [31]. The windswept deformity often leads to a leg length discrepancy (LLD) and dysfunction of the lower legs. The various abnormalities of the lower limb alignment cause various symptoms such as joint pain, bone pain, or joint laxity in the lower limbs as patients gain body weight via their skeletal growth and are subject to more weight-bearing stress on the lower extremities. Many researchers have suggested that severe residual deformities lead to degenerative changes in the joints of the lower limbs and impaired quality of life in adulthood [7,32–34].

Symptomatic deformities in the lower limbs should be treated as soon as possible and some asymptomatic deformities should also be treated via orthopedic procedures to prevent the patients from developing degenerative osteoarthritis of the lower limbs, spondylosis with functional scoliosis caused by LLD, and musculoskeletal pain in adulthood [35].

Most relatively mild cases with varus or valgus knee deformities are not corrected by osteotomies of the femur or the tibia in those periods but recently by temporary hemiepiphysiodesis using the guided growth method [15,36,37]. In guided growth surgery, a small plate is fixed on one side of a growth plate with two screws. These implants work as a tether system to the growth in one side of the epiphyseal plate and allow the lower limb alignment to improve with skeletal growth [38]. This method is less invasive, and the patients can relatively quickly return to their school life. However, severe deformities, which are not completely corrected by the guided growth method, are acutely or gradually corrected by osteotomies with internal implants (plate and screws) or external fixators. Gradual correction, which is based on distraction osteogenesis (the bone lengthening concept), can induce relatively accurate results and is a useful method. This surgical method is well established and usually applied to angular deformities or shortening of the tubular bones in various disorders. On the other hand, gradual correction puts a huge burden on the patients due to the long treatment period or many mild complications, such as pin site infections. In addition, one treatment precaution was pointed out in XLH patients receiving gradual correction [39]. Cho et al. reported the negative correlation between the regeneration of lengthened bone and serum phosphate levels and concluded that a serum phosphate level of 2.5 mg/dL as a cut-off point should be considered in deciding whether deformity correction alone or with concomitant leg lengthening should be undertaken [39]. The transition of MAD changes is monitored for the degree of improvement of lower limb deformities in both temporary hemiepiphysiodesis and correction by osteotomies. In addition, the orthopedic surgeons should consider the joint orientation angle (JOA) as an additional parameter during treatment planning. The JOA represents the angle between the mechanical axis and joint surface line of the knee or ankle [40]. A large deviation of the JOA from the normal range can cause an increase in shear stress on the joint cartilage and leads to early degenerative osteoarthritis. Therefore, lower limb deformities should be treated in adolescence, with an acceptable MAD and JOA achieved at skeletal maturity.

The guided growth method is also used for the correction of LLD in various diseases [41,42] and can be applicable to patients with XLH. A set of one plate and two screws is fixed on one side of a growth plate for the correction of angular deformities, whereas two sets are on fixed both sides of the growth plate in the longer lower limbs for the correction of LLD. On the other hand, bone lengthening of the shorter bones or shortening osteotomy of the longer bones is sometimes applied to patients with both angular deformities and LLD.

Rotational deformities of the lower limbs are also noticed as toe-in gait in late childhood and adolescence. Those rotational deformities in XLH include internal rotation of the lower leg (tibia and fibula) and external rotation of the femur. An internal rotational deformity of the tibia is more critical to toe-in gait [36]. Slight toe-in gait seldom causes symptoms and dysfunctions of lower limbs in everyday life. However, severe toe-in gait often gives rise to various symptoms such as joint pain of the knee or ankle, muscle and bone pain in the lateral lesions of the lower legs, or easier stumbling and spraining of the ankle, because the plane of motion of the knee joint is out of alignment with that of the ankle joint.

The correction of rotational deformities is less frequent than that of angular deformities and LLD, because there is not much impairment in daily life. However, the spontaneous correction of rotational deformities is less likely to occur compared to other deformities in late childhood and adolescence despite the use of conventional medication. An external rotational osteotomy is sometimes performed for the improvement of toe-in gait or pain of the joint and muscle.

These surgical procedures contribute to a reduction in burden and improvement of function in patients with XLH. However, the XLH patients are more predisposed to relapse of the corrected deformities or the development of adverse deformities, even in those periods, and these problems can provoke a further burden of treatment. The author also has experience with unexpected improvements of LLD and adverse deformities from guided growth surgery (Figure 3). The clinicians should make a cautious plan for treatment throughout the growth period and reduce the frequency of exposure to surgical procedures.

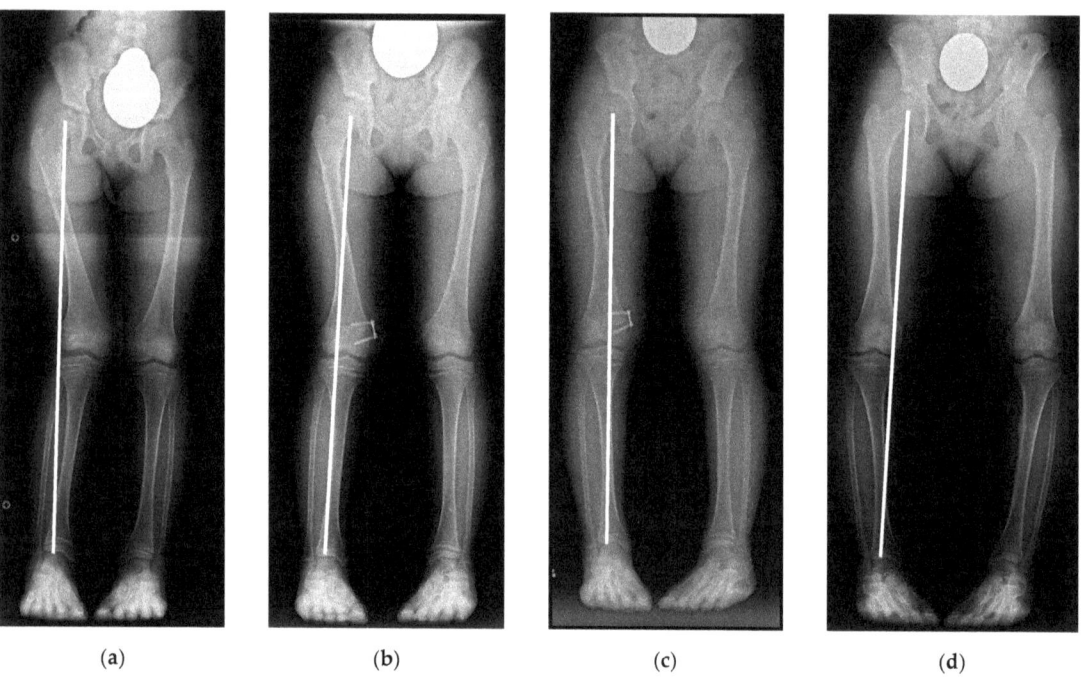

Figure 3. A case with varied deformities. White lines are the mechanical axis. (**a**) Preoperative; valgus deformity of the right lower limb and leg length discrepancy (LLD) (**b**) 1 year after guided growth surgery; valgus deformity and LLD was improving. (**c**) After deformity correction; only one side of guided growth surgery led to correction of both valgus knee deformity and leg length discrepancy (**d**) 1 year after implant removal; varus deformity of the corrected right lower limb emerged.

Recently, Mindler et al. reported persistent lower limb deformities in children with XLH receiving Burosumab for one year [5]. They concluded no positive effects of Burosumab on lower limb deformities. However, they suggested the limitation of a small study group and a short follow-up period and the necessity for further prospective studies with a large cohort and a longer follow-up. On the other hand, Insogna et al. showed the promotion of fracture healing by Burosumab treatment in adult patients [43]. This result suggests that Burosumab treatment might have an influence on osteotomy healing in patients with XLH. When the short-term and long-term effects of Burosumab on bones are clarified, this could modulate orthopedic treatments in XLH patients.

3.2. Fractures

A nontraumatic fracture is uncommon in children. Several groups have reported that the mean age at the first fracture was in the third decade [3,44]. The bone properties and morphology are important determinants of mechanical loading on the lower limbs. As the deterioration of these factors can lead to pathological fractures, they must be dealt with before skeletal maturity using medications and orthopedic interventions.

3.3. Scoliosis

Scoliosis, which is a condition involving a laterally curved deformity of the spinal column, can be caused by XLH in adolescence. Growth disturbances and a decrease in the bone properties of the vertebral bodies can lead to vertebral deformities, and these deformities can have a bad influence on the spinal alignment. A pediatric orthopedic book contains only one sentence stating that kyphoscoliosis is caused by rickets [12]. However, there are no papers on structural scoliosis, which is made up of vertebral bone deformities caused by XLH rickets in late childhood and adolescence. On the other hand, several groups have reported kyphoscoliosis in young adults with osteomalacia, who had experienced back pain and undergone spinal surgery [45,46]. Even though there is no evidence of a high incidence of scoliosis in XLH children, clinicians should pay attention to the presence of spinal deformities during the growth period considering the bone properties and the possibility of the deterioration of the spinal alignment after skeletal maturity in children with XLH. In addition, lower limb deformities, such as windswept lower limb deformities or large LLD, in childhood and adolescence cause functional scoliosis, which adjusts the trunk balance, and functional scoliosis can result in structural and degenerative scoliosis in adulthood [47,48]. Therefore, the spinal alignment should be carefully evaluated in patients with severe lower limb deformities in adolescence.

3.4. Musculoskeletal Pain

Several papers have indicated that the muscle density and strength are lower in patients with XLH than normal controls, while the muscle size is normal [49,50]. In addition, they reported that muscle functions are much lower in patients with severe leg deformities than those without deformities [51]. Low bone and muscle properties can lead to bone, joint, and muscle pain, which can impair physical functions. Furthermore, impairments of physical functions can cause muscle and bone weakness. Skrinar et al. demonstrated that many children with XLH had musculoskeletal pain as much as adult patients in spite of medication use [3]. Ito et al. also reported that Japanese and Korean children with XLH have pain in their lower limbs as adult patients [44]. These papers indicate that conventional therapies do not have enough effectiveness in terms of pain control of the musculoskeletal system. Recently, the efficacy of Burosumab has been reported in several papers, showing improvement in symptoms of rickets in children with XLH [30,51]. However, the efficacy of Burosumab for musculoskeletal pain is unclear. Further studies are expected in the near future.

4. Summary

This paper presented the orthopedic problems and interventions in children with XLH. The major issues in the orthopedic field are complicated lower limb deformities and their tendency to relapse. To resolve these problems, several surgical procedures are chosen for treatment and multiple surgeries are often performed until skeletal maturity (Figure 4). Therefore, orthopedic surgeons should make a cautious surgical plan for treatment throughout the growth period and reduce the burden of treatment in cooperation with pediatricians.

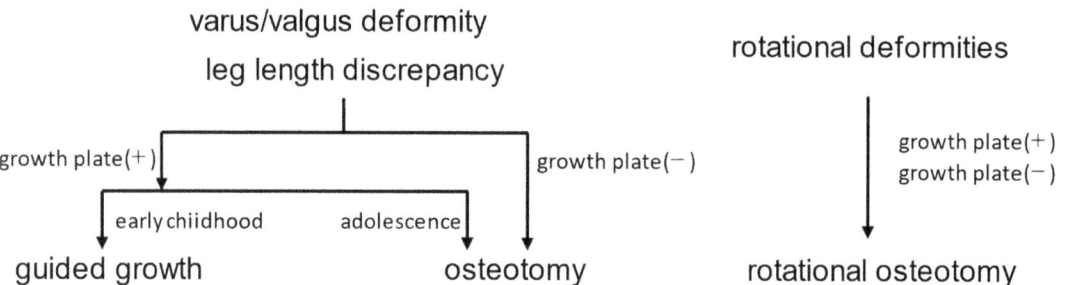

Figure 4. Brief algorithm of the surgical indication and method for varus or valgus deformities and leg length discrepancies, which are corrected by the guided growth method in early childhood and by osteotomy in adolescence. Rotational deformities are corrected by osteotomy in all patients.

Funding: This research received no external funding.

Institutional Review Board Statement: Not applicable.

Informed Consent Statement: Not applicable.

Data Availability Statement: No data availability.

Conflicts of Interest: The author declares no conflict of interest.

References

1. Read, A.P.; Thakker, R.V.; Davies, K.E.; Mountford, R.C.; Brenton, D.P.; Davies, M.; Glorieux, F.; Harris, R.; Hendy, G.N.; King, A.; et al. Mapping of human X-linked hypophosphatemic rickets by multilocus linkage analysis. *Hum. Genet.* **1986**, *73*, 267–270. [CrossRef] [PubMed]
2. Machler, M.; Frey, D.; Gai, A.; Orth, U.; Wienker, T.F.; Fanconi, A.; Schmid, W. X-linked dominant hypophosphatemia is closely linked to DNA markers DXS41 and DXS43 at Xp22. *Hum. Genet.* **1986**, *73*, 271–275. [CrossRef] [PubMed]
3. Skrinar, A.; Dvorak-Ewell, M.; Evins, A.; Macica, C.; Linglart, A.; Imel, E.A.; Theodore-Oklota, C.; Martin, J.S. The lifelong impact of X-linked hypophosphatemia: Results from a burden of disease survey. *J. Endocr. Soc.* **2019**, *3*, 1321–1334. [CrossRef] [PubMed]
4. Mindler, G.T.; Kranzl, A.; Stauffer, A.; Haeusler, G.; Ganger, R.; Raimann, A. Disease-specific gait deviations in pediatric patients with X-linked hypophosphatemia. *Gait Posture* **2020**, *81*, 78–84. [CrossRef]
5. Mindler, G.T.; Kranzl, A.; Stauffer, A.; Kocijan, R.; Ganger, R.; Radler, C.; Haeusler, G.; Raimann, A. Lower limb deformity and gait deviations among adolescents and adults with X-linked hypophosphatemia. *Front. Endocrinol.* **2021**, *12*, 754084. [CrossRef] [PubMed]
6. Steele, A.; Gonzalez, R.; Garbalosa, J.C.; Steigbigel, K.; Grgurich, T.; Parisi, E.J.; Feinn, R.S.; Tommasini, S.M.; Macica, C.M. Osteoarthritis, osteophytes and enthesophytes affect biomechanical function in adults with X-linked hypophosphatemia. *J. Clin. Endocrinol. Metab.* **2020**, *105*, e1798–e1814. [CrossRef] [PubMed]
7. Seefried, L.; Smyth, M.; Keen, R.; Harvengt, P. Burden of disease associated with X-linked hypophosphataemia in adults: A systematic literature review. *Osteoporos. Int.* **2021**, *32*, 7–22. [CrossRef] [PubMed]
8. Petersen, D.J.; Boniface, A.M.; Schranck, F.W.; Rupich, R.C.; Whyte, M.P. X-linked hypophosphatemic rickets: A study (with literature review) of linear growth response to calcitriol and phosphate therapy. *J. Bone Miner. Res.* **1992**, *7*, 583–597. [CrossRef]
9. Carpenter, T.O. New perspectives on the biology and treatment of X-linked hypophosphatemic rickets. *Pediatr. Clin. N. Am.* **1997**, *44*, 443–466. [CrossRef]
10. Carpenter, T.O.; Imel, E.A.; Holm, I.A.; Jan de Beur, S.M.; Insogna, K.L. A clinician's guide to X-linked hypophosphatemia. *J. Bone Miner. Res.* **2011**, *26*, 1381–1388. [CrossRef]
11. Fucentese, S.F.; Neuhaus, T.J.; Ramseier, L.E.; Ulrich Exner, G. Metabolic and orthopedic management of X-linked vitamin D-resistant hypophosphatemic rickets. *J. Child. Orthop.* **2008**, *2*, 285–291. [CrossRef] [PubMed]
12. Petje, G.; Meizer, R.; Radler, C.; Aigner, N.; Grill, F. Deformity correction in children with hereditary hypophosphatemic rickets. *Clin. Orthop. Relat. Res.* **2008**, *466*, 3078–3085. [CrossRef] [PubMed]
13. Evans, G.A.; Arulanantham, K.; Gage, J.R. Primary hypophosphatemic rickets: Effect of oral phosphate and vitamin D on growth and surgical treatment. *J. Bone Jt. Surg. Am.* **1980**, *62*, 1130–1138. [CrossRef]
14. European Medicines Agency. New Medicine for Rarebone Disease. *EMA* 2017. Available online: https://www.ema.europa.eu/en/news/new-medicine-rare-bone-disease_en.pdf (accessed on 1 August 2022).

15. US Food & Drug Administration. FDA Approves First Therapy for Rare Inherited Form of Rickets, X-Linked Hypophosphatemia. 2018. Available online: https://www.fda.gov/newsevents/newsroom/pressannouncements/ucm604810.htm (accessed on 1 August 2022).
16. Pharmaceutical Affairs and Food Sanitation Council. 2020. Available online: https://www.hospital.or.jp/pdg/14_20200825_02.pdf (accessed on 1 August 2022).
17. Stevens, P.M.; Maguire, M.; Dales, M.; Robins, A.J. Physeal stapling for idiopathic genu valgum. *J. Pediatr. Orthop.* **1999**, *19*, 645–649. [CrossRef]
18. Horn, A.; Wright, J.; Bockenhauer, D.; Van't Hoff, W.; Eastwood, D.M. The orthopaedic management of lower limb deformity in hypophosphataemic rickets. *J. Child. Orthop.* **2017**, *11*, 298–305. [CrossRef] [PubMed]
19. Thacher, T.D.; Fischer, P.R.; Pettifor, J.M.; Lawson, J.O.; Manaster, B.J.; Reading, J.C. Radiographic scoring method for the assessment of the severity of nutritional rickets. *J. Trop. Pediatr.* **2000**, *46*, 132–139. [CrossRef]
20. Whyte, M.P.; Fujita, K.P.; Moseley, S.; Thompson, D.D.; McAlister, W.H. Validation of a novel scoring system for changes in skeletal manifestations of hypophosphatasia in newborns, infants, and children: The Radiographic Global Impression of Change Scale. *J. Bone Miner. Res.* **2018**, *33*, 868–874. [CrossRef]
21. Lim, R.; Shailam, R.; Hulett, R.; Skrinar, A.; Nixon, A.; Williams, A.; Nixon, M.; Thacher, T.D. Validation of the Radiographic Global Impression of Change (RGI-C) score to assess healing of rickets in pediatric X-linked hypophosphatemia (XLH). *Bone* **2021**, *148*, 115964. [CrossRef]
22. Kim, H.K.W.; Seikaly, M.G. Metabolic and Endcrine Disorders of Bone. In *Tachdjian's Pediatric Orthopaedics*, 6th ed.; Herring, J.A., Ed.; Elsevier: Philadelphia, PA, USA, 2020; Volume 2, pp. 1928–1938.
23. Eguchi, Y.; Seki, A.; Uchikawa, S.; Tori, A.; Kimura, A.; Takayama, S. Kashisouguryouhou wo okonatta teirinnkesshousei-kurubyo (hypophosphatemic rickets) kannjinokeika. *Nippon Shouniseikeigeka Gakkai Shi* **2017**, *26*, 14–18.
24. Sharkey, M.S.; Grunseich, K.; Carpenter, T.O. Contemporary medical and surgical management of X-linked hypophosphatemic rickets. *J. Am. Acad. Orthop. Surg.* **2015**, *23*, 433–442. [CrossRef]
25. Rohmiller, M.T.; Tylkowski, C.; Kriss, V.M.; Mier, R.J. The effect of osteotomy on bowing and height in children with X-linked hypophosphatemia. *J. Pediatr. Orthop.* **1999**, *9*, 114–118. [CrossRef]
26. Nielsen, L.H.; Rahbek, E.T.; Beck-Nielsen, S.S.; Christesen, H.T. Treatment of hypophosphataemic rickets in children remains a challenge. *Dan Med. J.* **2014**, *61*, A4874. [PubMed]
27. Cagnoli, M.; Richter, R.; Bohm, P.; Knye, K.; Empting, S.; Mohnike, K. Spontaneous growth and effect of early therapy with calcitriol and phosphate in X-linked hypophosphatemic rickets. *Pediatr. Endocrinol. Rev.* **2017**, *15* (Suppl. S1), 119–122. [PubMed]
28. Makitie, O.; Doria, A.; Kooh, S.W.; Cole, W.G.; Daneman, A.; Sochett, E. Early treatment improves growth and biochemical and radiographic outcome in X-linked hypophosphatemic rickets. *J. Clin. Endocrinol. Metab.* **2003**, *88*, 3591–3597. [CrossRef] [PubMed]
29. Mao, M.; Carpenter, T.O.; Whyte, M.P.; Skrinar, A.; Chen, C.Y.; Martin, J.S.; Rogol, A.D. Growth curve for children with X-linked hypophosphatemia. *J. Clin. Endocrinol. Metab.* **2020**, *105*, 3243–3249. [CrossRef]
30. Ward, L.M.; Glorieux, F.H.; Whyte, M.P.; Munns, C.F.; Portale, A.A.; Högler, W.; Simmons, J.H.; Gottesman, G.S.; Padidela, R.; Namba, N.; et al. Impact of Burosumab Compared with Conventional Therapy in Younger Versus Older Children with X-Linked Hypophosphatemia. *J. Clin. Endocrinol. Metab.* **2022**, *107*, e3241–e3253.dgac296. [CrossRef]
31. Smyth, E.H. Windswept deformity. *J. Bone Jt. Surg. Br.* **1980**, *62*, 166–167. [CrossRef]
32. Che, H.; Roux, C.; Etcheto, A.; Rothenbuhler, A.; Kamanicky, P.; Linglart, A.; Briot, K. Impaired quality of life in adults with X-linked hypophosphatemia and skeletal symptoms. *Eur. J. Endocrinol.* **2016**, *174*, 325–333. [CrossRef]
33. Cheung, M.; Rylands, A.J.; Williams, A.; Bailey, K.; Bubbear, J. Patient-reported complications, symptoms, and experiences of living with X-linked hypophosphatemia across the life-course. *J. Endocr. Soc.* **2021**, *5*, bvab070. [CrossRef] [PubMed]
34. Lecoq, A.-L.; Brandi, M.L.; Linglart, A.; Kamenicky, P. Management of X-linked hypophosphatemia in adults. *Metabolism* **2020**, *103S*, 154049. [CrossRef]
35. Larson, A.N.; Trousdale, R.T.; Pagnano, M.W.; Hanssen, A.D.; Lewallen, D.G.; Sanchez-Sotelo, J. Hip and knee arthroplasty in hypophosphatemic rickets. *J. Arthroplast.* **2010**, *25*, 1099–1103. [CrossRef] [PubMed]
36. Mindler, G.T.; Stauffer, A.; Kranzl, A.; Penzkofer, S.; Ganger, R.; Radler, C.; Haeusler, G.; Raimann, A. Persistent lower limb deformities despite amelioration of rickets in X-linked hypophosphatemia (XLH)—A prospective observation study. *Front. Endocrinol.* **2022**, *13*, 866170. [CrossRef] [PubMed]
37. Novais, E.; Stevens, P.M. Hypophosphatemic rickets: The role of hemiepiphysiodesis. *J. Pediatr. Orthop.* **2006**, *26*, 238–244. [CrossRef]
38. Stevens, P.M. Guided growth for angular correction: A preliminary series using a tension band plate. *J. Pediatr. Orthop.* **2007**, *27*, 253–259. [CrossRef] [PubMed]
39. Choi, I.H.; Kim, J.K.; Chung, C.Y.; Cho, T.-J.; Lee, S.H.; Suh, S.W.; Whang, K.S.; Park, H.W.; Song, K.S. Deformity correction of knee and leg lengthening by Ilizarov method in hypophosphatemic rickets: Outcomes and significance of serum phosphate level. *J. Pediatr. Orthop.* **2002**, *22*, 626–631. [CrossRef]
40. Paley, D.; Herzenberg, J.E.; Tetsworth, K.; McKie, J.; Bhave, A. Deformity planning for frontal and sagittal plane corrective osteotomies. *Orthop. Clin. N. Am.* **1994**, *25*, 425–465. [CrossRef]

41. Lykissas, M.G.; Jain, V.V.; Manickam, V.; Nathan, S.; Eismann, E.A.; McCarthy, J.J. Guided growth for the treatment of limb length discrepancy: A comparative study of the three most commonly used surgical techniques. *J. Pediat. Orthop. B* **2013**, *22*, 311–317. [CrossRef]
42. Byyham, I.A.; Karatas, A.F.; Rogers, K.J.; Bowen, J.R.; Thacker, M.M. Comparing percutaneous physeal epiphysiodesis and Eight-Plate epiphysiodesis for the treatment of limb length discrepancy. *J. Pediatr. Orthop.* **2015**, *37*, 323–327.
43. Insogna, K.; Briot, K.; Imel, E.A.; Kamenicky, P.; Ruppe, M.D.; Portale, A.A.; Weber, T.; Pitukcheewanont, P.; Cheong, H.I.I.; Jan de Beur, S.; et al. A randomized, double-blind, placebo-controlled, phase 3 trial evaluating the efficacy of Burosumab, an anti-FGF23 antibody, in adults with X-linked hypophosphatemia: Week 24 primary analysis. *J. Bone Miner. Res.* **2018**, *33*, 1383–1393. [CrossRef]
44. Ito, N.; Kang, H.G.; Nishida, Y.; Evins, A.; Skrinar, A.; Cheong, H.I. Burden of disease of X-linked hypophosphatemia in Japanese and Korean patients: A cross-sectional survey. *Endocr. J.* **2022**, *69*, 373–383. [CrossRef]
45. Motosuneya, T.; Asazuma, T.; Yasuoka, H.; Tsuji, T.; Fujikawa, K. Severe kyphoscoliosis associated with osteomalacia. *Spine J.* **2006**, *6*, 587–590. [CrossRef] [PubMed]
46. Hensinger, R.N. Kyphosis secondary to skeletal dysplasias and metabolic disease. *Clin. Orthop. Relat. Res.* **1977**, *128*, 113–128. [CrossRef]
47. Brunk, M. The importance of rickets in childhood as a cause of scoliosis in adult age. *Acta Orthop. Scand.* **1951**, *9*, 3–114. [CrossRef]
48. Yang, X.; Zou, Q.; Song, Y.; Liu, L.; Zhou, C. A case report of severe degenerative lumbar scoliosis associated with windswept lower limb deformity. *BMC Surg.* **2020**, *20*, 195–200. [CrossRef] [PubMed]
49. Veilleux, L.-N.; Cheung, M.; Ben Amor, M.; Rauch, F. Abnormalities in muscle density and muscle function in hypophosphatemic rickets. *J. Clin. Endocrinol. Metab.* **2012**, *97*, E1492–E1498. [CrossRef] [PubMed]
50. Veilleux, L.N.; Cheung, M.S.; Glorieux, F.H.; Rauch, F. The muscle-bone relationship in X-linked hypophosphatemic rickets. *J. Clin. Endocrinol. Metab.* **2013**, *98*, E990–E995. [CrossRef] [PubMed]
51. Namba, N.; Kubota, T.; Muroya, K.; Tanaka, H.; Kanematsu, M.; Kojima, M.; Orihara, S.; Kanda, H.; Seino, Y.; Ozono, K. Safety and Efficacy of Burosumab in Pediatric Patients With X-Linked Hypophosphatemia: A Phase 3/4 Open-Label Trial. *J. Endocr. Soc.* **2022**, *6*, bvac021. [CrossRef]

MDPI
St. Alban-Anlage 66
4052 Basel
Switzerland
www.mdpi.com

Endocrines Editorial Office
E-mail: endocrines@mdpi.com
www.mdpi.com/journal/endocrines

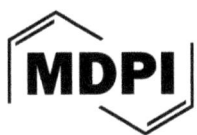

Disclaimer/Publisher's Note: The statements, opinions and data contained in all publications are solely those of the individual author(s) and contributor(s) and not of MDPI and/or the editor(s). MDPI and/or the editor(s) disclaim responsibility for any injury to people or property resulting from any ideas, methods, instructions or products referred to in the content.

www.ingramcontent.com/pod-product-compliance
Lightning Source LLC
LaVergne TN
LVHW070608100526
838202LV00012B/593